AF716435

Neurology and Religion

This innovative book examines what can be learnt about the role of the brain in religious belief and practice from studying people with neurological disorders, such as stroke, epilepsy and Parkinson's disease. Using a clinical case study approach, the book analyses the interaction of social influences, religious upbringing and neurological disorders on lived religious experience in a number of different faith traditions. The interdisciplinary contributors to the book ensure a variety of perspectives to help understand how the religious life is affected when different cognitive functions are impaired; how faith modifies the effects of neurological disorders; and how awareness of faith practices may assist in the treatment of these conditions.

Revd Professor Alasdair Coles is Professor of Clinical Neuroimmunology, University of Cambridge; Honorary Consultant Neurologist, Cambridge University Hospitals NHS Foundation Trust; and an ordained priest in the Diocese of Ely, Church of England.

Revd Canon Dr Joanna Collicutt is Karl Jaspers Lecturer in Psychology and Spirituality at Ripon College Cuddesdon and a Supernumerary Fellow of Harris Manchester College, University of Oxford. She is a clinical neuropsychologist and Anglican priest and was for many years head of the Oxfordshire neuropsychological rehabilitation service.

Contents

Contributors

Neil Krishan Aggarwal is Assistant Professor of Clinical Psychiatry at Columbia University Medical Center, a Member of the University's Committee on Global Thought and Research Psychiatrist at the New York State Psychiatric Institute. His research focuses on cultural psychiatry and psychiatric anthropology of South Asian populations.

Erik W. Asp is Assistant Professor of Psychology and Director of the Neuroscience Program at Hamline University. He completed his PhD at the University of Iowa in 2012 and was a Postdoctoral Research Fellow in the Center for Cognitive and Social Neuroscience at the University of Chicago from 2012 to 2013.

Roger A. Barker is Professor of Clinical Neuroscience at the University of Cambridge and is Honorary Consultant at Addenbrooke's Hospital. He trained in Oxford and London and has been leading research in Cambridge on Parkinson's and Huntington's diseases for the last twenty years.

Nikolas R. Block is a US resident in otolaryngology who is interested in the neural correlates of identity formation. His research at the University of California, San Francisco utilises neuroimaging and behavioural techniques to understand the neural basis of social behaviours. His research integrates principles from behavioural neurology, affective neuroscience and otolaryngology to ask novel questions that bridge these fields.

Warren S. Brown is Professor of Psychology and Director of the Travis Research Institute at the Graduate School of Psychology, Fuller Theological Seminary. Brown is a research neuropsychologist/neuroscientist interested in the cognitive impact of brain malformations. He has coauthored eighty scientific articles and five books on neuroscience and theology.

Aron S. Buchman is Professor of Neurological Sciences on staff at the Rush Alzheimer's Disease Center at Rush University Medical Center in Chicago. His research, funded by NIH, focuses on quantifying diverse behaviours of older adults participating in community-based cohort studies to explicate the neurobiology of age-related decline.

Sophie Grace Chappell is Professor of Philosophy at the Open University, Leverhulme Senior Research Fellow, 2017–20, and Visiting Fellow in the Universities of St Andrews and Glasgow. Her books include *Knowing What to Do*, *Ethics and Experience*, *The Inescapable Self* and *Reading Plato's Theaetetus*.

Kelly James Clark is Senior Research Fellow at the Kaufman Interfaith Institute at Grand Valley State University. He earned his PhD in philosophy and works on the philosophy of religion, cognitive science of religion and religion and compassion and peace. He has published more than twenty-five books, including *God and the Brain: Neuroscience and the Rationality of Belief* (2019).

Daniel De Haan is a Research Fellow at the Ian Ramsey Centre for Science and Religion, Oxford University. From 2015–2018 he was a postdoctoral researcher on the neuroscience strand of the Templeton World Charity Foundation's

Theology, Philosophy of Religion, and the Sciences project at Cambridge University. His research focuses on philosophical anthropology, philosophy of religion and the sciences.

Ashraf El-Mitwalli trained in Egypt and did stroke research at the University of Texas at Houston. He has worked in Egypt, Libya, Bahrain and Saudi Arabia. He is now Professor of Neurology at Mansoura University, Egypt.

Julian C. Hughes was until recently Professor of Old Age Psychiatry at the University of Bristol, having previously been Honorary Professor of Philosophy of Ageing at Newcastle University, UK. He remains an honorary professor at Bristol and a visiting professor at Newcastle, and he continues to write chiefly about ethics and philosophy in connection with ageing and dementia.

Stuart J. Judge held a Postdoctoral Fellowship at the US National Institutes of Health and was Research Fellow, Lecturer, Reader in Physiology and Fellow of St Anne's College at the University of Oxford. He is currently Associate of the Faraday Institute for Science and Religion, Cambridge, and Research Tutor at the Oxford Centre for Mission Studies.

Ian James Kidd is Assistant Professor at the Department of Philosophy, University of Nottingham. His research interests include the philosophy of religion and the spiritual life, phenomenology and philosophy of illness. He was co-editor (with José Medina and Gaile Pohlhaus, Jr) of *The Routledge Handbook to Epistemic Injustice* (2017) and is editing (with Heather Battaly and Quassim Cassam) *Vice Epistemology* (2020). His website is www.ianjameskidd.weebly.com.

Michael N. Marsh read medicine at Magdalen College, Oxford; became a university-based gastroenterologist; and studied theology (Oxford) on retirement. Then followed a doctorate on near-death experiences, with further publications on the ethical problems of disability, abortion, the human foetus, death and assisted suicide. He is now at Wolfson College.

Bruce Miller holds the A. W. and Mary Margaret Clausen Distinguished Professorship in Neurology at the University of California, San Francisco, where he directs the Memory and Aging Center. He is a behavioural neurologist whose work in neurodegenerative conditions emphasises brain–behaviour relationships and the genetic and molecular underpinnings of disease.

Gordon Pennycook is Assistant Professor of Behavioural Science at the Hill/Levene Schools of Business and Associate Member of the Department of Psychology at the University of Regina. He completed his PhD at the University of Waterloo in 2016 and was a Banting Postdoctoral Fellow at Yale University from 2016 to 2018.

Clare Redfern worked as a general practitioner in Manchester and Cambridge, then was a Research Associate at the Faraday Institute, and is now working as an Adlerian Counsellor. She is editor of *Green Christian* magazine.

Daniel Tranel is Clinical Neuropsychologist at the Department of Neurology, University of Iowa Hospitals and Clinics. He is also Professor in the Department of Psychological and Brain Sciences at the University of Iowa. He completed his PhD at the University of Iowa in 1982.

Ingela Visuri has a PhD in the Study of Religions, and her doctoral thesis deals with religious cognition and experience in high-functioning autistic individuals. She is especially interested in methodological and analytical issues relating to the study of atypical cognition, and combines mixed methods and theories from cognitive- and humanities oriented work on religion, cognition and autism in her research.

Kelsey Warner is a speech-language pathologist in Minneapolis, Minnesota. She specialises in assessment and functional treatment of patients with cognitive deficits following traumatic brain injury. Her research background is in psychology and behavioural and cognitive neuroscience at the University of Iowa, with graduate training completed at the University of Minnesota.

Giles Yeates is editor of the journal and book series *Neuro-Disability & Psychotherapy*, in addition to the Brain Injury book series. He is editor of the forthcoming book *Eastern Influences on Neuropsychotherapy*. As a clinical neuropsychologist in community neurorehabilitation, his clinical work and research focus on the innovation of psychological therapies and support of relationships following acquired brain injury. Giles is also a long-standing practitioner and teacher of Tai Ji and Kung Fu and studies under the Daoist Monks in Wudang Mountain, China. Giles is currently innovating the use of Tai Ji in neurorehabilitation (www.neuro-flowgroup.com).

Preface

We believe that careful observation of the lives of neurology patients can teach us useful things about human religious experience, belief and practice, especially when these observations are critically analysed by theologians and philosophers. But these worlds have rarely met; few health care professionals are interested in neurology patients' religious lives, and few theologians and philosophers have encountered the spiritual consequences of neurological disorders. This volume is an attempt to draw these disciplines together. We hope this book will be of interest to academics in the brain sciences, philosophy and theology; to ministers of religion; and to the interested layperson.

To those who say clinical observation has been made redundant by sophisticated brain scanning, we respond that imaging experiments are powerful but reductionist, methodologically limited (see Chapter 3) and with their ecological validity hampered by the paraphernalia of the scanning environment. Moreover, we argue that the encounter of the patient with a neurological clinician offers a unique perspective, as we observe how, in their spiritual lives, human beings overcome and respond to neurological deficits.

A straightforward and valuable outcome from this enterprise is increased understanding for patients, clinicians and pastors, on how faith might change with neurological conditions. But we also believe that there is academic value in observing how focal lesions fractionate the human experience of religion, just as our knowledge of the basis of language has thrived on the dissociative effects of brain lesions.

We affirm that religion involves multiple cognitive and affective domains, none of which may be exclusively 'religious'. Religion is also perhaps best understood not so much as an individual capacity as a social activity (after all, *religio* means to 'bind', and this connects with the idea of faith as social glue); thus it is more like cricket than binocular vision.[1]

For all these reasons, this book is not entitled the 'neuroscience of religion', which, as Warren Brown has argued, is an implausible topic (Jeeves and Brown 2009). Rather, we see the study of neurological patients as an opportunity to analyse the interaction between societal influences, prior conditioning, religious upbringing and metaphysical understanding with the primary effects of neurological lesions. What sort of religion emerges when this or that cognitive function is impaired, compensated for and made sense of?

Though the terms *religion* and *spirituality* are slippery, and variably understood, our preference is to favour 'religion', as it encompasses individual and communal behaviour, practice and belief as well as subjective experience. The relationship between religion and disease is complex and two-way. In this book we describe several ways in which brain disease may appear to diminish or distort human expressions of religion. But we also describe the positive role of religious practice in therapy and rehabilitation. We recognise that periods of enforced convalescence from illness may lead to a new attention to religious belief (as in the lives of Francis of Assisi and Ignatius of Loyola). Also the experience of suffering through illness can mature faith, through 'post-traumatic growth' (Tedeschi and Calhoun 1995), and a religious framework can provide meaning to disease and recovery. Being part of a worshipping congregation may be attractive to those living with illness

[1] An idea borrowed from Warren Brown (MacNamara 2006).

because of the offer of practical and emotional support. Conversely, illness may itself symbolise important internal religious conflicts, as in psychosomatic and dissociative disorders.

William James, in the first chapter of *The Varieties*, entitled 'Religion and Neurology', argues against the 'medical materialism' that 'finishes up Saint Paul . . . [as] an epileptic . . . snuffs our Saint Teresa as an hysteric, Saint Francis of Assisi as an hereditary degenerate' (James 1902, 14). It is not our intent to denigrate religion as pathological or to assume that the religious life of those with neurological disorders is inauthentic. We concur with James that the criteria of religious credibility lie outside of medicine, instead relating to 'immediate luminousness, . . . philosophical reasonableness and moral helpfulness' (James 1902, 17–18).

We originally envisaged a review of the interaction of a comprehensive range of neurological conditions and the beliefs and practices of the major religions. But we have inevitably ended up with a more modest volume, dominated by Western religious traditions and covering a representative sample of neurological conditions, which reflects the patchiness of the work in this area. Being very aware of its limitations, we offer this volume as the start of the conversation between neurology and religious studies rather than as its conclusion.

The book is in two parts. Part I explores basic issues of philosophy and methodology that need to be kept in mind in opening a conversation between neurology and religion. Following two chapters by the editors that describe the discipline of neurology and the history of treating religion as an object of scientific study, Chapter 3 by Stuart J. Judge discusses the practical and interpretative constraints and pitfalls in applying neuroscientific methods to religion. There are then five chapters on philosophical issues. Warren S. Brown (Chapter 4) addresses the old 'mind–body' problem, arguing against dualistic positions in favour of the notion of embodied cognition, in which the mind is understood to be an emergent property of an active and dynamic brain–body. Ian James Kidd (Chapter 5) argues for a phenomenological approach in which first-person accounts of illness experience (rather than clinical or scientific observations) are understood as the basic data set and treated accordingly. Daniel De Haan (Chapter 6) and Sophie Grace Chappell (Chapter 7) both interact with significant issues set out in Maxwell Bennett and Peter Hacker's influential work *Philosophical Foundations of Neuroscience* but take different positions. Finally, Neil Krishnan Aggarwal (Chapter 8) presents an approach to neuropsychiatry that is not founded on Western post-Enlightenment thought but located within an Islamic framework. This last chapter is in some ways an exemplar; other faith traditions have offered their own 'alternative' frameworks to medicine and psychology that have arisen largely in a northern European and American Protestant Christian framework, and this is picked up with a more practical focus in Giles Yeates' chapter in Part II (Chapter 17).

In this second part, which is likely to be more accessible to clinicians, the focus is on specific neurological disorders and therapy, using clinical observation and findings from empirical studies of patients to elucidate questions about the nature of religion.

Alasdair Coles (Chapter 9) writes on temporal lobe epilepsy and its association with mystical-like experience. Roger Barker and Clare Redfern (Chapter 10) present an empirical study of religion and spirituality in people living with Parkinson's disease. Working within a cognitive science of religion framework, Gordon Pennycook and colleagues explore in Chapter 11 the role of the prefrontal cortex in relation to strength of religious beliefs, drawing on studies of patients with prefrontal tumours. Ashraf El-Mitwalli (Chapter 12) examines the relationship between a religious practice – fasting – and brain function. Kelly James Clark and Ingela Visuri (Chapter 13) explore the expression and experience of religion in people with autism spectrum conditions. Julian Hughes (Chapter 14) opens up questions of personhood from the perspective of dementia studies, and Nikolas Block and Bruce Miller (Chapter 15) focus more specifically on frontotemporal dementia.

In a chapter on therapy and rehabilitation, Joanna Collicutt (Chapter 16) presents a model of rehabilitation that incorporates spiritual and religious issues, illustrating it with a detailed case study of memory rehabilitation in a minister of religion. Giles Yeates (Chapter 17) reviews a range of practices located in Eastern religion and philosophy that have been found to show promising effects in the treatment of patients with neurological disorders.

Finally, there are two chapters on death. Aron Buchman (Chapter 18) looks at the status of brain death in relation to Jewish law, while Michael Marsh (Chapter 19) offers a polemical essay on the causes and nature of near-death experiences.

We are very grateful to the John Templeton Foundation, which, through a grant to the Faraday Institute in Cambridge, funded a workshop in 2013 that was the catalyst for this volume.

References

James, W. 1904. *The Varieties of Religious Experience*. New York: Longmans, Green.

Jeeves, M. B., and W. S. Brown. 2009. *Neuroscience, Psychology and Religion: Illusions, Delusions, and Realities about Human Nature*. West Conshohocken, PA: Templeton Foundation Press.

McNamara, P., ed. 2006. *Where God and Science Meet: How Brain and Evolutionary Studies Alter Our Understanding of Religion*. Westport, CT: Praeger.

Tedeschi, R., and L. Calhoun. 1995. *Trauma and Transformation: Growing in the Aftermath of Suffering*. Thousand Oaks, CA: Sage.

Part I

The Neurological Study of Religion

Chapter 1

1.1 *The Natures of Neurology and Religion*

The Discipline of Neurology

Alasdair Coles

The History of Neurology

Neurology is the branch of medicine that deals with disorders of the nervous system. The subject started, in its modern form, with the work of Thomas Willis in seventeenth-century England, as mentioned by Joanna Collicutt in Chapter 2. Willis studied the effects of diseases (for instance stroke) of the brain in people in life, and compared these with their anatomical effects at post-mortem. From these observations, he systematically assembled an account of the hierarchical nature of the nervous system from the peripheral nerves to the spinal cord, and then on through an ascending series of structures in the brain. This clinico-pathological tradition reached its apogee in the work of Jean-Martin Charcot in late nineteenth-century Paris (Clifford Rose 1999). Since then, the imaging and laboratory sciences have increasingly informed our understanding of the normal function of the brain and its diseases.

A key concept, for the purposes of this volume, is that different parts of the brain are specialised for different functions. Thomas Willis proposed this, and since his time opinion has swung from the extremes of localisation (the idea, for instance, that one neuron in your brain is responsible for 'recognising' your grandmother) to the 'equi-potential view' (where all parts of the brain are equally involved in all brain function). The current view is that distinctive brain functions are subserved by separate networks of anatomical structures.

Most of the conditions described in this volume are due to damage of the brain. But day-to-day neurology also encompasses illnesses affecting the whole nervous system: the brain, the spinal cord, the nerves going to and from the muscles and sensory organs.

The Humdrum Neurological Consultation

At the heart of the practice of neurology is an encounter between two experts. The patient is an expert in his or her symptoms, their impact on his or her life and, in the light of this, their goals for treatment. And the neurologist is expert in interpreting symptoms, signs on examination and tests, to arrive at a diagnosis, prognosis and suggestions for treatment.

This encounter is a humdrum business. Behind the consultation door, the patient describes their experiences, not always completely and not always fluently, often hindered in this by anxiety. And the neurologist listens, sifts, probes and reassembles the story to create hypotheses about which part of the nervous system may be impaired (the 'where') and which pathological process might be occurring (the 'what'). These hypotheses are then tested in a focused physical examination. So, a story about difficulty walking may lead to a careful examination of the limbs and eye movements (which may reveal damage to the balance centres of the brain); whereas wasting in one hand leads to tests of sensation around the armpit (indicative of damage to the nerve root that supplies the muscles in the hands). Usually, at the end of this process, the neurologist has recognised a pattern of symptoms and signs that points to one or two possible diagnoses. Tests may be needed to confirm the diagnosis or discriminate between alternatives, but their importance is usually overestimated by patients; for instance, it is perfectly possible to diagnose three prevalent neurological conditions (Parkinson's disease, multiple sclerosis and epilepsy) by modern criteria, without doing a single test. There follows a discussion about the diagnosis, and its implications for the future, and possibilities for cure or control of the underlying health condition and amelioration of its symptoms.

This process is not restricted to doctors. Any professional treating someone with diseases of the nervous system will go through the same process. Physiotherapists, occupational therapists, speech and language therapists and clinical psychologists, must start by understanding their patient's experiences, before interpreting how they relate to the underlying disorder and whether they might be alleviated. In so doing, whether consciously or not, they are also neuroscientists.

Learning from Experiments of Nature

We have learnt much about brain function from studies of animals in the laboratory, for instance about visual pathways from experiments in cats and motor control from monkeys. But there are some distinctive human capacities and experiences that cannot be studied in this way. Consider, for example, language. For several hundred years, the mechanism by which the brain mediated language could only be studied by observation of focal brain disorders. Tumours and strokes which lead to problems with speech, reading or writing – though personally disastrous – illuminate how language is organised in the human brain. Another sad source of information for neurologists is the consequences of accident, such as the tamping iron of Phineas Gage (Harlow 1868) (teaching us about the role of the frontal lobe in personality), and war, for instance the gunshot wounds of the First World War (revealing the anatomy of vision) (Holmes 1945). As John Hughlings Jackson, the great nineteenth-century British neurologist, put it: neurologists 'alone witness the results of experiments of disease on the nervous system of man' (quoted in Penfield 1955).

And so, an 'atlas' of patients' experiences following damage to different parts of the brain has been accumulated. This is of interest to the anatomy enthusiasts, but others might reasonably ask: so what? It is non-controversial to say that the brain is involved in experience, so what is there to learn from the distorted experiences of people with acquired brain injury?

The first lesson to be learned from such patients is how humans fractionate experience and function. To return to language, it is perhaps not surprising that brain segregates the understanding of language (the temporal lobe) from the production of speech (close to the tongue area of the motor cortex). But it is profoundly interesting that the memory for names of inanimate objects seemed to be stored separately from the names of living things and foods (Warrington and Shallice 1984). And bizarrely, a stroke may lead to someone speaking their native language perfectly – but in a foreign accent (Tomasino et al. 2013). These observations raise questions about why humans would distinguish tools and accents in this way.

Another important lesson is the lived experience, over decades sometimes, of patients with neurological deficits. In the last 20 years, structural and functional imaging of the brain has provided an exciting way to study the healthy brain at work, but this can only document changes that occur over minutes. But the neurology clinic can report on literally a lifetime's experience of living with a neurological deficit. Philosophers can do the 'thought experiment' of contemplating life without memory, and functional images can study the anatomy of memory in a healthy brain. But only the life of people like 'HM' – who had parts of both temporal lobe removed in an attempt to treat his epilepsy – can teach us what it is like to live without the ability to lay down new memories for decades (Augustinack et al. 2014).

A Neuroanatomy Primer

For those unfamiliar with the brain, a little anatomy is needed. The basic unit is a 'neuron' or nerve cell (Figure 1.1A). There are 100 billion of these in the brain. The nerve cell sends out little fibres ('dendrites') to receive signals from other nerves (possibly up to several thousand) and sends out one long branching fibre ('axon') to carry electrical signals to other nerve cells. The longest of these fibres connect the top of the brain to the muscles of the feet. Making some big assumptions about the average length of axons, if you laid out all the neurons in the brain in a row, they would stretch for 1 million kilometres.

Where nerve fibres meet, there are specialised connections for the flow of electrical and chemical signals called 'synapses'. These are like signal boxes in a complicated railway network indicating 'go' or 'no go'. There are 10 trillion synapses in the human brain.

The varied functions of the brain are achieved by specialisation in two domains. Firstly, nerve cells themselves come in all sorts of shapes and sizes, with tiny little nerve cells extending a few micrometres to do the relatively simple job of connecting nerve cells in the same region ('interneurons') to the favourite, the majestic oak-like Purkinje cell of the

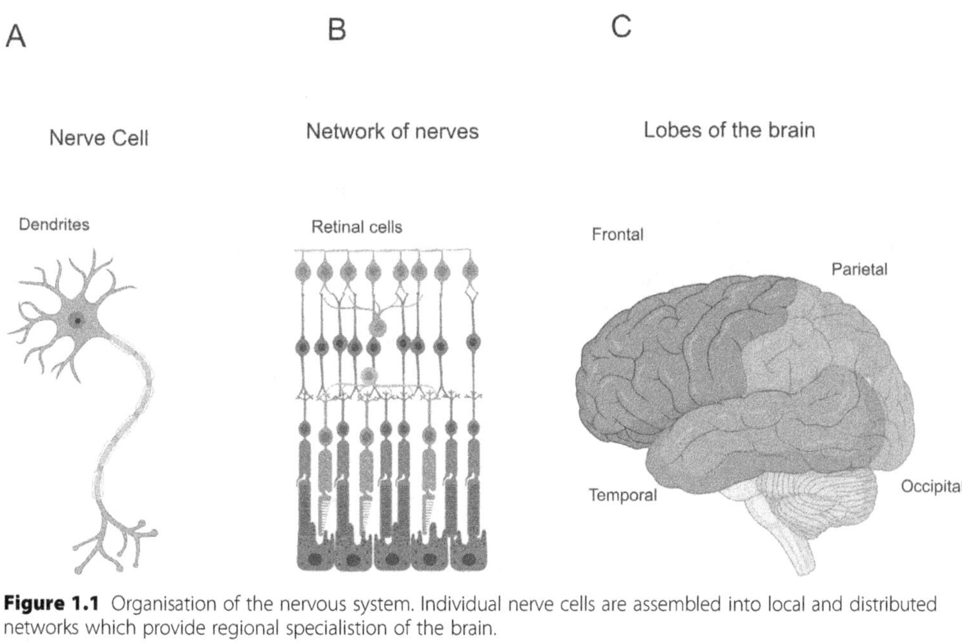

Figure 1.1 Organisation of the nervous system. Individual nerve cells are assembled into local and distributed networks which provide regional specialistion of the brain.

cerebellum, whose complex and systematic connections subserve the difficult task of coordinating movements. Secondly, different areas of the brain specialise in different tasks; so a neuron in one part of the brain can mediate some aspect of vision whereas a similar-looking nerve cell a few centimetres away is preoccupied with hearing. In this case, it is the sources of information to the neuron and its regional connections that determine its function.

The next level of organisation of the brain are 'networks': the local or regional arrangement of nerve cells. For instance, in the retina (Figure 1.1B) the receptors are connected to the retinal ganglion cells, which carry the output of vision, by a series of intermediary neurons which modulate the activity of neighbouring ganglion cells. Thus there is some processing of the photoreceptor signalling within the retina itself. The ganglion cells then send out their axons in a bundle, called the optic nerve, which then connects, via some relay nerves, to the part of the brain which mediates the perception of vision (the occipital cortex). The complex interweaving of nerves and fibres, making up these networks, are then folded in upon themselves into larger structures.

We can subdivide the gross structure of the brain. There are two 'hemispheres' which connect by a broad strap of nerves (the corpus callosum). Mostly these hemispheres are mirror-opposites: the right hemisphere controls movements of the left side of the body and vice versa. However, there is specialisation between the hemispheres; for instance, usually the brain mechanisms underlying language are in the left hemisphere. Each hemisphere can be divided into four: the frontal, parietal, occipital and temporal 'lobes' of the brain (Figure 1.1C).

Localisation and the Mereological Fallacy

The experienced neurologist is aware that symptoms can arise from any level of the nervous system: from a molecular defect, overstimulation of a neurotransmitter receptor, damage to nerve fibres, compression of the spinal cord, stroke affecting one region of the brain, psychological stress, psychiatric disorders, malingering and social dysfunction. As Daniel De Haan kindly says in this volume (Chapter 6), neurologists often traverse these layers competently, searching for the most fruitful point of intervention, which might be – among others – medication, an operation, counselling, cognitive-behavioural therapy or simply reassurance. But, not all are so skilful. As Roger Barker and Clare Redfern point out in Chapter 10, there is a literature which suggests that Parkinson's disease may reduce scores in measures of religiosity. This has been wrongly interpreted as indicating that the disease affects a 'spirituality centre'; more cautious investigators have considered that lower scores may be because impaired mobility from the disease leads to reduced attendance at religious services.

The principle of 'double dissociation' allows complex functions – such as language – to be fractionated and localised. For example, lesions of part of the frontal lobe rob people of the power of speech, but they can understand others perfectly; whereas damage to the superior temporal lobe means people can speak fluently, but there is no understandable content and they cannot comprehend others. But that does not mean that speech production depends only on the frontal lobe, nor does understanding solely reside in the temporal lobe.

Consider a lesion in *structure X* which means people cannot do *function Y*, so *function Y* is mediated by *structure X*. This is as logical as this statement: without the key, a car cannot move, therefore it is the key which moves a car.

A philosophical corrective to the localisations of the clumsy neurologist comes from an important book, *Philosophical Foundations of Neuroscience* by Bennett and Hacker (2003), to which several authors in this volume refer. They argue that the *mereological fallacy* is the mistake of attributing psychological qualities to specific anatomical structures rather than to the whole person. Experience from treating neurological diseases supports this view. As well as correcting any biochemical or anatomical disruption, if possible, the therapist will also seek to promote repair, regeneration and plasticity, to minimise impairment; and also encourage the patient to reframe their disability and adapt their life to minimise its impact. In this way, the whole person can re-establish healthy living despite significant impairment.

Humility and the Boundaries of Neurology

Like any discipline, neurology is circumscribed. The neurologist rightly has much to say about the business of diagnosing and treating a neurological disease. And he or she has a duty to report back to neuroscientists observations which enlighten our understanding of brain function.

But neurologists are neither philosophers nor theologians. Occasionally, however, chutzpah and hubris drive neurologists to misuse their expertise to support (for instance Andrew Newberg) or denigrate (Michael Persinger) religious and spiritual claims. The self-defined field of 'neurotheology' is largely made up of such embarrassments. The most a neurologist should and can comment on is the human business of believing, experiencing and practising religious lives.

References

Augustinack, J. C., A. J. van der Kouwe, D. H. Salat, T. Benner, A. A. Stevens, J. Annese, B. Fischl, M. P. Frosch and S. Corkin. 2014. H.M.'s contributions to neuroscience: a review and autopsy studies. *Hippocampus* 24: 1267–86.

Bennett, M. R., and P. M. S. Hacker. 2003. *Philosophical Foundations of Neuroscience*. Hoboken, NJ: Blackwell.

Clifford Rose, F., ed. 1999. *A Short History of Neurology*. Oxford: Butterworth-Heinemann.

Harlow, J. M. 1868. Recovery from the passage of an iron bar through the head. *Publications of the Massachusetts Medical Society* 2: 327–47.

Holmes, G. 1945. The organization of the visual cortex in man. *Proceedings of the Royal Society, Series B* 132: 348–61.

Penfield, W. 1955. The twenty-ninth Maudsley Lecture: the role of the temporal cortex in certain psychical phenomena. *Journal of Mental Science* 101: 451–65.

Tomasino, B., D. Marin, M. Maieron, T. Ius, R. Budai, F. Fabbro and M. Skrap. 2013. Foreign accent syndrome: a multimodal mapping study. *Cortex* 49, no. 1: 18–39.

Warrington, E. K., and T. Shallice. 1984. Category specific semantic impairments. *Brain* 107: 829–54.

Chapter 2

I.I *The Natures of Neurology and Religion*

The Scientific Study of Religion

Joanna Collicutt

Is it possible to study religion scientifically, and if so does it make any sense? This chapter briefly explores the relationship between scientific and religious accounts of reality before setting out some of the key historical landmarks and current issues in the scientific study of religion.

Science and Religion

In the history of Western thought science and religion are often presented as at war; after all everyone knows that the Roman Catholic Church put Galileo in prison. Yet as is often the case, the reality is more complex and nuanced. Religion and science have always been engaged in essentially the same endeavour, attempting to understand human beings and the world in which they are set, and often evolving in their different ways to fit the constraints imposed by a common cultural context.

Sometimes they come very close together, as in the development of the modern discipline of neurology. The word 'neurology' was coined by Thomas Willis (1621–75). A contemporary of John Locke, Willis took a radically empirical approach to the study of the nervous system and its functions, setting aside received wisdom in favour of close observation and systematic experimentation. Crucially his work made it clear that many of the psychological functions previously attributed to the existence of an immaterial soul that – as it were – inhabited the brain, actually had their basis in the brain itself. As Willis was a Christian believer and much of his work was funded by the Church, this presented him with an intellectual and political dilemma. Human capacities that had previously come firmly within the scope of theology had now been brought into the province of neurology. Willis' solution to the dilemma was not very satisfactory. He posited two souls, a 'corporeal soul', firmly based in the brain and shared with non-human animals, and an immaterial 'rational soul', unique to humans and which continued to exist after death.

Yet the dilemma was more apparent than real (Green 2003). A dualistic model of the human person is not inherent to Christian theology; in fact it is at odds with it. It had developed because the church had uncritically hitched its wagon to an earlier unsatisfactory science and metaphysics. The new science of neurology (and the other emerging branches of modern science) prompted theologians to return to first principles, to re-appropriate the embodied and integrated models of the human person found in the Hebrew Bible, and re-examine many of their assumptions in ways that proved to be creative and fruitful. As it turned out, they did not need Willis' well-meaning two-soul model.

If 'soul functions' are agreed to have their basis in the material world, to arise through the activity of the human brain and, more broadly, the human body, then it makes sense to study at least some aspects of them using the concepts and methods of the biological sciences. If 'soul functions' include the areas of relationships with other creatures and what we might loosely call 'the transcendent', then it makes sense also to involve the concepts and methods of the social sciences. A scientific account of the human soul (literally the human psyche) is not an exhaustive account. Nor does it provide a scientific account of God (this is a category error made most famously by Sigmund Freud (1928) and, more recently, by Richard Dawkins (2006)).

The Nature of Scientific Accounts

In his 2013 book *Why Religion Is Natural and Science Is Not*, the cognitive scientist of religion Robert McCauley offers a simple and helpful way of distinguishing between religious and scientific accounts of phenomena. This relates to the rules for invoking agents. Both religious and scientific accounts employ causal rules; both refer to invisible causal factors. But the nature of these factors is different. Religious explanations can invoke intentional agents (angels, spirits, deities) as causal factors along with non-intentional processes such as the passage of electric current. Science consciously restricts itself to non-intentional, non-agentic, factors in constructing its explanations.

McCauley first distinguishes academic approaches that require conscious reflection and the use of critical analytic faculties from more natural and plausible but often misleading intuitive approaches. Training in any academic field requires that this pre-reflective intuitive thinking be set aside, and is therefore effortful and unnatural. This is the nature of academic rigour, characteristic of both academic theology (for example studying theories of the Trinity) and science (for example studying quantum mechanics).

He then draws a second distinction between the types of explanatory framework invoked, arguing that science is particularly unnatural in that it requires the setting aside of the deeply ingrained natural human tendency to explain things in terms of intentional agents. This is so natural that even sophisticated scientists will lapse into agentic language, talking about evolution 'designing' things, impersonal forces 'trying to' do things, and so on. Both academic scientists and theologians are equally prone to praying for a parking space when under stress. When this happens they have lapsed back into the natural thinking typical of popular religion.

McCauley's analysis (summed up in Table 2.1) is helpful because it does not simply pit religious and scientific explanations against each other, portraying one as developed and the other as primitive and superstitious, but does better justice to the nature of their differences. Either type of explanation can be rigorous or unreflectively intuitive. The difference between a rigorous scientific account and a rigorous religious account is simply in their conventions for invoking agents as explanations.

Table 2.1 The natures of religious and scientific explanation

	Unrestricted use of agency	Restricted use of agency
Reflective cognition	Theology (unnatural)	Science (highly unnatural)
Intuitive pre-reflective cognition	Popular religion (highly natural)	Common sense (natural)

Source: Adapted from McCauley (2013, 231).

A scientific account of human religion does not rule out other accounts. It does not necessarily claim to give the best account. It is simply and most fundamentally an account that refuses to admit invisible intentional agents as valid explanations, while remaining agnostic as to their existence.

The Nature of Religion

The focus of this book is religion. The study of people doing religion or being religious is surely easier to delineate than the study of the human soul discussed in the first section of this chapter. Yet the scientific study of religion still faces some significant challenges. While religion is a human social phenomenon often said to be recognisable by the presence of creed, code and cult (Swidler and Mojzes 2000), its existence as a distinct and unitary phenomenon has been questioned by many on both empirical and ideological grounds (for a helpful review, see Chaves 2010). It has proved to be an elusive concept that defies tight definition. Is football a religion? Is psychoanalysis a religion? Are atheist Sunday Assemblies religious?[1] Are civic acts of remembering the fallen religious? Are Christianity and Buddhism recognisably the same sort of thing?

Definitions of religion usually acknowledge the complexity of the (contested) phenomenon by presenting it as multifaceted, with an increasing recognition that its different facets may be only very loosely associated with each other. Writing in 1965, Charles Glock and Rodney Stark proposed five dimensions to all world religions: affiliation, practice, consequences, experience and belief. More recently Michael Argyle (2002) focused on the individual psychological aspects of religion, using the related term 'faith' (also favoured by David Wulff [1996]), and argued that this is best conceived as an attitude (enduring disposition) with cognitive, behavioural and emotional components. In contrast, Kenneth Pargament treats individual faith as more fluid – something that emerges at times of crisis (Pargament 1997), but agrees that it has multiple facets or components.

The consensus on the aggregate nature of 'religion' leads to a requirement for multiple ways of operationalising it and multiple methods of capturing it: quantitative and qualitative; self and observer report; experiment, correlation and naturalistic ethnographic observation; single-case series, large samples and population surveys; physiological and psychosocial measures; a focus on the mundane and a focus on the extreme or pathological. All of these can be found in classic and contemporary studies in the field (Hill and Hood 1999; Emmons and Paloutzian 2003; Kapuscinski and Masters 2010).

The Scientific Study of Religion

Modern systematic study of religion began with the rise of anthropology in the eighteenth and nineteenth centuries, culminating in influential works such as James Frazer's (1890) *The Golden Bough: A Study in Comparative Religion*. The first recognisably psychological study of religion is probably Edwin Starbuck's (1899) autobiographical questionnaire survey of development and religious conversion. It is representative of the early work by American psychologists in this area in its aspiration to empirical rigour and its focus on conversion (a particular concern of Protestant Christians). James Leuba (1925) also stood in

[1] www.sundayassembly.com.

this tradition and attempted to construct an entirely psycho-biological account of mystical experience in his book *The Psychology of Religious Mysticism.*

The approach in Europe was more diverse. There was a particular interest in the pathological religiosity of patients (mainly women) with neuropsychiatric health conditions, for example in the work of Jean-Martin Charcot that would later be drawn on by Freud. Rudolf Otto's (1917/1958) *The Idea of the Holy* is a phenomenological account of mystical experience, interwoven with theological reflection. This more phenomenological approach is also a feature of William James' famous Gifford Lectures of 1900–1902, published as *The Varieties of Religious Experience* (James 1902). Here James takes a broadly scientific approach to different aspects of human religiosity, focusing on extreme experience, in a series of descriptive case studies and psychological reflections.

The US-based Society for the Scientific Study of Religion was founded in 1949, with its journal of the same name established 12 years later. Its website describes its aims and activities:

> The Society for the Scientific Study of Religion (SSSR) is an interdisciplinary academic association that stimulates, promotes, and communicates social scientific research about religious institutions and experiences . . . Today SSSR fosters interdisciplinary dialogue and collaboration among more than a thousand scholars from sociology, religious studies, psychology, political science, economics, international studies, gender studies, and many other fields.[2]

In Europe, the International Association for the Psychology of Religion has its origins as far back as the beginnings of the twentieth century, with the establishment of the Archiv für Religionspsychologie and describes itself as:

> an international organization promoting scientific research and exchange within the field of the psychology of religion.[3]

In 1976 the American Psychological Association established Division 36, then known as 'The society for religion' but since 2008 'The society for religion and spirituality', with a journal of the same name:

> The Society facilitates the interchange of ideas between science and clinical and applied practice, and seeks through its activities to increase public awareness of psychological dimensions of religion and spirituality.[4]

There is a focus on practice here, as in the Spirituality and Psychiatry Special Interest Group within the British Royal College of Psychiatrists, and with it a move towards a more dialogical model in which scientific studies of human religiosity might inform theological understandings and vice versa. Nevertheless, the use of scientific language and concepts remains central.

With the rapid development of structural and functional neuroimaging techniques in the last 20 years interest in the neuroscientific study of religious experience and cognition has developed apace, with the launch of the specialist journal *Religion, Brain, and Behavior* in 2011. Despite the proliferation of journals devoted to the study of religion, researchers also continue to publish in generic journals in their particular scientific field. This is especially the case where practical clinical applications beyond the religious sphere have been identified (e.g. Exline et al. 2011, 2012).

---

2 https://sssreligion.org/about/history/.
3 www.iaprweb.org/about.html.
4 www.apadivisions.org/division-36/about/index.aspx.

Questions of Method and Strategy

Much of the scientific study of religion has suffered from a lack of theoretical framework to support it. The dominant approach remains that of correlational studies that can appear to be fishing exercises, for example exploring the association between religiosity and health, moral behaviour, patterns of cerebral activity and so on. However, certain theoretical approaches drawn from cognitive science, attachment theory, coping (especially meaning-making) theory, are beginning to emerge as dominant in the field (Hill and Gibson 2008; Barrett and Burdett 2011). Experimental and quasi-experimental methodologies are also becoming somewhat more common (e.g. Saroglou et al. 2009).

In his Gifford Lectures James set out some of the key issues of method and strategy in the scientific study of religion. They remain challenges for today:

- Identifying more precisely the range of human experience and behaviours that come under the umbrella 'religious'
- Identifying the distinctive features of religious versus non-religious ideologies or aesthetic experiences and creative enterprises, and the related question of whether the study of religion requires a distinct methodology
- Identifying the differences and similarities between individual spirituality and communal institutional religion and its role as 'social glue'
- Deciding whether religion can be studied as a universal human phenomenon or whether there are only locally contextualised religions
- Avoiding reductionism – what James terms 'medical materialism'
- Delineating differences between what he terms 'healthy minded religion' and the 'sick soul' – the nature of the relationship between religion and psychopathology
- Understanding the relationship between the exceptional extreme case and the statistically normal in the area of human religiosity

The last three challenges are particularly pertinent to the subject of this book: religion in people with neurological conditions. They set an agenda, impose some constraints, yet may also, it is hoped, be illuminated by the material and perspective offered by each author.

References

Argyle, M. 2002. State of the art: religion. *The Psychologist* 15: 22–6.

Barrett, J., and E. Burdett. 2011. The cognitive science of religion. *The Psychologist* 24: 252–5.

Chaves, M. 2010. Rain dances in the dry season: overcoming the religious congruence fallacy. *Journal for the Scientific Study of Religion* 49: 1–14.

Dawkins, R. 2006. *The God Delusion*. London: Random House.

Emmons, R., and R. Paloutzian. 2003. The psychology of religion. *Annual Review of Psychology* 54: 377–402.

Exline, J., C. Park, J. Smyth and M. Carey. 2011. Anger toward God: socialcognitive predictors, prevalence, and links with adjustment to bereavement and cancer. *Journal of Personality and Social Psychology* 100: 129–48.

Exline, J., M. Prince-Paul, B. Root, K. Peereboom and E. Worthington Jr. 2012. Forgiveness issues at the end of life: a study with family members of hospice patients. *Journal of Palliative Medicine* 15: 1113–19.

Frazer, J. 1890. *The Golden Bough: A Study in Comparative Religion*. London: Macmillan.

Freud, S. 1928. *The Future of an Illusion*. Trans. James Strachey. London: Hogarth Press.

Glock, C., and R. Stark. 1965. *Religion and Society in Tension*. Chicago: Rand McNally.

Green, J. 2003. Science, religion and the mind–brain problem: the case of Thomas Willis (1621–1675). *Science and Christian Belief* 15: 165–85.

Hill, P., and N. Gibson. 2008. Whither the roots? Achieving conceptual depth in psychology of religion. *Archive for the Psychology of Religion* 30: 19–35.

Hill, P., and R. Hood Jr. 1999. *Measures of Religiosity*. Birmingham, AL: Religious Education Press.

James, W. 1902. *The Varieties of Religious Experience*. New York: Longmans, Green.

Kapuscinski, A., and K. Masters. 2010. The current status of measures of spirituality: a critical review of scale development. *Psychology of Religion and Spirituality* 2: 191–205.

Leuba, J. 1925. *Psychology of Religious Mysticism*. New York: Harcourt, Brace.

McCauley, R. 2013. *Why Religion Is Natural and Science Is Not*. Oxford: Oxford University Press.

Otto, R. 1917/1958. *Das Heliege/The Idea of the Holy*. Trans. J. W. Harvey. Oxford: Oxford University Press.

Pargament, K. 1997. *The Psychology of Religion and Coping*. New York: Guilford Press.

Saroglou, V., O. Corneille and P. Cappellen. 2009. Speak, Lord, your servant is listening: religious priming activates submissive thoughts and behaviors. *International Journal for the Psychology of Religion* 19: 143–54.

Starbuck, E. 1899. *The Psychology of Religion: An Empirical Study of the Growth of Religious Consciousness*. New York: Scribner.

Swidler, L., and P. Mojzes. 2000. *The Study of Religion in an Age of Global Dialogue*. Philadelphia: Temple University Press.

Wulff, D. 1996. *Psychology of Religion: Classic and Contemporary*. New York: John Wiley.

Chapter 3

I.I *The Natures of Neurology and Religion*

Methodological Hazards in the Neuroscientific Study of Religion

Stuart Judge*

The purpose of this chapter is to survey the various approaches and methods that have been employed in the attempt to study the extent to which religious beliefs, practices and experiences are associated with activity in different parts and pathways of the human brain. This includes not only the neurology of religion in the sense of how damage to the brain affects aspects of religious practice and belief, but also studies of neurotypical subjects. My aim has been to cover the full range of modern studies. For good measure I have mentioned some techniques that although not so far used for this purpose, could be used in future.

My purpose in spreading the net more widely than studies of patients is to highlight the substantial amount of research that has been done recently on neurotypical subjects, to assess its strengths and weaknesses, and to indicate its implications for neurology. Some topics are dealt with elsewhere in the book and in those cases I have simply referred the reader to the appropriate chapter. I have tried to keep in mind that many readers of this book are likely to be practitioners in neurology, neuropsychology and related professions caring for those with damage or disease of the brain, and to draw attention to the implications of the studies cited for such readers.

The approach I take is that of a 'Systems Neuroscientist'. My interest for many years was the study of movements of the eyes – one small, well-defined and easily measured aspect of behaviour whose neural control is now understood in some detail (Leigh and Zee 2015). By using the term 'behaviour' I do not wish to indicate a commitment to the dogma that the only proper data in the scientific study of humans is observable behaviour. On the contrary I take the view that both what can be observed, and what a person can tell one (signs and symptoms, in the usual medical usage) are evidence. Moreover I do not accept the common view among scientists that 'objective' observations trump 'subjective' reports. Rather, my view is that the aim of unbiased neuroscience is to investigate the relationships between the account given by third-person observers of what is going on in the brain with the account (in very different terms) of the first-person owner of the brain. I will use the term 'correlate' as a noun to refer in relatively neutral terms to the neural processes that are thought to underlie or accompany a particular first-person experience or activity.

Schjoedt's (2009) article 'The Neuroscience of Religious Experience' is a valuable critical review. As Schjoedt remarks, 'neuroscience has unwittingly become an effective tool for myth creation and wild speculations about religious brain processes and God modules'.

* I am grateful to the University of Oxford for access to the Bodleian Library.

Measuring Religion

Questionnaires

Questionnaires ('instruments') are one way of capturing the religious beliefs and practices of subjects. There are numerous scales that claim to capture some aspect of the religious life, with varying degrees of validity and reliability. Emmons and Paloutzian (2003) note that Moberg (2002) doubted that valid, universal measures of spirituality can be constructed because of differing conceptions of spirituality in different religious traditions. As in all scales, but especially perhaps for religious terminology, careful use of language is important. For instance, in a scale to be used assessing the spirituality of an unselected population, including those who do not profess a faith, the words 'God', 'Divine Power' or 'Higher Being' may be differently understood by different subjects.

The splendidly entitled *Religion and Spirituality: Unfuzzying the Fuzzy* by Zinnbauer et al. (1997) is a good place to start. The most comprehensive survey of the literature would appear to be *Measures of Religiosity* by Hill and Hood (1999). Emmons and Paloutzian (2003) surveyed the subject and reduced a voluminous literature to selected citations. One particular instrument worth mentioning is the World Health Organisation Quality of Life question (WHOQOL). This includes a spirituality section (SRPB) that has been validated in a large and diverse population (WHOQOL SRPB Group 2006). A more recent update is given by Kapuscinski and Masters (2010) in a careful technical review. Like Emmons and Paloutzian they commend the Expressions of Spirituality Inventory (ESI) developed by MacDonald (2000).

Monod et al. (2011) give a careful analytical review of questionnaires measuring spirituality that they deemed useful in a clinical context (in the sense of being suitable for use with patients), and recommended the FACIT-sp (Brady et al. 1999) and the Spirituality Index of Well-Being (Ellison 1983) as the best validated instruments for this purpose. The authors have some experience of the Brief Multidimensional Measure of Religion and Spirituality (BMMRS), as modified by Johnstone et al. (2009). It has been used in studies evaluating the effect of religion on health, and on the effects of neurological disease on religion (McNamara et al. 2006).

Kapogiannis et al. (2009b) used a questionnaire-based approach to investigate neural correlates of religion (and they do mean religion rather than a broader sort of spirituality). At this point I only describe their questionnaires. I will deal later with their use. The approach they take begins with the most comprehensive recent survey of US religious practice: the Institute for Studies of Religion Survey of the Baylor Institute for the Study of Religion (2006). A representative sample of 1721 respondents was surveyed by the Gallup Organisation in 2005. Both the complete questionnaire and a summary of the findings are available online. The survey included 29 questions about God's character and behaviour. Factor analysis on the responses to these questions revealed two factors, the first related to perception of God's level of engagement in the world, and the second to perception of God's level of anger.

Kapogiannis et al. (2009b) followed up this finding by constructing and validating a set of 70 brief statements about God or religion, drawing the questions from Hill and Wood (1999) or the Baylor Religion Survey. Twenty-six subjects of varying degrees of self-reported religiosity were then asked to carry out two tasks. The first task was to rate the dissimilarity of pairs of these questions on a 7-point Likert scale. The second task was to rate (again on 7-point Likert scales) each of the 70 statements according to six criteria: the extent to which the statements indicated (1) God's level of involvement (from high to low), (2) God's emotion (from anger to love), (3) religious knowledge source (from doctrinal to experiential), (4) exposure to the concept (from high to low), (5) prospective reward (from punishment to reward) and (6) time horizon (from present to afterlife). Multi-dimensional scaling showed that the results could be accounted for by three dimensions: one negatively correlated with God's perceived level of involvement, a second negatively correlated with God's perceived anger and positively with God's perceived love, and a third dimension correlated positively with doctrinal and negatively with experiential religious content. They used this approach in order to simplify the phenotyping of individuals' religiosity into three vectors, which they then correlated with changes in brain activation on various tasks. In a second study (Kapogiannis et al. 2009a), an entirely different questionnaire was used. Factor analysis of this questionnaire found four components, described as 'experiencing an intimate relationship with God', 'religiosity of upbringing', 'non-religious pragmatism' and 'experiencing fear of God's anger'. Supplementary online information with each paper includes the complete questionnaires.

Tasks

An alternative approach is to compare brain activity during tasks, either ones that form a natural feature of religion (e.g. prayer or meditation), or tests that have been constructed to discriminate in some way between non-religious and religious subjects. An example of the latter is the implicit association test used by Crescentini et al. (2015).

Neurological Studies

Temporal Lobe Epilepsy

Probably the best-known case of brain disorder that is associated with experience described as religious is Dostoyevsky temporal lobe epilepsy. This was memorably described by Dostoyevsky in *The Idiot*:

> He was thinking, incidentally, that there was a moment or two in his epileptic condition almost before the fit itself (if it occurred in waking hours) when suddenly amid the sadness, spiritual darkness and depression, his brain seemed to catch fire at brief moments . . . His sensation of being alive and his awareness increased tenfold at those moments which flashed by like lightning. His mind and heart were flooded by a dazzling light. All his agitation, doubts and worries, seemed composed in a twinkling, culminating in a great calm, full of understanding . . . but these moments, these glimmerings were still but a premonition of that final second (never more than a second) with which the seizure itself began. That second was, of course, unbearable.

The condition is discussed in Chapter 9 by Alasdair Coles. One key point is that it is very rare.

Parkinson's Disease

A number of studies of patients with Parkinson's Disease (Butler et al. 2010, 2011a, 2011b) have shown disturbances of religiosity (as defined by questionnaires or a semantic priming task). It is not clear to me that the effects demonstrated are specific to religion. It would be useful to know whether the loss of religiosity is part of a wider diminution of interests. For example, do PD patients who had a strong interest in politics lose their political passion? Modestino et al. (2016) used the methods of Kapogiannis et al. (2009b) on Parkinson's disease patients fMRI imaged in both ON and OFF medication states. The disturbance of religiosity in Parkinson's disease is discussed in Chapter 10 by Barker and Redfern.

Surgical Lesions

Gordon Pennycook, Daniel Tranel, Kelsey Warner and Erik W. Asp describe their work in Chapter 11.

Urgesi et al. (2010) studied the spirituality of 88 patients (assessed by their self-transcendence score on the Temperament and Character Inventory (TCI) of Cloninger et al. (1994) and Cloninger (1994)) before and after surgery for gliomas or meningiomas. They divided patients into those who had undergone frontotemporal cortex surgery ('anterior' patients) and those who had undergone occipitotemporoparietal cortex surgery ('posterior' patients). They found that anterior patients had common scores before surgery, regardless of the pathology, and their scores were unaltered by surgery. The same was true for those with posterior meningiomas. On the other hand those with high-grade posterior gliomas had significantly higher scores pre-surgery which rose significantly after surgery. Those with low grade gliomas had significantly higher scores only after surgery, and those with recurrent gliomas had significantly higher scores than other patients that were unchanged by surgery. Urgesi et al, suggest these findings 'hint at the active, crucial role of left and right parietal systems in determining self-transcendence'.

This is one of the most careful studies in the field. One matter of concern with the study is the scale used to assess spirituality. This is part of Cloninger's TCI scale. Unfortunately the validity of this instrument is contested. Farmer and Goldberg (2008) find many weaknesses of the instrument and summarise their findings as follows:

> Overall there is not strong support for the main assumptions of Cloninger's theory, nor is there solid support for the hypothesized structure of personality traits as measured in several versions of this inventory . . . the model and the measures used to operationalize its main elements have several significant flaws, and have limited utility in exploring and explaining important processes related to personality and psychopathology.

Hayward et al. (2011) reported in a longitudinal study of 306 subjects given repeated structural MRI every two years for up to eight years that the left orbitofrontal cortex (OFC) atrophied less in those who reported a life-changing spiritual or religious experience during the study, and in members of Protestant religious groups who reported being 'born again' when entering the study. On the other hand greater atrophy of the left OFC was associated with more frequent participation in public worship.

Neuropsychological Studies

Johnstone and Glass (2008) and Johnstone et al. (2012) have carried out what one might call purely neuropsychological studies in which they assessed patients with traumatic brain injury on tests of frontal, parietal and temporal lobe function, and of religiousness/spirituality – without reference to anatomical assessments of the pathology. They summarise their principal finding as showing a correlation between decreased right parietal lobe functioning and 'increased spiritual transcendence' as measured by the Inspirit and BMMRS tests. Examination of the data shows that the significant correlations are restricted to that between one specific test of right parietal lobe function – the JOLO test of line orientation – and the 'forgiveness' dimension of the Inspirit test. There is also a positive correlation between the Trail Making Test of frontal function and private religious practice.

Electrophysiological Patient Studies

Stimulation of the Brain during Surgery

At least since Penfield, neurosurgeons attempting to gain control over medically intractable epilepsy have stimulated the brain prior to surgery in the attempt to avoid damaging brain regions whose loss might be more of a handicap than severe epilepsy. It is possible that such stimulation might have induced religious or quasi-religious experiences (as described by Fabienne Picard, reviewed in Alasdair Coles' Chapter 9). Penfield and Erickson (1941) reported,

> Patient G.A. suffered habitual epileptic attacks that never evoked hallucinations. Yet upon electrical stimulation of her right superior temporal gyrus at point 0 . . . , she spontaneously exclaimed: 'I have a queer sensation as if I am not here . . . As though I were half here and half not here'. She reported that she had never felt this way before. Stimulation of point 1 elicited the response that she felt queer again, as if she were floating away. Similar responses occurred for point 3 and for point 5 in the neighboring parietal lobe. Penfield noted that these out-of-body experiences appeared to be linked to vestibular illusions rather than to visual or auditory hallucinations. Also, the patient seemed to have 'mental diplopia' – an understanding of her current surroundings superimposed on illusory impressions of being elsewhere. Penfield proposed that such resulting conflict in sensory impressions might account for her sense of remoteness and unreality.
>
> (quoted in Tong 2003, 105)

More recently, Blanke et al. (2002) found that stimulation of certain areas at the parieto-temporal junction induces a sensation of being outside of one's body, and this has been offered as support to the theory that the out-of-body experiences sometimes reported by those surviving severe trauma could be caused by the re-activation of this part of the brain as the subject recovers consciousness.

Electrophysiological Recordings

Electrical recordings have been made of single neurons in humans as part of assessment for surgical treatment of epilepsy. I am not aware of any such studies that investigated how neurons behave during religious activity.

Near-Death Experiences

The subject of near-death experiences is discussed in Chapter 19 by Marsh.

Structural Brain Variations with Religiosity

Kapogiannis et al. (2009b) carried out *structural* MRI imaging using a 3T scanner on 40 healthy adult subjects whose religiosity was assessed by the instrument described above, which could be understood as assessing the four components described:

> Experiencing an intimate relationship with God and engaging in religious behavior was associated with increased volume of the right middle temporal cortex, BA21. Experiencing fear of God was

> associated with decreased volume of the left precuneus, and left orbitofrontal cortex, BA11. A cluster of traits related with pragmatism and doubting God's existence was associated with increased volume of the right precuneus.
>
> (E7180)

The analysis included age, gender, education and total intracranial volume as covariates, and it was particularly important to include age.

Detailed results show that non-religious pragmatism is correlated with the size of the BA17: the primary visual cortex. It is very hard to see what role primary visual cortex could play in pragmatism, and one suspects that this is either a spurious result or has a very indirect explanation. Either way one worries about the meaning of the other correlations. It would have been very interesting to know the absolute magnitude of the differences in volume, together with measures of the noise level of the imaging and analysis procedure.

Fundamentally these data are hard to interpret primarily because it is unknown whether these differences in size of brain areas are functionally significant.

Electromagnetic Stimulation of the Brain in Healthy Volunteers

There are two established techniques of non-invasive transcranial stimulation of the brain.

Transcranial Magnetic Stimulation (TMS)

TMS was introduced by Barker et al. (1985). It applies a very large transient magnetic field, typically in a direction approximately normal to the cortical surface. Pascual-Leone et al. (2000) reviewed applications of TMS to cognitive neuroscience. Crescentini et al. (2014) studied how TMS altered performance on an implicit association test (IAT). The main effect they report is that TMS to the inferior parietal cortex improved performance on the IAT.

One of the original uses of IATs was to investigate racial stereotyping. Subjects were asked, for example, to indicate by pressing one or other button whether personal names were more likely to be of black or white individuals. In separate trials subjects indicated whether descriptive words such as 'happiness' were pleasant or unpleasant. Subjects were then asked in a new block of trials to indicate whether words fell into categories defined as either black or unpleasant, or white or pleasant. Finally subjects were asked to indicate whether words fell into conjoint categories defined as black or pleasant, or white or unpleasant. Responding more quickly and accurately in the black or unpleasant versus white or pleasant task than in the opposite task suggested racial stereotyping in a white subject.

Cresentini et al. used an IAT in which the first discrimination was religious/spiritual versus physical words. The second discrimination was self versus other where all the items were pronouns or possessives, e.g. I, you, mine, yours. It is not clear that this task is a sensible IAT, because for that one needs a category one pole of which is tied to one pole of the religious/physical domain – preferably opposite poles in religious and on-religious subjects. Perhaps what the experimenters had in mind was that the self/other distinction would serve as a proxy for subjects identifying as religious or anti-religious.

Transcranial Direct Current Stimulation (tDCS)

The second technique is transcranial direct current stimulation. Nitsche and Paulus (2000) revived interest in this approach by showing that the excitability of human motor cortex could be altered by this means. The technique was reviewed by Nitsche et al. (2008). I have not been able to find tDCS studies of religiosity or spirituality, but there are a number of interesting demonstrations of effects on cognition such as the work by Ruff et al. (2013) showing that 1mA transcranial currents applied to the human right lateral prefrontal cortex altered normal compliance behaviour, with anodal currents and cathodal currents having opposite effects.

Persinger's Helmet

A series of experiments (e.g. Persinger et al. 2001; Cook and Persinger 2001; Hill and Persinger 2003) were carried out using a custom-designed helmet that delivered very weak magnetic fields (many magnitudes smaller than in TMS) to the scalp overlying the temporal lobes. The claim was that these induced a 'sensed presence'. Granqvist et al. (2005) studied 89 subjects using Persinger's apparatus in a double-blind design, in which on half the trials the stimulator was not activated, and found no effect of stimulation. Such effects as were found correlated with suggestibility of subjects.

Functional Brain Imaging of Religion

Psychedelic Drugs

Psychedelic drugs are of interest because one of their effects is to induce a sense of ego-dissolution described in terms such as 'feeling at one with the universe', and this has some similarity with experiences reported by religious mystics. Swanson (2018) summarises recent work using fMRI to study the effects of administration of various psychedelic drugs:

> First, functional connectivity between key 'hub' areas – medial prefrontal cortex (mPFC) and posterior cingulate cortex (PCC) – is reduced. Second, the 'strength' or oscillatory power of the default mode network (DMN) is weakened and its intrinsic functional connectivity becomes disintegrated as its component nodes become decoupled under psilocybin (Carhart-Harris et al. 2012, 2013), ayahuasca (Palhano-Fontes et al. 2015) and LSD (Carhart-Harris et al. 2016; Speth et al. 2016). Third, brain networks that normally show anticorrelation become active simultaneously under psychedelic drugs. This situation, which can be described as increased between-network functional connectivity, occurs under psilocybin (Carhart-Harris et al. 2012, 2013; Roseman et al. 2014; Tagliazucchi et al. 2014), ayahuasca (Palhano-Fontes et al. 2015) and especially LSD (Carhart-Harris et al. 2016; Tagliazucchi et al. 2016).

It is worth realising that in such studies 'functional connectivity' means simply that activity in the two or more areas concerned is correlated in time.

There are two established techniques of non-invasive transcranial stimulation of the brain.

Meditation

Schjoedt et al. (2009) observed that the majority of studies on the relation between neural activity and religious behaviour have focused on meditation (see review by Cahn and Polich 2006). He argues that the difficulty of drawing any general conclusions about the neuroscience of religion from these studies are that mediation is at best only one dimension of religious experience, and moreover there is room for doubt that meditation as practised in different religions is a universal rather than variable concept. More recently the functional neuroanatomy of meditation has been reviewed by Fox et al. (2016).

Prayer

Schjødt et al. (2008) carried out a study of 20 devout Danish Christians who prayed silently in a 1.5T fMRI scanner. Brain activation was compared under five conditions: praying the Lord's Prayer, improvised personal prayer, silently recalling a well-known rhyme, wishing to Santa Claus and counting backwards from 100. The right (but not left) caudate nucleus was activated when praying the Lord's Prayer. Moreover, this was not so in other subjects, who though self-reported as religious did not pray regularly. Schjoedt et al. (2009) reported whole brain findings from the same study, summarising their findings as that areas of social cognition were recruited in personal prayer.

Cognitive Tasks That Differentiate Religious from Non-religious Subjects

Han et al. (2008) imaged 28 subjects (half of whom were Christians) using 3T fMRI while the subjects distinguished (yes or no) whether adjectives presented visually described (1) themselves, (2) Jesus, (3) Sakyamuni or (4) Zhu-Rongji (the former Chinese premier). There was also a control trial when the subjects distinguished whether the word was in bold-face or not. The main result was that the ventromedial prefrontal cortex (vmPFC) of the Christian subjects did not respond differentially whether an adjective was deemed to describe oneself or any other person, whereas in the non-religious subjects the vmPFC was activated when adjectives were deemed to apply to self and suppressed when they were deemed to apply to others. The dorsomedial prefrontal cortex, on the other hand, was not differentially activated in non-religious subjects distinguishing adjectives relating to self versus those relating to others but was differentially activated in the Christian subjects.

Kapogiannis et al. (2009b) used event-related 3T fMRI to measure 'activity' while 40 subjects indicated whether they mostly agreed or not with the 70 statements about God and religion described above. There was a control condition where the subjects simply reported the font of the statement:

> Statements reflecting *God's lack of involvement* modulated activity within 2 right-sided anterior-posterior networks, one lateral, consisting of
>
> > Right (R) inferior frontal gyrus (IFG), Brodmann area (BA) 45,
> > R middle occipital gyrus, BA 19,
> > R middle temporal gyrus (MTG), BA 21,
> > R inferior temporal gyrus (ITG), BA 20,
>
> and one medial, consisting of
>
> > R superior medial frontal gyrus, BA 8 and 10,
> > R precuneus, BA 7),
> > Left (L) IFG, BA 45.
>
> Statements reflecting *increasing involvement by God* did not produce a reliable pattern of activity.
>
> Statements reflecting *God's love* modulated activity within the R middle frontal gyrus (MFG), BA 11. Statements reflecting God's anger modulated activity within the L MTG, BA 21
>
> Statements reflecting *doctrinal religious knowledge* modulated activity within the R ITG and MTG, BA 20 and 21, and the R inferior parietal gyrus, BA 40, the L middle cingulate gyrus, BA 23 and the L superior temporal gyrus, BA 22.

> Statements reflecting *experiential religious knowledge* modulated activity within a large area in bilateral occipital lobes, with main foci at bilateral calcarine gyri, BA 17 and 18, with activation extending to the L fusiform gyrus, BA19, and the L precuneus, BA 7. They also modulated activity within L frontal areas, such as the L IFG, pars triangularis, BA 45/47, and the premotor cortex, BA 6.
>
> *Religiosity* covaried across dimensions with activity within the L precuneus, BA 23, the L temporoparietal junction area (BA 39) and the L MFG, BA 47.

The authors discuss to what extent these complex results can be understood in terms of other evidence for the functional role of the various brain areas. For example, they assert that 'statements reflecting God's lack of involvement engaged a lateral network concerned with understanding agents' actions, with main foci of activation within bilateral IFG, pars triangularis, BA 45'.

That the primary visual cortex (BA 17) and the secondary visual cortex (BA 18 and 19) should be involved in understanding statements about experiential religious knowledge seems to me to be so wildly implausible that it leads me to worry about how many of the results are spurious.

Limitations of Functional Imaging

Ecological Validity

Like standard clinical MRI machines, fMRI scanners are very noisy and cramped, and the head needs to be kept accurately still. The first limitation is therefore the extent to which a rather constrained and unpleasant environment like this is appropriate for what one might term natural religious activity. Schjoedt (2009) refers to this as the issue of ecological validity.

Uncertainty about What Is Being Measured

Most fMRI experiments cited use the Blood Oxygen Level Dependent (BOLD) signal. This is a measure of the susceptibility of the blood, which depends very slightly on the degree of oxygenation of the haemoglobin. The BOLD signal is probably a function both of the degree of oxygenation and the blood flow rate. Despite a substantial effort (e.g. Logothetis 2003, 2008), it is not known how this signal relates to more fundamental aspects of neuronal transactions such as firing rate or synaptic activity. Furthermore it is clear that there is not a spatially constant relationship between changes in neuronal activity and the changes in the BOLD signal (David et al. 2008; Friston 2009). There is therefore a very complex relationship between changes at the neuronal level and changes in the BOLD signal.

Statistical Issues

Each scan contains ~100 000 voxels, and the statistical analysis typically involves a large number of comparisons. A substantial minority of older imaging studies (25 to 30 per cent of those published in 2008, according to Bennett et al. (2009)) use rules of thumb that look plausible but can be shown to give false positive results on random data. For example, the studies of Azari et al. (2001) and Beauregard and Paquette (2006) appear not to have been corrected for multiple comparisons and are therefore likely to include spurious claims. More recent studies of religion using functional imaging seem generally to have been corrected for multiple comparisons.

Difficulties with Claims about Causal Flow in Networks

Kapogiannis et al. (2014) re-analysed the data from Kapogiannis et al. (2009b) with the aim of revealing the causal flow within the network of areas they previously identified as related to statements about religious beliefs. They use an approach called Granger causality. The validity of the technique has been criticised by Friston (2009), drawing on data of David et al. (2008), and it would seem likely that the results need to be treated with caution.

Conclusion

Perhaps it is only to be expected that it would be hard to make progress in understanding what happens in the human brain, one of the most complex entities in the universe, as subjects practice and believe religion, one of the most varied and complex of human social activities. That no very simple story has emerged seems to me to be what one might have expected if one took the view that living out religious beliefs involves a wide range of social behaviour. Some obvious examples would be altruistic behaviour, group support and solidarity and maintenance of authority. Moreover it is notoriously the case that not all religion is practised consistently (across time in an individual, and between individuals within any particular religious group). These two factors, that religion has multiple dimensions of out-working, and that the consistency of this out-working between individuals and across societies is variable, seem to me to lead one to expect that 'religion' would have a complex footprint in the brain.

References

Azari, N. P., J. Nickel, G. Wunderlich, M. Niedeggen, H. Hefter, L. Tellman, H. Herzog, P. Stoerig, D. Birnbacher and R. J. Seitz. 2001. Neural correlates of religious experience. *European Journal of Neuroscience* 13: 1649–52.

Barker, A. T., R. Jalinous and I. L. Freeston. 1985. Non-invasive magnetic stimulation of human motor cortex. *The Lancet* 325: 1106–7.

Baylor Institute for Studies of Religion. 2006. *American Piety in the 21st Century: New Insights to the Depth and Complexity of Religion in the US.* Houston, TX: Baylor Institute for Studies of Religion.

Beauregard, M., and V. Paquette. 2006. Neural correlates of a mystical experience in Carmelite nuns. *Neuroscience Letters* 405: 186–90.

Bennett, C. M., G. L. Wolford and M. B. Miller. 2009. The principled control of false positives in neuroimaging. *Social Cognitive and Affective Neuroscience* 4: 417–22. doi:10.1093/scan/nsp053.

Blanke, O., S. Ortigue, T. Landis and M. Seeck. 2002. Stimulating illusory own-body perceptions. *Nature* 419: 269–70.

Brady, M. J., A. H. Peterman, G. Fitchett, M. Mo and D. Cella. 1999. A case for including spirituality in quality of life measurement in oncology. *Psycho-oncology* 8: 417–18.

Butler, P. M., P. McNamara and R. Durso. 2010. Deficits in the automatic activation of religious concepts in patients with Parkinson's disease. *Journal of the International Neuropsychological Society* 16: 252–61. doi:10.1017/S1355617709991202.

Butler, P. M., P. McNamara, J. Ghofrani and R. Durso. 2011a. Disease-associated differences in religious cognition in patients with Parkinson's disease. *Journal of Clinical and Experimental Neuropsychology* 33: 917–28.

Butler, P. M., P. McNamara and R. Durso. 2011b. Side of onset in Parkinson's disease and alterations in religiosity: novel behavioral phenotypes. *Behavioral Neurology* 24: 133–41.

Cahn, B. R., and J. Polich. 2006. Meditation states and traits: EEG, ERP and neuroimaging studies. *Psychological Bulletin* 132: 180–211.

Carhart-Harris, R. L., D. Erritzoe, T. Williams, J. M. Stone, L. J. Reed, A. Colasanti et al. 2012. Neural correlates of the psychedelic state as determined by fMRI studies with psilocybin. *Proceedings of the National Academy of Sciences of the United States of*

America 109: 2138–43. doi:10.1073/pnas.1119598109.

Carhart-Harris, R. L., R. Leech, D. Erritzoe, T. M. Williams, J. M. Stone, J. Evans et al. 2013. Functional connectivity measures after psilocybin inform a novel hypothesis of early psychosis. *Schizophrenia Bulletin* 39: 1343–51. doi:10.1093/schbul/sbs117.

Carhart-Harris, R. L., S. Muthukumaraswamy, L. Roseman, M. Kaelen, W. Droog, K. Murphy et al. 2016. Neural correlates of the LSD experience revealed by multimodal neuroimaging. *Proceedings of the National Academy of Sciences of the United States of America* 113: 4853–8. doi:10.1073/pnas.1518377113.

Cloninger, C. R. 1994. Temperament and personality. *Current Opinion in Neurobiology* 4: 266–73.

Cloninger, C. R., T. R. Przybeck, D. M. Svrakic and R. D. Wetzel. 1994. *The Temperament and Character Inventory (TCI): A Guide to Its Development and Use*. St. Louis, MO: Center for Psychobiology of Personality, Washington University.

Cook, C. M., and M. A. Persinger. 2001. Geophysical variables and behavior: XCII. Experimental elicitation of the experience of a sentient being by right hemispheric, weak magnetic fields: interaction with temporal lobe sensitivity. Percept. *Motor Skills* 92: 447–8.

Crescentini, C., S. M. Aglioti, F. Fabbro and C. Urgesi. 2014. Virtual lesions of the inferior parietal cortex induce fast changes of implicit religiousness/spirituality. *Cortex* 54: 1–15. doi:10.1016/j.cortex.2014.01.023.

Crescentini, C., M. Di Buccahinacio, F. Fabbro and C. Urgesi. 2015. Excitatory stimulation of the right inferior parietal cortex lessens implicit religiousness/spirituality. *Neuropsychologia* 70: 71–9. doi:10.1016/j.neuropsychologia.2015.02.016.

David, O., I. Guillemain, S. Saillet, S. Reyr, C. Deransart et al. 2008. Identifying neural drivers with functional MRI: an electrophysiological validation. *PloS Biology* 6: 2683–97. doi:10.1371/journal.pbio.0060315.

Ellison, C. W. 1983. Spiritual well-being: conceptualization and measurement. *Journal of Psychology and Theology* 11: 330–40.

Emmons, R. A., and R. F. Paloutzian. 2003. The psychology of religion. *Annual Review of Psychology* 54: 377–402.

Farmer, R. F., and L. R. Goldberg. 2008. A psychometric evaluation of the Revised Temperament and Character Inventory (TCI-R) and the TCi-140. *Psychological Assessment* 20: 281–91.

Fox, K. C. R., M. L. Dixon, S. Nijeboer, M. Girna, J. L. Floman, M. Lifshitz, M. Ellamild, P. Sedlmeier and K. Christoff. 2016. Functional neuroanatomy of meditation: a review and meta-analysis of 78 functional neuroimaging investigations. *Neuroscience and Biobehavioral Reviews* 65: 208–28. doi:10.1016/j.neubiorev.2016.03.021.

Friston, K. 2009. Causal modelling and brain connectivity in functional magnetic resonance imaging. *PLoS Biology* 7: e1000033. doi:10.1371/journal.pbio.1000033.

Friston, K. J. and R. J. Dolan. 2010. Computational and dynamic models in neuroimaging. *Neuroimage* 52: 752–65.

Granqvist, P., M. Fredrikson, P. Unge, A. Hagenfeldt, S. Valind, D. Larhammar and M. Larsson. 2005. Sensed presence and mystical experiences are predicted by suggestibility, not by the application of transcranial weak complex magnetic fields. *Neuroscience Letters* 379: 1–6.

Han, S., L. Mao, X. Gu, Y. Zhu, J. Ge and Y. Ma. 2008. Neural consequences of religious belief on self-referential processing. *Social Neuroscience* 3: 1–15. doi:10.1080/17470910701469681.

Hayward, R. D., A. D. Owen, H. G. Koenig, D. C. Steffens and M. E. Payne. 2011. Associations of religious behavior and experience with extent of regional atrophy in the orbitofrontal cortex during older adulthood. *Religion, Brain and Behavior* 1: 103–18.

Hill, P. C., and R. W. Hood Jr. 1999. *Measures of Religiosity*. Birmingham, AL: Religious Education Press.

Hill, D. R., and M. A. Persinger. 2003. Application of transcerebral, weak (1 microT) complex magnetic fields and mystical experiences: are they generated by field-induced dimethyltryptamine release from the pineal organ? Percept. *Motor Skills* 97: 1049–50.

Johnstone, B., and B. A. Glass. 2008. Support for a neuropsychological model of spirituality in persons with traumatic brain injury. *Zygon* 43: 861–74. doi:10.1111/j.1467-9744.2008.00964.x.

Johnstone, B., D. P. Yoon, K. L. Franklin, L. Schopp and J. Hinkebein. 2009. Re-conceptualizing the Factor Structure of the Brief Multidimensional Measure of Religiousness/Spirituality. *Journal of Religion and Health* 48: 146–63. doi:10.1007/s10943-008-9179-9.

Johnstone, B., A. Bodling, D. Cohen, S. E. Christ and A. Wegrzyn. 2012. Right parietal lobe-related 'selflessness' as the neurophysiological basis of spiritual transcendence. *International Journal for the Psychology of Religion* 22: 267–84. doi:10.1080/10508619.2011.657524.

Kapogiannis, D., A. K. Barbey, M. Su, F. Krueger and J. Grafman. 2009a. Neuroanatomical variability religiosity. *PLoS One* 4(9): e7180.

Kapogiannis, D., A. K. Barbey, M. Su, G. Zamboni, F. Krueger and J. Grafman. 2009b. Cognitive and neural foundations of religious belief. *Proceedings of the National Academy of Sciences of the United States of America* 106: 4876–81. doi:10.1073/pnas.0811717106.

Kapogiannis, D., G. Deshpande, F. Krueger, M. P. Thornburg and J. H. Grafman. 2014. Brain networks shaping religious belief. *Brain Connectivity* 4: 70– 79. doi:10.1089/brain.2013.0172.

Leigh, R. J., and D. Zee. 2015. *The Neurology of Eye Movements*. 5th edn. Oxford: Oxford University Press.

Logothetis, N. K. 2003. The underpinnings of the BOLD functional magnetic resonance imaging signal. *Journal of Neuroscience* 23: 3963–71.

Logothetis, N. K. 2008. What we can do and what we cannot do with fMRI. *Nature* 453: 869–78. doi:10.1038/nature06976.

MacDonald, D. A. 2000. Spirituality: description, measurement and relation to the five factor theory of personality. *Journal of Personality* 68: 153–97.

McNamara, P., R. Durso and A. Brown. 2006. Religiosity in patients with Parkinson's disease. *Neuropsychiatric Disease and Treatment* 2: 341–8.

Moberg, D. 2002. Assessing and measuring spirituality: confronting dilemmas of universal and particular evaluative criteria. *Journal of Adult Development* 9: 47–60.

Modestino, E. J., P. O'Toole and A. Reinhofer. 2016. Experiential and doctrinal religious knowledge categorization in Parkinson's disease: behavioral and brain correlates. *Frontiers in Human Neuroscience* 10: 113. doi:10.3389/fnhum.2016.00113.

Monod, S., M. Brennan, E. Rochat, E. Martin, S. Rochat and C. J. Büla. 2011. Instruments measuring spirituality in clinical research: a systematic review. *Journal of General Internal Medicine* 26: 1345–57. doi:10.1007/s11606-011-1769-7.

Nitsche, M. A., and W. Paulus. 2000. Excitability changes induced in the human motor cortex by weak transcranial direct current stimulation. *Journal of Physiology* 527: 633–9.

Nitsche, M. A., L. G. Cohen, E. M. Wassermann, A. Priori, N. Lang, A. Antal, W. Paulus, F. Hummel, P. S. Boggio, F. Fregni and A. Pascual-Leone. 2008. Transcranial direct current stimulation: state of the art 2008. *Brain Stimulation* 1: 206–23. doi:10.1016/j.brs.2008.06.004.

Palhano-Fontes, F., K. C. Andrade, L. F. Tofoli, A. C. Santos, J. A. S. Crippa and J. E. C. Hallak et al. (2015). The psychedelic state induced by ayahuasca modulates the activity and connectivity of the default mode network. *PLoS One* 10: e0118143. doi:10.1371/journal.pone.0118143.

Pascual-Leone, A., V. Walsh and J. Rothwell. 2000. Transcranial magnetic stimulation in cognitive neuroscience – virtual lesion, chronometry, and functional connectivity. *Current Opinion in Neurobiology* 10: 232–7.

Penfield, W., and T. C. Erickson. 1941. *Epilepsy and Cerebral Localization*. Oxford: Charles C. Thomas.

Persinger, A. M., S. A. Koren and R. P. O'Connor. 2001. Geophysical variables and behavior: CIV. Power-frequency magnetic field transients (5 microtesla) and reports of haunt experiences within an electronically dense house. *Perceptual and Motor Skills* 92: 673–4.

Roseman, L., R. Leech, A. Feilding, D. J. Nutt and R. L. Carhart-Harris. 2014. The effects of psilocybin and MDMA on between-network resting state functional connectivity in healthy volunteers. *Frontiers in Human Neuroscience* 8: 204. doi:10.3389/fnhum.2014.00204.

Ruff, C. C., G. Ugazio and E. Fehr. 2013. Changing social norm compliance with noninvasive brain stimulation. *Science* 342: 482–4. doi:10.1126/science.1241399.

Schjødt, U., H. Stødkilde-Jørgensen, A. W. Geertz and A. Roepstorff. 2008. Rewarding prayers. *Neuroscience Letters* 443: 165–8.

Schjoedt, U. 2009. The religious brain: a general introduction to the experimental neuroscience of religion. *Method and Theory in the Study of Religion* 21: 301–39.

Schjoedt, U., H. Stødkilde-Jorgensen, A. W. Geertz and A. Roepstorff. 2009. Highly religious participants recruit areas of social cognition in personal prayer. *Social Cognitive and Affective Neuroscience* 4: 199–207. doi:10.1093/scan/nsn050.

Speth, J., C. Speth, M. Kaelen, A. M. Schloerscheidt, A. Feilding, D. J. Nutt and R. L. Carhart-Harris. 2016. Decreased mental time travel to the past correlates with default-mode network disintegration under lysergic acid diethylamide. *Journal of Psychopharmacology* 30: 344–53. doi:10.1177/0269881116628430.

Swanson, L. R. 2018. Unifying theories of psychedelic drug effects. *Frontiers in Pharmacology* 9: 172.

Tagliazucchi, E., R. L. Carhart-Harris, R. Leech, D. Nutt and D. R. Chialvo. 2014. Enhanced repertoire of brain dynamical states during the psychedelic experience. *Human Brain Mapping* 35: 5442–56. doi:10.1002/hbm.22562.

Tagliazucchi, E., L. Roseman, M. Kaelen, C. Orban, S. Muthukumaraswamy and K. Murphy et al. 2016. Increased global functional connectivity correlates with LSD-induced ego dissolution. *Current Biology* 26: 1043–50. doi:10.1016/j.cub.2016.02.010.

Tong, F. 2003. Out-of-body experiences: from Penfield to present. *Trends in Cognitive Sciences* 7: 104–6.

Urgesi, C., S. M. Aglioti, M. Skrap and F. Fabbro. 2010. The spiritual brain: selective cortical lesions modulate human self-transcendence. *Neuron* 65: 309–19. doi:10.1016/j.neuron.2010.01.026.

WHOQOL SRPB Group. 2006. A cross-cultural study of spirituality, religion, and personal beliefs as components of quality of life. *Social Science and Medicine* 62: 1486–97.

Zinnbauer, B. J., K. I. Pargament, B. Cole, R. S. Rye, E. M. Butter, T. G. Belavich, K. M. Hipp, A. B. Scott and J. L. Kadar. 1997. Religion and spirituality: unfuzzying the fuzzy. *Journal for the Scientific Study of Religion* 36: 549–56.

Chapter 4

I.II *Philosophical and Historical Aspects*

Embodied Cognition and the Neurology of Religion

Warren Brown

An objective psychologist, hoping to get at the physiological side of behavior, is apt to plunge immediately into neurology trying to correlate brain activity with modes of experience. The result in many cases only accentuates the gap between the total experience as studied by the psychologist and neuronal activity as analyzed by the neurologist.

(Sperry 1939, 295)

This statement by Nobel laureate Roger Sperry encourages us to consider the sort of information that is necessary to bridge the conceptual gap between psychological phenomena (such as religious behaviours and experiences) and the phenomenology of neurology. But what is it that needs to be taken into account in the gap between basic neurophysiology and the social and psychological phenomena of religiousness? Are religiousness and spirituality embodied physical phenomena at all? Answers to such questions are critical to establishing the basis upon which one should approach study of the impact of neurological disorders on religiousness and spirituality. What model of the relationship between body and mind is most fruitful for such study?

This chapter argues that questions about the nature of religiousness entail a larger question regarding the nature of the human mind. Building a bridge over the gap between psychology and neurology requires one to be explicit about the mind–body relationship. Substantial progress in understanding the neurology of religion must begin with a robust theory of mind that comprehends the science of neurophysiology, the clinical practice of neurology and the psychology of human life.

Theories of the Nature of Mind

Over the centuries during which neurology has emerged as a science and practice, a number of philosophical positions have held sway for different periods of time and within different disciplines. These are worth summarising, if for no other reason than to serve as contrasts with the position to be asserted in this chapter. The following is a very 'broad-brush' summary of these models of mind.

For many centuries, primarily in the Christian West, the *Cartesian* mind – that is, body-soul (or body-mind) dualism – was the dominant view.[1] While its origins were in the philosophy of Plato, this view became most explicit in Western Christian thought in the writings of Augustine and later René Descartes. In this view, the mind is a non-material entity that interacts with the body in an inexplicable way. For the present discussion, the important point is that, since religious faith and experience were considered primarily phenomena of the non-material soul, there was not much ground for talking about the neurology of religiousness. Nevertheless, correlations between body and mind/soul could not be avoided. For example, the relationship between the epileptic seizures of some individuals and intense mystical experiences were known from the time of the early Greeks (see Chapter 9 by Alasdair Coles in this volume).

This sort of mind–body dualism bred an empirical methodology in the early development of the field of psychology called *introspectionism* in which persons provided information about their minds by reporting their subjective experiences. However, in the early part of the twentieth century there arose a reaction to the lack of scientific rigour of this methodology that spawned *behaviourism*. This view argued that nothing could be learned scientifically about the 'mind' (if in fact there was such a thing). The only thing that could be known or studied was outward behaviour. All that existed was the body and its actions; any speculation about processes of mind where just that – speculation.

Neurology of religiousness could not flourish much under either Cartesian or behaviourist views. If the mind was immaterial and only accessible via introspection, then neurological disorders should have little impact. If behaviour was all that existed, then religiousness was reduced to the conditioning of bodily responses in certain contextual circumstances, leaving, at best, only a neurophysiology of learning and conditioning to be considered.

The dominant model of mind in the latter half of the twentieth century has been the information processing model (also called the *computational* model). Emergence of the computational model led to what is referred to as the Cognitive Revolution. This model began to explore systematically the nature of human cognition (language, memory, emotion, spatial ability, perception, motor control etc.), as well as the specific neural systems subserving these properties of mind. The function and architecture of a computer provided the basic metaphor. Thus, within the computational model, mental life is based on the inner manipulation of abstract symbols. Sensory and motor systems (and the body itself) are merely input and output buses (detectors and effectors) for a central processor. To be processed, information must be converted into a non-bodily form, that is, into abstract symbols (like strings of bits in a computer). Therefore, stimulus information must be 'encoded', i.e. altered to suit the brain's computational processes, in order to enable thought and decision-making. Thinking is distanced from perceiving or doing. Bodily, contextual and social influences on mind are reduced to internal computational processes involving relationships between the abstract entities that encode these phenomena.

Interestingly, the computational model leads to another sort of dualism, not entirely unlike the Cartesian view – that is, the dualism of disassociating the *outer* body from *inner* brain processes, which is sometimes referred to as *Cartesian materialism* – that is, brain–body dualism (Dennett 1991). In this view, mind is a computational process that is entirely

[1] Until recent times there was little or no distinction between the terms 'soul' and 'mind'.

internal to the brain, with the Cartesian corollary that the real self is not the whole embodied person, but something inside.

In this view, religious cognitions (experiences, behaviours, beliefs) were considered the outcome of computations in specialised modules within the brain. Thus, the idea of a 'God module' has arisen – that is, a specialised neural computational system underlying religious experience (Ramachandran et al. 1997; a similar conclusion can be found in Joseph 2001, 105). Whether or not a specialised computational module exists, this view nevertheless sees religiousness as the outcome of manipulations and computations of abstracted, encoded information that is only distantly related to the body and its ongoing interactions with the environment. Thus, Cartesian materialism views religious belief and religious experiences as entirely inward, symbolic and many processing (encoding) steps removed from bodily interactions with the physical and social world.

Embodied Cognition

Over the last two decades a new perspective has emerged in thinking about the nature of mind and the physical systems that constitute it. *Embodied Cognition* presumes that all mental processes are rooted in sensory-motor interactions of the body with the world.[2] Thus, all aspects of 'minding' (cognition) are shaped by the nature of the body and records of ongoing sensory-motor interactions of the body with the physical and social worlds. Most importantly, embodied cognition gives a very robust and explicit explanation of how the mind of an individual can be a developmental emergent of the ongoing life of the brain/body in the world.[3]

As an illustration of the theory of embodied cognition, consider the nature of the knowledge of, let us say, a pen. Within a computational model, knowing about a pen would be constituted by having an abstract encoding of 'pen' situated within a network of other semantically related abstractions relevant to 'pen-ness'. The actual sensory (visual, tactual etc.) nature of the pen or the motor knowledge of what might be done with a pen would be replaced by the abstract symbol for 'pen'. However, in embodied cognition, to know what is a pen when you see it would be constituted by an immediate link to sensory-motor knowledge of what can be done with a pen – that is, recall of the sensory-motor contingencies of past interactions with a pen. This form of knowing based on recall of relevant sensory-motor interactions is what Gibson referred to as *affordances* (Gibson 1979). To know about the visual world is to know what can be done – what interactional possibilities are afforded (offered, implied) by what is being sensed in the environment. To know the semantics of the word 'pen' is to have had linguistic (sensory-motor) interactions about pens using the *word* 'pen'. Language itself is a form of bodily sensory-motor social interaction, and the semantics of language are formed in what the philosopher Wittgenstein (1953) referred to as 'language games'. Thus, the theory of embodied cognition argues that the fundamental roots and origins of the human mind are constructed from embodied interactions with the world. While this view of mind has always been implicit in theories of

2 Advocates of Embodied Cognition include Lawrence Barsalou, Andy Clark, Raymond Gibbs, Douglas Hofstadter, Mark Johnson, George Lakoff, Alva Noë, Rafael Núñez, Donald MacKay and others.

3 Embodied cognition and its implication for religious life are also covered in Brown and Strawn (2012).

child development, it has been replaced by an abstract computational model in the understanding of the adult mind.

Two phenomena seem to be problematic in the description thus far of embodied cognition: *internal modes of thought* (i.e. thinking not expressed in current ongoing sensory-motor interactions), and *abstract thinking* (e.g. thinking about an abstract idea like 'democracy'). In the embodied view, internal, non-active thought is contingent on the capacity to run offline simulations of actions and interactions with an imagined physical or social environment (more of this later) (see e.g. Barsalou 2008). Abstract ideas or thoughts are metaphorical extensions of embodied experience (Johnson 2007). For example, 'time' is an abstract idea. However, our concepts of time are based on embodied spatial knowledge: time passes, there is the past (what is behind) and the future (what is in front of us), intervals of time are long or short etc. We also have quantitative metaphors for time based, it would seem, on the hour glass: time runs out, is sufficient for this purpose, is spent doing something etc.

What Does Embodied Cognition Assert?

In order to deepen our understanding of embodied cognition, it is useful to consider the following list of claims made by this theory of mind:

Cognition is for action. The basic problem of mind is what to do next – how to adjust ongoing behaviour to be more effective; whether to shift to another behaviour; what to do in the immediate or distant future; what can and should be said.

Cognition is situated. Actions (current, remembered or anticipated) which constitute mind cannot be extracted from situational contexts. The content of mind is what one can do in particular situations and, thus, the processes of mind are always in some sense situated. Knowing is inseparable from doing in particular physical, social, cultural contexts. Mind is built upon sensory-motor contingencies between agent and world.[4]

Cognition is time-pressured. Thinking is on-the-fly, rather than a temporally disengaged retrieval of stored abstract, symbolic knowledge. The basic problem of mind is what to do *now or next*, even if current thinking is primarily internal and decoupled (for now) from direct physical interactivity.

Action (and therefore cognition) is enmeshed in recurrent situational feedback. Mind is what is going on *between* the body and the world, not what is going on in disengaged abstract space in the head. Thus, mind is engaged in cycles of action and feedback. The ongoingness of mind cannot be stopped as if awaiting the next conscious decision regarding what to do. Consciousness can be shifted to internal modes of action-simulation, but never ceases to be ongoing.

Offline cognition is body-based (simulation). To seemingly 'stop and think', or ruminate, or meditate is to run emulations and simulations of physical and social engagements and interactions. Running behavioural simulations in our sensory-motor neural systems constitutes 'offline' thought.[5]

Meaning of language is rooted in sensory-motor experiences. Semantic content is constituted by *linguistic* interactions with the social world. For a word to have meaning is

[4] The theory that mind is constituted by sensory-motor contingency between agent and world is sometimes referred to as 'Enactivism'. See e.g. Regan and Noë (2001).

[5] The idea of thought a simulation is often referred to as 'grounded cognition'; see Barsalou (2008).

for it to have some linkage to action in the world – that is, meaning is primarily constituted in prior language interactions with persons in particular contexts. The 'intentionality' of a word is how it is used in embodied social interactions – that is, the stored memories of interactions involving the word.

Mind is primarily constituted in communities of practice. Human communities provide contexts for social, cultural and linguistic interactional learning. Communities embody understandings of how the physical and social world functions and can be successfully manipulated. Knowing is expressed in, and constituted by, the agent's ability to act as an increasingly competent participant in a community of practice.

Emotions are indices of the dynamics of bodily attunement with the environment. Ease, distress, frustration, anger, joy, happiness, positive or negative feedback are all means of attuning the body to the contingencies of the current (and sometimes imagined) physical and social context. Emotions are not primarily inner subjective experiences, although these often accompany.

Some cognitive work is offloaded into the environment. If mind is constituted by situated sensory-motor interactions, then situations themselves, and the artefacts they contain, become a part (a catalyst and necessary element) of intelligent, high-level cognitive activity. Philosopher of mind Andy Clark has commented that 'we make the world smart so that we can be dumb in peace' – e.g. a smartphone (Clark 1997, 180).

The above tenets of embodied cognition suggest the following about the nature of human religiousness: it is a whole-person property formed out of and expressed in ongoing situated action. It is assimilated in communities of practice that include acquisition of certain linguistic semantics rooted in the life of the community. Meditation, prayer and other contemplative practices are offline simulations of religiously understood actions and interactions that are rooted in the religious life of the community. To the degree that religiousness is experienced as subjective feelings and emotions, these are indicators of qualities of attunement with the religious events of one's life, whether the events are current or remembered. Some of religiousness is offloaded into artefacts of the community, whether written texts, visual art, rituals, architecture or modes of life together. Whether or not a particular form of embodied religiousness is a *true* reflection of the metaphysical nature of the universe and nature of divine presence is a question for reflection of another kind. But for the purposes of neurology of religiousness, viewing religiousness as a form of embodied cognition seems most fertile and productive.

Evidence for Embodied Cognition

The idea that cognition and mind are built on bodily experience has been given strong support by the now-familiar (and extensive) research on mirror neurons. Mirror neurons are neurons in sensory-motor systems that respond in the same way while *viewing* the activity of another individual as they do when the observer is *doing* the same motor activity. Understanding the actions of another person appears to require modelling the activity being observed within one's own motor control systems. Besides action comprehension, neural mirroring of sensory-motor experience has been used to account for such high-level cognitive and social capacities as:

- Action anticipation – when noting the onset of an action, we use out body memories to model the completion of the action.

- Speech perception – recognition of the phonemes contained within the rapidly ongoing speech being heard is contingent on being able to model the making of those particular sounds within our own articulatory neural systems. We perceive the speech sounds that we are well practised at making ourselves.
- Empathy – to have empathy for the pain or distress (or joy or pleasure) of another person is to activate neural systems involved in our own bodily experience of the same physical or emotional states.
- Theory of mind – to know what is likely going on in the mind of another person (their intentions and experiences) is contingent on being able to model (mirror) the actions and experiences of the other person within our own sensory-motor systems.
- Imitation – having understood the actions of another by modelling them in our own action systems, these systems are now primed, increasing the likelihood of doing the same activity if circumstances are sufficiently similar.

Thus, these very high-level understandings of the world are inherently perceptual-motor – that is, cognition based on sensory-motor mirroring.

The theory of embodied cognitions is also supported by a wide range of research. Examples abound in research on child cognitive development. For example, motor exploration in infants (embodied motor activity) initiates a cognitive developmental cascade that enhances intellectual and academic achievement (Bornstein et al. 2013). School-aged children learn words and math better when encouraged to gesture while learning (Goldin-Meadow 2003). In adults, imaginary rotation of a visual object is enhanced by the same direction of rotation of the hand, and inhibited by the opposite direction of hand rotation (Wexler et al. 1998). Thus, the mental activity of visual rotation appears to be done by the same motor systems used for controlling rotational movement of the hands. Reading or imaging qualities of other persons tends to induce motor mimicry, such that reading words related to elderly persons caused research participants to walk more slowly when leaving the lab (Bargh et al. 1996). Using functional brain imaging, it was found that naming tools activates sensory-motor areas of the brain that would be involved in using the tools (Grabowski et al. 1998). The fact that some cognition (e.g. memory) is offloaded into the environment is suggested by the fact that expert bar tenders line up distinctive glassware to remember multiple orders needing to be filled. Their facility at simultaneously filling a large number drink orders is considerably impaired by forcing them to use the same glassware for all orders.

The close relationship between motor and cognitive systems is illustrated by congenital disruption of a gene transcription factor know as FOXP2. This condition results in abnormal development of the movements of the face and mouth necessary for speech (called developmental verbal dyspraxia). Associated with this disruption of orofacial movements are cognitive problems in both receptive and expressive language, including difficulties in reading, writing and grammatical knowledge. This condition suggests that the systems used to organise the facial and oral movements of speech also play an important role in the cognitive processes of language.

Embodied Cognition and the Nature of Religiousness

From the point of view of embodied cognition, religiousness would be the outcome of a process of self-organisation and learning arising out of action in the world, and would continue to be rooted in sensory-motor memories and representations. From this point of view, with respect to its human participants (apart from its transcendent truth), the religiousness of persons is not the function of a non-material mind or soul, nor merely behavioural, nor the expression of internal computational manipulations of abstract symbols and propositions. Rather, religiousness is formed in persons by sensory-motor participation within a community of practice, and continues to be primarily this sort of phenomenon (even when religious ideas metaphorically extended beyond rudimentary sensory-motor experiences). Privately practised religiousness (including private meditation and prayer) is an offline bodily remembrance, simulation and rehearsal of community-learned practices, in the same way that internal processes of thought are simulations of embodied action (including simulations of linguistic acts).

Consistent with this view of religiousness is Donald MacKay's description of the nature of belief. In his Gifford Lectures, MacKay argues that belief is a 'conditional readiness to reckon' (MacKay 1991, 66–7). That is, believing something to be true is constituted by being physically *ready* to interact (*reckon*) with the subject of that belief should the relevant *conditions* arise. Thus, belief (including religious belief), according to MacKay, is an action readiness, not an abstract idea credited with a high degree of truth value. While 'reckoning' might be at times internalised, religious belief is constituted for MacKay in its implications for action readiness.

Embodied cognition implies a particular understanding of ritual in religious observances. There are bodily postures that are present in many religious observances which have universal embodied meaning – that is, the meaning is constituted by the body position itself. For example, kneeling, bowing the head, prostration and looking upwards are nearly ubiquitous in religious participation and have an obvious embodied meaning. These are acts which physically signify humility and honouring of a higher power. Thus, the meanings of these ritual acts are not abstract, but inherent in the acts themselves. Similarly, many religious rituals are performances of a core narrative of that particular religion. For example, Eucharist within Christianity is an embodied re-enactment of the core narrative of the Last Supper. From the point of view of embodied cognition, the significance of this ritual is primarily constituted by the physical re-enactment itself. Likewise, a spoken or read narration of the Last Supper engenders simulations of these events within the sensory-motor systems of listeners, which are reinforced by the embodied action of the Eucharist. Again, the meaning of the ritual would not be entirely abstract or symbolic, but would carry deep meaning that is constituted by the bodily action of the participants.

Implications of Embodied Cognition for the Neurology of Religion

The view of human cognition argued herein implies that the implications of neurological disorder for religiousness will involve brain systems and processes that are in common with many other domains of human life and entail sensory-motor processing in some manner. It is not likely that a 'God module' exists such that there is an area of the brain that is involved in religiousness, and only religiousness. Neural systems that are activated during events or activities with extremely high levels of personal significance may be activated in contexts other than a particular person's religious life, but the neural process itself would nevertheless be general and only the current content religiously specific. Thus, we should find a great deal of overlap between neurological disorders of religiousness and disorders of other aspects of a patient's life.

Alzheimer's disease (AD) is one example of the impact of more general neurological disorder on a patient's religiousness. Glen Weaver (2004) has written about embodied spirituality in individuals suffering from this form of dementia. Weaver relates how cognitive symptoms such as forgetfulness, agitation, depression and suspiciousness/paranoia create forms of spiritual disorientation and suffering for these patients. According to Weaver, the impact of AD on religiousness is found in the following areas:

- loss of one's spiritual life narrative
- fear of sinister spiritual forces
- diminished participation in spiritual practices
- difficulty experiencing God's presence, comfort and security
- experienced guilt about the loss of close relationships
- inability to initiate acts of service to others.

The breadth and complexity of life experience involved in religiousness, as well as the impact that a neuro-cognitive disorder not specific to religiousness has on a wide variety of religious experiences and behaviours, is clear from Weaver's list. Similar points are made by Julian Hughes (Chapter 14). It can also be seen that these domains of religious disruption are linked to disruptions of embodied cognition in that they all implicate mental life that is rooted in current or recalled actions and interactions with the physical or social world: loss of the record of one's past agency, emotive responses to anticipated interactions (fear), reduced religious participation, and disruption of possibilities for ongoing social interactions (service, social relationships). In this view, the religious impact of dementia is not a manifestation of problems with recall and manipulation of abstract, disembodied symbols or propositions, but rather an inability to recall and reinstate episodic records of one's embodied, interactional history.

A similar story is told by Roger Barker and Claire Redfern regarding the impact of Parkinson's disease on religiousness (Chapter 10). As Barker and Redfern summarise, Parkinson's disease has both direct and indirect impact on the religious behaviours and experiences of these patients. Direct effects include the impact of apathy and cognitive changes, as well as the possibility of a less robust theory of mind as the patient becomes less able to readily emulate the actions of others (with possible implications for capacities assumed to depend on a theory of mind such as empathy and inference of the personhood of God). Indirect effects include reduced ability to participate in religious services and religious fellowship. From the perspective of embodied cognition, it is noteworthy that, in Parkinson's disease, motor slowing is accompanied by cognitive slowing.

A somewhat different, but equally relevant, story comes from the account of mystical experiences associated with seizures – that is, deeply significant sensory experiences that the patient recognises as religious.[6] It is perhaps revealing that sensori-motor experiences at times carry meaning for persons that may have more veracity than any secondary and more abstract attributions. Some individuals with these seizures regard them as authentic spiritual experiences even though they clearly recognise that the experiences were caused by disease. Due to their sensory, motor and emotive richness, the experience of the seizure

[6] A good description of the religious experiences of a patient with temporal lobe seizures can be found in Naito and Matsui (1988).

carries meaning that is not readily altered by anything said or known secondarily regarding the neurobiological causes that may have been involved.

A similar conundrum exists with experiences created by psilocybin. An example of the impact that this drug can have on religious experiences is found in the famous 'Good Friday experiment' done many years ago by Walter Pahnke as his Harvard doctoral dissertation (Pahnke 1963; see also Pahnke and Richards 1969). In this experiment, a group of students were given either a placebo or a hallucinogenic drug (psilocybin) – without them knowing which – just prior to listening to a Good Friday service from the basement of a church. Both groups were interviewed immediately after the service and six months later. The group that was given the hallucinogenic drug rated their experiences during the service as significantly more intense and mystical than the group without the drug. At the six-month follow-up, the drug group was even more likely to recall the experience as deeply mystical and to have integrated the experience into their lives in a positive manner even though they realised they had been in the group that received the drug. Perhaps the religious veracity of both such seizure-related and drug-induced religious experiences is due to the fact that they are neither conjured up intentionally by the person nor related to events in the physical environment, and thus create a strong attribution of agency that can only be mysterious. Therefore, the meaning of the experience *is* the sensory-motor memory, not any later abstract information about neural disease, however convincing.

In the end, the solution to the abstract versus embodied debate in philosophy of mind will likely end up somewhere in between. Nevertheless, it is important to consider the embodied cognition position on its own merit, and to consider the neurology of religiousness in this light.

References

Bargh, J. A., M. Chen and L. Burrows. 1996. Automaticity of social behavior: direct effects of trait construct and stereotype-activation on action. *Journal of Personality and Social Psychology* 71: 230–44.

Barsalou, L. W. 2008. Grounded cognition. *Annual Review of Psychology* 59: 617–45.

Bornstein, M. H., C. Hahn and T. D. Suwalsky. 2013. Physically developed and exploratory young infants contribute to their own long-term academic achievement. *Psychological Science* 24: 1906–10.

Clark, A. 1997. *Being There: Putting Brain, Body, and World Together Again*. Cambridge, MA: MIT Press.

Dennett, D. C. 1991. *Consciousness Explained*. Boston: Little, Brown.

Gibson, J. J. 1979. *The Ecological Approach to Visual Perception*. Boston: Houghton Mifflin.

Goldin-Meadow, Susan. 2003. *Hearing Gesture: How Our Hands Help Us Think*. Cambridge, MA: Harvard University Press.

Grabowski, T. J., H. Damasio and A. Damasio. 1998. Premotor and prefrontal correlates of category-related lexical retrieval. *Neuroimage* 7: 232–43.

Johnson, M. L. 2007. *The Meaning of the Body: Aesthetics of Human Understanding*. Chicago: University of Chicago Press.

Joseph, R. 2001. The limbic system and the soul: evolution and neuroanatomy of religious experience. *Zygon* 36: 105–36.

MacKay, D. M. 1991. *Behind the Eye*. Hoboken, NJ: Basil Blackwell.

Pahnke, W. N. 1963. Drugs and mysticism: an analysis of the relationship between psychedelic drugs and the mystical consciousness. Doctoral dissertation, Harvard Univeristy.

Pahnke, W. N., and W. A. Richards. 1969/1990. Implications of LSD and experimental nysticism. In *Altered States of Consciousness*, ed. C. T. Tart, 399–428. New York: John Wiley.

Ramachandran, V. S., et al. 1997. The neural basis of religious experiences. In *Society for Neuroscience Conference Abstracts*, 1316. New York.

Sperry, R. W. 1939. Action current study in movement coordination. *Journal of General Psychology* 20: 295–313.

Weaver, G. 2004. Embodied spirituality: experiences of identity and spiritual suffering among persons with Alzheimer's dementia. In *From Cells to Souls – and Beyond: Changing Portraits of Human Nature*, ed. M. A. Jeeves, 77–99. Grand Rapids, MI: Eerdmans.

Wexler, M., S. M. Kosslyn and A. Berthoz. 1998. Motor processes in mental rotation. *Cognition* 68: 77–94.

Wittgenstein, L. 1953. *Philosophical Investigations*. Malden, MA: Blackwell.

Chapter 5

Phenomenology, Neurology, Psychiatry and Religious Commitment

Ian James Kidd*

This chapter offers a phenomenological analysis of changes in the structure of experience that fundamentally characterise both several main forms of neuropsychiatric illness and the nature of religious commitment. The use of the portmanteau term 'neuropsychiatric' acknowledges the fact that many of the conditions discussed in this chapter do not fit neatly within the shifting and unclear professional boundaries of psychiatry and neurology, a problem with which other chapters in this volume engage. In this chapter, in fact, I propose that these conditions are best understood phenomenologically in a way that challenges those professional partitions. Specifically, neuropsychiatric illness and religious commitment both involve distinctive changes to the structure of first-person experience that can be characterised phenomenologically in terms of altered *existential feelings* – a neglected set of affective states, currently a topic of research by philosophers, psychiatrists and cognitive scientists. Later in the chapter, I go on to make the further, stronger claim that the fundamentally phenomenological character of neuropsychiatric and religious experience assigns investigative and interpretive priority to phenomenology rather than to neuroscience. As a caveat before beginning, my claim is not that neuropsychiatric illness and religious commitment are identical or that religiosity is pathological, though doubtless they can be, and indeed surely are, complexly related in many cases.[1] Instead, the claim is that what a person experiences during neuropsychiatric illness and in religious commitment ought to be understood phenomenologically in terms of alterations in their existential feeling.

Existential Feeling and Neuropsychiatric Illness

The term 'existential feeling' was introduced in a 2005 paper by the philosopher Matthew Ratcliffe to refer to a set of neglected affective experiences that are argued to be distinct from, but often conflated with, the more familiar set of emotions, feelings and moods.[2] Given this fact, it is useful to begin a characterisation of existential feeling by explaining how they differ from emotions and moods, and how this makes them significant to our understanding of neuropsychiatric illness.

The philosophical literature on emotions has tended to construe them either as intentional states, bodily feelings or some combination of these two.[3] (This is rather different from the psychological literature which construes emotions as biopsychosocial responses.) An emotion is an *intentional state* in the sense that it is directed towards particular objects,

* I offer my thanks to Matthew Ratcliffe for helpful discussions of existential feelings and to the editors for their invitation and guidance. This chapter was written during an Addison Wheeler Fellowship.

persons or situations – as when I am angry at my broken laptop, or a lazy colleague or an instance of social injustice. Such emotions can also take the form of bodily feelings, as when a person is 'shaking with rage' or 'angry to the core' – indeed, most cases of emotion will plausibly have both intentional and bodily aspects. There is a standard philosophical list of emotions that usually includes anger, fear, grief, guilt, joy and sadness and the attention and interest of philosophers has usually been directed at these. Ratcliffe argues, however, that this focus has tended to occlude a range of other affective states that are distinctive by virtue of their being *pre-intentional* – they are not directed *at* particular things, but rather allow things to appear *as* things, which can then become the objects of intentional thoughts and attitudes.

Such feelings are *existential feelings* and they pertain to our sense of being or belonging to the world, and therefore provide the essential background to the more familiar set of explicit intentional emotions. Consider once again the emotion of *anger*. To experience anger – at an object, person or situation – is already to find oneself within a world of structured activities, projects and purposes because it is only against this background that specific intentional attitudes become possible and intelligible. An object can after all only anger or frustrate us, or delight and please us, against the background of a sense of the world as a space of significant possibilities. Otherwise there is no reason why any particular object, person or situation could elicit anger, joy or any other emotion – they would not 'stand out' as features of our experience.[4] It is this typically taken-for-granted sense of being in a world that the more familiar range of emotions and moods become possible – a sense of belonging to a world of significant possibilities for experience, thought and action.

It is this elusive sense of being in, and belonging to, a world that is captured by the concept of existential feeling. A useful way to characterise these feelings further is to consider the different ways in which people often try to describe their relationship to the world. Ratcliffe notes that use of the term 'feeling' is not restricted to emotions, given that it is also used to 'articulate various ways of experiencing one's relationship to the world that would not ordinarily be regarded as . . . emotional'.[5] A person might feel distant, detached or estranged from the world, such that it appears strange, oppressive or forbidding; or one might feel in tune with, part of, or in harmony with the world, which might the feel homely, expansive and peaceful.[6]

Such remarks are clearly not descriptions of particular features of the world – of *this* object or *that* situation – even if it might be certain objects or situations that prompt a person to recognise and report these feelings. These feelings are 'world-directed' in the sense that they structure our relationship with the world as a whole, and thereby provide the experiential basis for our specific intentional and emotional experiences of specific objects, persons and situations. An existential feeling therefore structures all experience, thought and activity and constitutes a tacit and implicit sense of reality, in a way that constitutes our sense of *being in a world* at all. So characterised, existential feelings may sound like moods in the psychological sense, but there are crucial differences. Existential feelings concern ways of experiencing or 'finding oneself within' a world, that shape the more specific types of emotions and moods that one might experience and so 'constitute a variable sense of the possibilities that the world incorporates'.[7] To be in a bad mood, for instance, presupposes the prior phenomenological achievement of *finding oneself in a world* – a world of projects that can be frustrated, persons who can dismay us, or experiences that can anger us. Second, existential feelings are intimately related to how we experience possibilities. If I'm in a bad mood with you for letting me down, that presupposes my inhabiting a world inclusive of such core possibilities as forming and sustaining intersubjective relationships, completing or terminating shared projects, and so on. Such possibilities are structured by existential feelings, making them prior to more specific moods, emotions and affects.[8]

The task of describing existential feeling is difficult for two closely related reasons. The first is that because they pre-structure all thought, experience and activity, including our explicit practices of reflection and enquiry, they do not usually appear as objects of thought and experience. Generally a person is absorbed in their experiences and activities – enjoying a sunset, writing a book chapter, laughing with friends – such that the background conditions for their possibility do not appear at the level of conscious awareness and attention.[9] It generally takes special types of interest, practice or experience to achieve such recognition, a point emphasised throughout the writings of the founding figures of the phenomenological tradition.[10]

Consider, for instance, how during our everyday linguistic activity – arguing, chatting, negotiating – we are not usually conscious of the grammatical rules and norms that are constantly and automatically pre-structuring that activity – except during special situations (such as engaging in linguistic analysis or after a deliberate misuse of grammar for comedic purposes). Since existential feelings underlie and shape our experience, thought and activity as a whole, it takes special effort and skill to recognise and explore them; indeed, phenomenology has to be practised.

The second reason why it is difficult to describe existential feelings is that they are inextricable from our *sense of reality*, our typically implicit sense of the world as a space of meaningful practical and experiential possibilities.[11] Consider, for instance, my experience of being in my office as I am typing. This rather small and drab room appears as being filled with objects that are significant in various ways – a keyboard for typing, pens for writing, biscuits for nibbling – and these objects are experienced as being *available*, *usable*, as being ready and 'on-hand' for practical use. These objects can, however, only appear as available and ready for use because they enjoy a more basic sense of reality: before an object can be available, usable or significant it must first be experienced as being real, being there and located within a structured array of other objects that collectively and holistically constitute a space of meaningful experience, thought and activity. Since this sense of reality is usually quite stable it remains invisible and unrecognised, but in certain cases it can change and become conspicuous, such that once-familiar objects and situations seem *strange* or *unreal*, in a sense that can be hard to articulate, and the world somehow *feels* different or altered.

A rich source of descriptions of alterations in a person's sense of reality is the vast body of first-person accounts of a variety of neuropsychiatric conditions. Much of the literature in phenomenological neuropsychiatry and psychopathology is devoted to case studies of a range of specific neuropsychiatric conditions, including major depression, schizophrenia, depersonalisation disorder and the Cotard and Capgras delusions (which involve the conviction that one is dead, damned or unreal, or that one's intimates have been replaced by imposters or duplicates, respectively).[12] As I suggest later in the chapter, many forms of religious or mystical experience likely also involve changes in the sense of reality. These case studies use phenomenological methods to describe changes in the structure of experience that characterise these conditions. Consider, for instance, the following accounts offered by persons with major depression. The first:

> I awoke into a different world. It was as though all had changed while I slept: that I awoke not into normal consciousness but into a nightmare.[13]

The emphasis here is on *change*, whereas in the second it is on a felt sense of *loss*:

> You know that you have lost life itself. You've lost a habitable earth. You've lost the invitation to live that the universe extends to us at every moment. You've lost something that people don't even know it.[14]

These two testimonies describe alterations in the overall structure of a person's relationship to the world, rather than to a shift in the experience of specific objects or situations within that world; indeed, what is different is 'the world', 'the universe' or 'life itself'. Ratcliffe suggests that these experiences can be understood in terms of the erosion of a formerly taken-for-granted sense of reality that ordinarily discloses the world as a structured space of significant experiential and practical possibilities. The loss of this sense is experienced, by the two persons quoted, as an emergence into a new and understandably 'nightmarish' world. A third account is offered by a woman who describes the experience of melancholic depression as being akin to 'falling into a deep black pit' in which gradually enters a 'state of non-being' in which the 'ability to live recedes'.[15]

Such remarks are typical of first-person accounts of a variety of neuropsychiatric conditions and can be interpreted as reports of alterations in existential feeling and the sense of reality. What changes is fundamentally one's experience of the world, the way one finds oneself within a wider reality; as the world itself becomes 'nightmarish', 'a deep black pit', the range and types of mood, emotion and affect to which one will be disposed shifts, too. The entire character of the world changes, as it becomes *alien, strange, different*, often in a way that is difficult to express and even more difficult to endure; especially since our capacity to identify and describe objects and experiences will depend upon a sense of reality that, in these cases, has suddenly changed. The interpretive utility of a phenomenological analysis of neuropsychiatric conditions in terms of altered existential feeling is further demonstrated in cases where a person reports the temporary restoration of a sense of reality. Ratcliffe quotes the following remark by 'Renee', the eponymous subject of the *Diary of a Schizophrenic Girl*:

> When we were outside I realised that my perception of things had completely changed. Instead of infinite space, unreal, where everything was cut off, naked, and isolated, I saw Reality, marvellous Reality, for the first time. The people whom we encountered were no longer automatons, phantoms, revolving around, gesticulating without meaning; they were men and women with their own individual characteristics, their own individuality. It was the same with things. They were useful things, having sense, capable of giving me pleasure. Here was an automobile to take me to the hospital, cushions I could rest on . . . What an unknown joy, to have an influence on things; to do with them what I liked and especially to have the pleasure of wanting the change.[16]

A striking feature of this rich and poignant passage is the restoration of Renee's sense of the world as a space of significant practical and experiential possibilities – of cushions for sitting, cars for driving, of people as concrete individuals – and of her consequent 'joy' at an experience of the world with a restored sense of reality.

During this fleeting moment, Renee again had the feeling of being in and belonging to the world, where a *world* is understood to consist not simply of recognisable objects – *chair, car, man, woman* – but as objects that constitute a meaningful structure of practical and interpersonal possibilities. It is not difficult to see why the restoration of this sense of being in and belonging to a world should be accompanied by a sensation of joy. Indeed, *anhedonia*, or diminished capacity to experience pleasure, is a typical feature of depression.[17]

I have argued that one can provide a phenomenological analysis of changes in the structure of experience in neuropsychiatric conditions in terms of altered existential feeling, and consequent changes in the sense of reality. Such an analysis has the double virtue of being empirically adequate of fidelity to the body of first-person testimonies and explanatory powerful. In the case of Renee, for instance, explanation of the transformed experience of the world falls short if it were treated in perceptual or cognitive terms alone: what changes, here, is that for that golden moment, she was able to experience the world as a rich, dynamic space of attractive, enticing practical, perceptual and intersubjective possibilities – she didn't suddenly *remember* or *notice* that cushions are for sitting or cars for travelling. Such perceptual and other changes presupposed a more fundamental transformation of her experience, as she was no longer 'cut off, naked and isolated' from the world. The phenomenology of existential feeling offers the resources better to understand aspects of the experience of neuropsychiatric illness – such as loss of hope, things 'seeming strange', and so on – in terms of radical changes in the structure of one's experience of the world. But what is not yet clear is the question of the relative merits of phenomenology and neuroscience in the context of understanding neuropsychiatric illness, and specifically of the contested question of the priority of the one over the other.

The relationship between phenomenology and empirical science has been a topic of debate throughout the history of the phenomenological tradition, and of course is the subject of lively debate in other areas of contemporary philosophy. Certainly it is clear that the founding figures of the phenomenological tradition all maintained, albeit for slightly different reasons and in different ways, that the empirical sciences were a second-order form of enquiry. There are several different ways to make this claim, depending upon the particular figures and arguments one might prefer to employ, but a very general form of the argument is that scientific enquiry can only proceed upon the basis of a more fundamental sense of the world that cannot, itself, be an object of scientific enquiry.[18]

Scientific enquiry is directed to particular objects within the world that are judged to be significant in light of our purposes or projects, and so relies upon a taken-for-granted sense of being in the world. Since the objects of scientific enquiry are selected from a pre-existing structure of experience, thought and activity which does not itself usually appear as an object of scientific enquiry – and does not figure in scientific descriptions of reality – the claim that science is an epistemically fundamental discipline is untenable. It obliviously presupposes a background sense of reality that cannot be an object of scientific enquiry, and so has a derivative or second-order status. As phenomenologists often put it, scientific enquiry is not fundamental because it cannot account for the conditions of its own possibility, though this is a rejection, not of the epistemic utility of science, but rather of a claim about its epistemic status relative to other kinds of enquiry.

Since this is a complex claim, I will focus upon the specific case of neuroscience, phenomenology and neuropsychiatry.[19] It is uncontroversial to say that any enquiry must begin with a working account of its subject matter, on the basis of which one could develop appropriate investigative strategies, select relevant objects and so on. In the case of neuropsychiatric illness, for instance, a neuroscientist might seek to identify the neural correlates of various specific conditions, such as major depression (and for present purposes I will set aside the difficult and contested issues about the nosological descriptions for neuropsychiatric illnesses).

Ratcliffe asks us to consider the case of a patient who 'complains that nothing seems real anymore, that her body feels peculiar and that the world is drained of significance', and warns against the temptation to distinguish three distinct phenomena: *bodily feelings*, *altered experience* and certain consequent *beliefs*.[20] A neurobiologist who then began to investigate the neural correlates of such feelings, experiences and beliefs would break up a phenomenologically unitary experience in three abstracted components: even though the altered sense of things being 'unreal' diminishes our sense of being bodily situated within a space of practical possibilities.

In this case, the utility of neuroscientific enquiry can evidently proceed only on the basis of descriptions of the structure of experience provided by a first-person account. As Ratcliffe puts the point:

> The phenomenologist studies aspects of experience that are presupposed by all empirical, scientific investigation into what the world contains . . . Hence scientific practices do not escape existential backgrounds and then confront them as objects of empirical study. Rather, scientific practices and scientific conceptions of the world arise within the space of possibilities that the phenomenologist describes.[21]

A general form of the argument for the explanatory priority of phenomenology is therefore that it provides the subject matter for investigation by neuroscience.

There is a further, related sense in which neuroscience ought to cede explanatory priority to phenomenology. The epistemic contribution of neuroscience is to identify the neural correlates of behavioural performance in neuropsychiatric conditions, but this is neither identical with, nor reducible to, the phenomenological task of describing alterations in the structure of those experiences. Even a complete description of the neural correlates of the experiences that accompanies neuropsychiatric illness, such as estrangement or of loss of hope, would still not provide a description of the *structure* of those experiences.[22] If so, then to assign privileged status to neuroscience would be to needlessly deprive ourselves of a richer range of investigative resources for understanding the experiential complexity of neuropsychiatric illness.

In this section, I have argued that neuropsychiatric illness ought to be understood in terms of altered existential feeling; in the next section, I make a parallel claim about religious commitment.

The Phenomenology of Religious Commitment

A central debate in analytic philosophy of religion is the nature of religious belief and a wider set of issues concerning the nature of religiosity itself. Such debates have typically operated on the basis of what one might call a 'belief model', according to which to be religious is to hold a set of beliefs, typically drawn from doctrinal and creedal structures of religious traditions. Such beliefs can then be appraised in terms of their rational and evidential credentials, hence the vigour of debates concerning faith and evidence, the rationality of religious belief and the merits of arguments for the existence and attributes of god.[23]

A standard complaint about the belief model and its variants has been that it arguably fails to capture certain distinctive, if not essential aspects of the nature of religious commitment. Central among there are the roles of *feeling* and a range of related affective states and experiences, including a foundational sense of belonging to the world that unmistakably recalls Ratcliffe's remarks on existential feeling. Such a sense might be tacit and inarticulate, but no less genuine for that reason, and several testimonies could be offered for this claim. It was, for William James, a feeling of 'spiritual excitement' that animated religious reflection; or took the form of the 'impulses' that for John Dewey constitute a 'religious attitude'; or perhaps the 'feeling of participation in the ultimate reality' described by Leszek Kolokowski.[24] Such remarks merit close and careful analysis, not least given the differing concerns of the figures cited, but an obvious theme is that religiosity is grounded in an affectively charged experiential relationship to the world.[25]

Many other testimonies could be offered and interpreted profitably as instances of what the philosopher Paul Moser calls *kardiatheology*: 'a theology of the heart', to be contrasted with cognitivist theologies that tend to be more narrowly focused upon argument, belief and theory.[26] Such claims gather around the conviction that it is a mistake to construe religious commitment in terms of a set of rationally determined and evidentially warranted doctrinal and doxastic commitments, usually for the reason that – as the philosopher of religion John Cottingham puts it – the cognitivist stance 'does not capture what is at stake when someone gives, or refuses, their allegiance to a religious worldview'.[27] Certainly argument, belief and doctrine are only certain components of a religious life, alongside practices, communities, institutions, texts, soteriological projects, a spiritual heritage, aesthetic experiences, each complexly related to one another in what can be concisely and complexly described as a *way of life*.[28]

The practical and experiential dimensions of religious commitment that tend to be absent from much mainstream analytic philosophy of religion are much better served within the psychology of religion. The phenomenology of religion is therefore partly an effort to bridge the philosophical and psychological studies of experiences of religious commitment.[29] Doing this requires an investigation of the phenomenological conditions for the possibility of religious experience, thought and activity. Any conscious experience, thought, or activity can only become possible against the background of a taken-for-granted sense of being in the world – of belonging to a world that appears as a structured space of possibilities, of being among objects, persons and situations that appear as *real*, *significant* and so on. This is just as true of a religious person as of the secular atheist humanist, given that existential feeling and a sense of reality is a precondition for the possibility of experience, thought and activity. The study of the structure of experience in the context of religious belief, practice and experience is called *phenomenology of religion*.

The starting point for a phenomenological study of religion is the core idea that our thought, experience and activity presuppose a lived relationship to the world, which can be understood in terms of existential feeling and a sense of reality. Indeed, the phenomenologist Mark Wynn suggests that existential feelings might provide the experiential basis for the consciously articulate systems of concepts, beliefs and practices upon which typical philosophical interest has tended to focus.[30] There are several closely related aspects to this claim, the first of which being that existential feeling will be implicated very generally within the life of a religious person. After all, if our existential feelings constitute our sense of being in a world of significant practical and experiential possibilities, then the possibility of religious belief and practice will depend upon certain existential feelings. A person who engages in religious practices, such as thanksgiving or praying, and who believes in the goodness of god and the providential structure of his creation, can only do so on the basis of their sense of being in the world – of, for instance, their being in a world in which thanksgiving and praying appear as significant practical possibilities.

Since this is true whether a person is religious or not, the second aspect of Wynn's claim is that certain existential feelings might predispose a person towards the practical and doctrinal resources provided by the historical religious traditions. Given that existential feelings comprise both a 'generalised sense of the nature of reality', inclusive of some sense of its 'existential import' for human life, then one might judge that certain existential feelings could count as forms of religious experience.[31] Such religiously tinged existential feelings are not, of course, associated with specific beliefs or doctrines, but rather act to predispose a person towards certain broad types of metaphysical or ethical conviction. A person who feels the world to be dark, empty and forbidding is not thereby *required* to adopt a mystical doctrine coupled to a pessimistic estimate of the human condition, but they would certainly have experiential justification for finding such doctrines cogent, if not compelling.

Indeed, Wynn speculates – quite plausibly, in my view – that, at least in cases of religious commitment, 'many believers take their tradition to be plausible . . . because they find that there is a "fit" between the defining concepts of that tradition and the world as it is presented to them in experiential terms'.[32] Certain beliefs and doctrines about the nature of reality, and the existential situation of human beings within it, can enjoy a pre-reflective degree of intelligibility and plausibility, not on the basis of careful rational deliberation, but because at a deep, often inarticulable sense, they cohere with one's foundational sense of how the world is. And in case this seems to entail that religious commitment is, ultimately, irrational or 'subjective', it should be emphasised that these claims also apply to non-religious doctrines and claims. It is clear that many critics of religion are, in fact, equally reliant upon a taken-for-granted sense of what the world is like, even if they fail to recognise it.[33] Indeed, our capacity to provide robust rational justification for our fundamental convictions is actually quite limited, especially since we must take certain facts about the world for granted even to begin projects of enquiry.

So far, I have suggested that existential feeling plays a general role in a religious life, given that such a life will presuppose a way of being in the world, and also the more specific role of shaping a person's predispositions towards the articulated beliefs and doctrines contained in the world's historical religious traditions. There is no necessary causal chain from having a certain existential feeling and adopting the beliefs and doctrines of a particular religious tradition. Rather, we do better to think of existential feelings as contributing to tacit sense of the nature of reality and of our situation in it – perhaps one of estrangement from a dark, alien realm – that can be explored and articulated using the socially deployed, historically inherited resources of religious traditions.

Indeed, Wynn suggests that 'certain cultural and religious traditions' could, perhaps, 'contribute to the formation of a correlative existential feeling', and, through 'ongoing interchange', even arrive at a 'state of equilibrium'.[34] This is not an individual achievement, of course, since so many religious practices and projects are shared, co-operative ones, often extending across generations. Underlying so many of the world's religious and spiritual traditions is a deep imperative to seek some form of intimacy or integration with the world, although this takes many different specific, merging forms.[35] All of these presuppose, however, the possibility of an experientially and existentially complex relationship with reality, and obviously this is an imperative that presupposes a certain sense of *being in*, or *belonging to*, the world – for instance, a world to which one feels one could or does belong, in some suitably integrated and intimate way, and not 'dark', 'cold', or 'forbidding'.

Wynn brings these points about existential feeling and religious commitment together in a way that include bodily feeling, experience and what I called the deep imperative that animates the world's religious traditions:

> The religions are interested in a deeper transformation of the person ... aim not simply, if at all, at doctrinal conformity, and outward conformity of the body to various religious practices. They also aim at engendering in the person a new sensibility, where this sensibility does not, in the normal case, float free from doctrinal affirmations or bodily practices, but nonetheless transcends them insofar as it is a condition of the whole person, and extends not simply to what they do and what they, in all sincerity, say, but to what they feel and, crucially, how the sensory world is presented to them.[36]

It should be clear from these remarks that there are complex phenomenological preconditions for the possibility of a life of religious commitment. Such a life only partly involves reflective adoption of certain beliefs, robust performance of certain practices or regimented participation in certain social and historical communities. Instead, such experiences, thoughts and practices all presuppose a background sense of being in the world – of being in, and perhaps belonging to, the world – that should be understood in terms of existential feeling and a sense of reality. A life of religious commitment begins in a felt sense of one's being in the world, upon the basis of which beliefs can be adopted, and activities undertaken.

Certainly, something like this phenomenological account is evident in the writings of many leading spiritual writers and religious authorities, of which I will offer just two. The first is a beautiful passage by the eighteenth-century German theologian, Friedrich Schliermacher, describing a type of 'mysterious moment' – both profound and indescribable' – that is 'the natal hour of everything living in religion'. Such moments are experienced as 'feelings or intuitions' rather than articulable insights, and occur when some particular 'event' – a church service, say, or sunset – 'develops quickly into an image of the universe'.[37] These religious experiences are bodily feelings and involve an altered, intensified experiential relationship with the world, and commentators have interpreted them in terms of changes in existential feeling.[38]

The second example of altered existential feeling in religious life is taken from the nineteenth-century German theologian, Rudolf Otto, who describes, in his book *The Idea of the Holy*, certain experiences involving awareness of 'the presence of that which is a Mystery inexpressible'. Such experiences need not be profound and periodic, for they can underlie 'sudden, strong ebullitions of personal piety' and the 'fixed and ordered solemnities of rites' – *belief* and *practice*, one might say – and they bring with them a sense of the world as a whole as 'something beautiful and pure and glorious'.[39] These remarks by Schleiermacher and Otto both testify to the core claim of phenomenologists of religion, such as Wynn, that a fundamental experiential relationship to the world underlies the articulated beliefs and structured practices of a religiously committed life – a form of life shared among a community of the fellow faithful.

If religious commitment ought to be understood phenomenologically in terms of existential feeling, then it will be useful to consider potential cases of radical alterations in existential feeling. An obvious place to look for altered existential feeling in religion is *conversion experience*, defined by Wynn as an experience of 'fundamental and in principle dateable shift in religious outlook'.[40] Though existential feelings are changeable, they will naturally be more conspicuous when they alter rapidly or radically, or indeed when a person has rich descriptive or introspective capacities.

A good example is the experienced described by the Russian author, Leo Tolstoy, in the autobiographical essay *A Confession*, especially since it is discussed by both Ratcliffe and Wynn.[41] The *Confession* describes an experience that might today be classed as major depression, during which Tolstoy struggles with a profound state of existential despair, despite reflecting on the positive course of his life until that point. After failing to find solace in religion, philosophy or learned culture, Tolstoy finally came to a new religious conviction, and in chapter 13 he reflects on his altered 'relations to faith':

> Formerly life itself seemed to me full of meaning and faith presented itself as the arbitrary assertion of propositions to me quite unnecessary, unreasonable, and disconnected from life. I then asked myself what meaning those propositions had and, convinced that they had none, I rejected them. Now on the contrary I knew firmly that my life otherwise has, and can have, no meaning, and the articles of faith were far from presenting themselves to me as unnecessary – on the contrary I had been led by indubitable experience to the conviction that only these propositions presented by faith give life a meaning. Formerly I looked on them as on some quite unnecessary gibberish, but now, if I did not understand them, I yet knew that they had a meaning, and I said to myself that I must learn to understand them.

In the richness of this passage there are three broadly discernible stages that could be interpreted as reflections of altering existential feeling. The first stage is that of a comfortably taken-for-granted sense of existentially secure being in a world, with no felt sense of any need for religious solace. The second stage, by contrast, involved a radical loss of a sense not only of the meaningfulness of Tolstoy's life, but also the loss of the possibility of its ever being meaningful. A person might, after all, feel that their life currently lacks meaning, but still feel that it could come to have meaning, perhaps if one changed it in some substantive way. The third stage involved a partial restoration of the sense of the possibility that a life could be meaningful, albeit newly accompanied by a felt need that actualising this possibility required spiritual effort.

At this third stage, we might say that Tolstoy gained, to recall Wynn's words, a 'new sensibility' – or way of being in the world – that incorporated a felt sense of need for the practical and doctrinal resources of, in this case, the Russian Orthodox Church. Although this is far from a complete analysis, I suggest that Tolstoy's conversion experience can be understood in terms of a radical alteration of existential feeling, especially when contrasted with the more positive experiences described by Schleiermacher and Otto. These three figures each testify, albeit in different ways, to the conviction that certain ways of experiencing the world can be religiously significant, but which are not 'religious experiences', for two reasons. The first is that they do not necessarily have as their object anything specifically *religious* – such as God or a prophet – and the second is that they are not, strictly speaking, experiences *of* any specific object at all; for sure, they may be occasioned by religious activities, such as prayer or worship, and might be interpreted using the conceptual resources of a given religion, but they are, on close analysis, ways of being in the world that can be articulated and perhaps cultivated using the practical and conceptual resources of the world's historical religious traditions. In fact, one might speculate that those traditions emerged partly as responses to felt need by persons with requisite existential feelings to express them practically and conceptually. James, in fact, suggested that 'dispassionate intellectual contemplation of the universe' by itself could not have 'resulted in religious philosophies such as we now possess'.[42]

In this section I have argued that religious commitment should be understood phenomenologically in terms of particular forms of existential feeling, though the relationship between such feelings and explicit systems of religious belief and practice is very complex. It should also be clear that, if that claim is correct, then neuroscience can play only a limited explanatory role where religious commitment is concerned. An essential precondition for religious commitment will be finding oneself in the world as a theatre of possibilities, including such specific and complex possibilities as achieving a degree of intimacy with the world of a sort that lends structure and salience to those beliefs, doctrines, emotions and practices constitutive of the religious life. A religious sense of the world is a way of finding oneself within a world, something that has to be in place before more specific beliefs, moods and behaviours can become possible.

Conclusion

This chapter has offered a phenomenological analysis of the structure of experience in neuropsychiatric illness and religious commitment in terms of altered existential feeling. The core idea is that the possibility of experience, thought and activity presuppose our having a typically tacit, unrecognised sense of being in, and belonging to, a world, and that this can be disclosed through phenomenological analysis. During certain forms of neuropsychiatric illness, such as major depression, this background sense of being in the world is eroded and a person loses their sense of inhabiting a space of significant possibilities – hence reports of objects, people or the world itself seeming to be different, altered or unreal, and of a consequent sense of emptiness, despair or estrangement. Such transient alterations in the background sense of the world are to be found in both pathological and non-pathological experiences, even if they become particular acute, and therefore conspicuous, in cases of grief, despair, sin, moral abjection or during conditions such as temporal lobe epilepsy. Moreover, the focus on experiences of altered existential feeling can also be used to interpret cases of religious conversion, including either the loss or the gain of religious faith, and so in turn illuminate the nature of religious commitment. Indeed, the case of Tolstoy's experience – of despair, conversion and faith, as one prefers – could be classified as either religious or neuropsychiatric, or it could be taken more usefully as an illustration of the interpretive complexity of human experience. A central claim of the chapter has been that experience, thought and activity rely upon a tacit sense of being in the world. Since scientific enquiry takes those experiences, thoughts and activities as they are given as its subject matter, and is therefore confined to particular aspects of certain experiences rather than the conditions of possibility for experience as such. If so, then phenomenology enjoys priority in the task of exploring and understanding of neuropsychiatric illness and religious commitment.

Endnotes

1. W. James, *The Varieties of Religious Experience: A Study of Human Nature: Being the Gifford Lectures on Natural Religion Delivered at Edinburgh in 1902* (London: Longman, Green, 1902); J. Carrette, *William James and 'The Varieties of Religious Experience'* (London: Routledge, 2004); C. Taylor, *Varieties of Religion Today: William James Revisited* (Cambridge, MA: Harvard University Press, 2003).
2. M. Ratcliffe, 'The Feeling of Being', *Journal of Consciousness Studies* 12 (2005): 43–60; Ratcliffe, *Feelings of Being: Phenomenology, Psychiatry, and the Sense of Reality* (Oxford: Oxford University Press, 2008); Ratcliffe, 'The Phenomenology of Existential Feeling', in *The Feeling of Being Alive*, ed. S. Marienberg and J. Fingerhut (Berlin: de Gruyter, 2012), 23–54.
3. P. Goldie, ed., *The Oxford Handbook of Philosophy of Emotion* (Oxford: Oxford University Press, 2010).
4. The main writers include Antonio Damasio, Peter Goldie and Robert Solomon.
5. Ratcliffe, 'Feeling of Being', 45.
6. For examples, see Ratcliffe, *Feelings of Being*, chapter 2.
7. M. Ratcliffe, *Experiences of Depression: A Study in Phenomenology* (Oxford: Oxford University Press, 2015), 2.
8. The differences between existential feelings, moods, emotions and affects is more fully discussed in M. Ratcliffe, 'Why Mood Matters', in *The Cambridge Companion to Heidegger's 'Being and Time'*, ed. M. Wrathall (Cambridge: Cambridge University Press, 2013), 157–75; Ratcliffe, *Experiences of Depression*, chapter 2.
9. Martin Heidegger, *Being and Time*, trans. J. Macquarrie and E. Robinson (Oxford: Blackwell, 1980), 80.
10. A useful introduction to phenomenology is Shaun Gallagher and Dan Zahavi, *The Phenomenological Mind: An Introduction to Philosophy of Mind and Cognitive Science* (London: Routledge, 2008).
11. See e.g. Ratcliffe, 'Phenomenology of Existential Feeling', sections 3 and 5.
12. See e.g. Ratcliffe, *Experiences of Depression*; Ratcliffe, 'Interpreting Delusion', *Phenomenology and the Cognitive Sciences* 3, no. 1 (2004): 25–48.
13. Quoted by Dorothy Rowe, *The Experience of Depression* (London: Wiley, 1978), p. 269
14. Quoted by Gail A. Hornstein, *Agnes's Jacket: A Psychologist's Search for the Meanings of Madness* (Emmaus, PA: Rodale Books, 2009), p. 213
15. P. C. Whybrow, *A Mood Apart: Depression, Mania, and Other Afflictions of the Self* (New York: HarperCollins/ Basic Books, 1997), p. 23
16. Marguerite Sechehaye, *Autobiography of a Schizophrenic Girl* (New York: Signet, 1970), pp. 105–6.
17. A recent review of research on anhedonia and depression is S. J. Rizvi, D. A. Pizzagalli, B. A. Sproule and S. H. Kennedy, 'Assessing Anhedonia in Depression: Potentials and Pitfalls', *Neuroscience and Biobehavioural Reviews* 65 (2016): 21–35.
18. The phenomenological critique of the primacy of science takes different form, but a sophisticated 'synthetic' account is offered by David E. Cooper, *The Measure of Things: Humanism, Humility, and Mystery* (Oxford: Clarendon, 2002), chapters 5, 9 and 10.
19. M. Ratcliffe, 'Phenomenology, Neuroscience and Intersubjectivity', in *The Blackwell Companion to Phenomenology and Existentialism*, eds. H. Dreyfus and M. Wrathall (Oxford: Blackwell, 2006), 327–43.
20. Matthew Ratcliffe, 'Understanding Existential Changes in Psychiatric Illness: The Indispensability of Phenomenology', in *Psychiatry as Cognitive Neuroscience: Philosophical Perspectives*, eds. Matthew Broome and Lisa Bortolotti (New York: Oxford University Press, 2009), 239.
21. Ibid., 241.
22. A lively study is Raymond Tallis, *Aping Mankind: Neuromania, Darwinitis and the Misrepresentation of Humanity* (Durham, UK: Acumen, 2011).

23. A useful critical survey of the 'belief model' and its status within contemporary philosophy of religion is John Cottingham, *The Spiritual Dimension: Religion, Philosophy, and Human Value* (Cambridge: Cambridge University Press, 2005).

24. I. J. Kidd, 'Emotion, Religious Practice, and Cosmopolitan Secularism', *Religious Studies* 50 (2014): 139–56; Kidd, 'A Phenomenological Challenge to "Enlightened Secularism"', *Religious Studies* 49 (2013): 377–98.

25. See e.g. Mark Wynn, *Emotional Experience and Religious Understanding: Integrating Perception, Conception and Feeling* (Cambridge: Cambridge University Press, 2005).

26. P. Moser, *The Evidence for God: Religious Knowledge Reexamined* (Cambridge: Cambridge University Press, 2010).

27. John Cottingham, *The Spiritual Dimension: Religion, Philosophy and Human Value* (New York: Cambridge University Press, 2005), 2.

28. See Cottingham, *Spiritual Dimension*, and Cottingham, *Why Believe?* (London: Continuum, 2009).

29. A useful starting point is Mark Wynn, 'Phenomenology of Religion', in *The Stanford Encyclopedia of Philosophy*, ed. E. N. Zalta, http://plato.stanford.edu/entries/phenomenology-religion/.

30. Mark Wynn, *Renewing the Senses: A Study of the Philosophy and Theology of the Spiritual Life* (Oxford: Oxford University Press, 2013), 64–70.

31. Ibid., 67.

32. Ibid., 107.

33. I. J. Kidd, 'Is Naturalism Bleak?', *Environmental Values* 22 (2013): 689–702.

34. Wynn, *Renewing the Senses*, 68, 65.

35. The plurality of forms of religious or spiritual aspiration are explored by D. E. Cooper, 'Sense, Mystery, and Practice', *International Journal of Philosophy and Theology* 79 (2018): 425–36 and by I. J. Kidd, 'Spiritual Exemplars', *International Journal of Philosophy and Theology* 79 (2018): 420–4.

36. Wynn, *Renewing the Senses*, 74.

37. Friedrich Schliermacher, *On Religion: Speeches to Its Cultured Despisers*, trans. Richard Crouter (1799; repr., Cambridge: Cambridge University Press, 1976), 31–2.

38. G. Andrejč, 'Bridging the Gap between Social and Existential-Mystical Interpretations of Schleiermacher's "Feeling"', *Religious Studies* 48 (2012): 377–401.

39. Rudolf Otto, *The Idea of the Holy: An Inquiry into the Non-rational Factor in the Idea of the Divine and Its Relation to the Rational*, trans. J. W. Harvey (London: H. Milford/Oxford University Press, 1923), 12–13.

40. Wynn, *Renewing the Senses*, 16.

41. M. Ratcliffe, 'Evaluating Existential Despair', in *Emotion and Value*, ed. S. Roeser and C. Todd (Oxford: Oxford University Press, 2014), 229–46.

42. W. James, *The Varieties of Religious Experience* (New York: Longmans, Green, 1902), 431.

Chapter 6

I.II *Philosophical and Historical Aspects*

Philosophical Hazards in the Neuroscientific Study of Religion

Daniel De Haan

To deny the truth of our own experience in the scientific study of ourselves is not only unsatisfactory; it is to render the scientific study of ourselves without a subject matter.
F. Varela et al., The Embodied Mind

Given that common sense recommends a world view with physical and psychological elements, the neuroscientific eliminativist about everyday psychology . . . changes the subject when he speaks of states of the brain: he fails to bring a concept of *person* to bear when he says that commonsense psychology merits elimination.
Jennifer Hornsby, Simple Mindedness

I am tasked with addressing philosophical hazards in the neuroscientific study of religion. As a philosopher concerned with the well-being of neuroscientists studying religion, I am inclined to begin with the philosophical hazards of philosophy. I am well aware of the extraordinary difficulties of both tasks, for the hazards are many and it is easy to miss the forest for the trees or the trees for the forest. Instead of focusing on one issue in great detail, I shall hang a number of warning signs around a forest of issues that identify various philosophical hazards which deserve particular caution when it comes to neuroscience and religion. Since I am aiming for breadth over depth, my brief remarks on each issue shall be synoptic, non-exhaustive, contentious and suggestive for additional consideration and reflection. To redress such deficits, I have provided references for further reading.[1]

Hazards of Identifying Hazards

I begin with a few hazards concerning the project of identifying hazards. First, most of the philosophical hazards I discuss are general problems for philosophy and neuroscience that are foundational with respect to the specific issues pertaining to scientifically studying religion. I start with these general hazards before touching on a few hazards specific to religion. Second, the dominant or 'standard' stories in philosophy are not difficult to find; one can consult the online versions of the *Internet Encyclopedia of Philosophy* and *Stanford*

Encyclopedia of Philosophy (*SEP*), or the fine handbooks and companions published by University Presses. I aim to draw attention to hazards not often flagged by these approaches. Many of these hazards challenge prevailing – sometimes merely fashionable – philosophical and scientific views, views that range from being false, to misleading, or merely require self-criticism or cautious charitable investigation of rival views. Sometimes it is important to remember that: default positions have their own uncritical assumptions; that the default view owes as much to historical contingency as it does to the cogency of its arguments; and, that there are persuasive *alternative ways* of seeing matters related to neuroscience and religion which cannot be ignored. Finally, due to limitations of space I am forced to make unqualified generalisations about various *hazards*, but the reader must recognise that there do not exist any nice and neat cookie-cutter shaped positions – *hazards* or otherwise – held by philosophers, scientists and religious persons. Reality is much more complex than our abstractions, idealisations, and claims to knowledge sometimes suggest, including my own.

Hazards of a Neuroscientific Explanation of Religion

The target of explanation for us is religion, the means by which it is to be investigated, studied, described and explained is by neuroscience. What hazards might a philosopher draw attention to here? My central claim is this: The most fundamental philosophical hazard for the neuroscientist studying religion to avoid vigilantly is the failure to appreciate adequately the unified and integrated whole that is religious, namely the human person. Human persons are religious, not their minds or brains. Neuroscience can only provide a *partial* explanation of religion insofar as the brain can only be but a *partial* – even if a *sine qua non* – factor in anything approximating a complete description and explanation of human persons, including those who are religious. Claims to explanatory comprehension that outstrip these limitations imperialistically exceed what is reasonable and true. The investigation of human persons and religion should be holistic and aim to illuminate, explain and integrate the vast multi-level interconnections to be found from *subpersonal level* attributes like molecules, genes, organelles, cells, organic systems (e.g. cardiovascular, immune, endocrine, neuronal and glial systems), organs, organisms, to the ways these causally and constitutionally enable but neither eliminate nor provide explanatory substitutes for the complex *personal level* psychosomatic, rational, social and historical factors that figure into the lives of human persons.[2]

This distinction between *personal level* and *subpersonal level* descriptions and explanations of human persons provides a helpful heuristic for demarcating and integrating the aforementioned diverse forms of enquiry, description and explanation in the neuroscientific study of religious persons.[3] The expansive concepts of common-sense psychology – pain, sensation, perception, emotion, memory, imagination, enquiry, understanding, beliefs, desires, practical reason and voluntary action – belong to the personal level insofar as the paradigmatic meanings and attribution of these concepts essentially involves mention of persons. A proper understanding of these personal level psychological attributes must integrate their distinct manifestations from first-, second- and third-person perspectives. Understanding the many *ways* we accurately attribute the concepts of *belief* and *pain*, for instance, requires appreciating a host of behavioural, epistemic, social, linguistic, logical and other criteria exhibited in the contrasts between *I believe X, you believe X, this person believes X* and *I am in pain, you are in pain, this person is in pain.*[4] Subpersonal level phenomena fall under the purview of psychological, cognitive and neurological enquiries, descriptions and explanations that address what factors underlie, constitute, enable and cause phenomena at the personal level. Whereas the first- and second-person perspectives are essential and exclusive to personal-level attributes, subpersonal level attributes are exclusively approached from a *distinctive form* of the third-person perspective, namely one that looks to the non-personal, non-conscious, non-rational, non-linguistic and principally biological factors that enable and make a difference to personal level attributes. The subpersonal level pertains to enquiry, descriptions and explanations that are unavailable to the perspectives of first-, second- and third-person interactions with other persons *as* persons; it concerns what we can know about the human being's subpersonal psychology and biology by observations and inductive correlations achieved through invasive and non-invasive techniques, e.g. blood tests, X-ray, EMG, EEG, fMRI.

The personal/subpersonal distinction is not another version of the mental–physical dichotomy; most *personal level* descriptions – e.g. someone intentionally going to the store to buy milk – require putative mental *and* physical attributes. Indeed, the conceit behind the view I am urging recommends abandoning the mental–physical dichotomy in philosophy, psychology and neuroscience, and adopting the integrated way of understanding human persons illuminated by the personal/subpersonal distinction. Significantly, the personal and subpersonal are not to be conceived as two independent things, they illuminate two ways of describing and explaining the complex and integrated features that constitute our embodied form of life as rational animals. Consider episodic or experiential memory; it admits of both personal level and subpersonal level accounts that are not in conflict or competition, but which can and should be integrated. Insofar as episodic memory shows up in enquiries, descriptions or explanations that involve or require first-person, second-person and third-person interactions – like narrating how someone met their spouse – then we are addressing the personal level features of episodic memory. So, the personal level pertains to both ordinary and clinical interactions and discourse concerning whether *I remember*, *you remember* or *this person remembers* experiencing when, where or what something or other happened. But insofar as we draw upon the resources of neurology, neuropsychology or cognitive neuroscience – which concern medial temporal lobe damage and models of information processing, encoding, consolidation and retrieval – we are looking to subpersonal level factors. Clinicians are especially adept at bringing together the resources of the personal and subpersonal level to provide a holistic account of, for instance, the symptoms of anterograde amnesia experienced by a patient and their family with imaging evidence of damage to the medial temporal lobe, and integrating both resources to find a holistic way to treat or cope with disorders.

The personal/subpersonal distinction is not a conceptual panacea; it is a heuristic or rough rule of thumb that helps us situate distinct but complementary forms of enquiry, description and explanation about human persons. It shows one of several ways forward that allows us to reject the presumption that the only starting place for understanding ourselves is to adopt either dualism or reductive physicalism. Not only do these two metaphysical frameworks fail to exhaust the range of metaphysical views, they should not purport to be first principles of investigation; at best, they are among its possible conclusions. Prior to such investigations, there is no need to pigeon hole the human person into the conceptual straight jacket of either one of these restrictive frameworks.

Philosophy, Science and Conceptual Frameworks

From Socrates to the present, philosophers have been concerned with asking questions, understanding and reflectively arriving at knowledge of the truth about the nature of reality. Philosophy draws attention to the fact that we all employ a worldview (*Weltanschauung*) – a conceptual framework that includes many concepts and categories – in our ordinary and scientific discourses about the world and ourselves. The collaborative human endeavour to know the truth about reality requires serious reflection on the overt and tacit ways in which we employ concepts and language to describe and explain the reality we experience. Unsurprisingly, there can be many subtle mistakes in the coherence and logical structure of our categories, arguments and ways of thinking and speaking that can mislead our philosophical and scientific understandings of the world. Philosophy in particular challenges us to draw critical attention to the ways we use and understand such fundamental polysemous concepts as being, entity, identity, reality, phenomenon, nature, essence, kind, substance, property, relation, constitution, whole, part, datum, fact, concrete, abstract, modalities (necessity, possibility, contingency, and impossibility), state, event, action, passion, process, activity, agent, ability, disposition, power, capacity, manifestation, space, time, laws of nature, causation, supervenience, emergence, teleology, reduction, elimination and many other concepts that are ubiquitously employed by us in a variety of ways to understand and arrive at knowledge of reality.

I introduce these polysemous concepts at the outset to draw attention to the fact that without many of them, reality would be unintelligible and the practice of science and its clinical applications impossible. Given the fundamental importance of these concepts in science there is a *desideratum* for scientists to cultivate and practice a disciplined use of concepts by reflecting on what they intend to mean when using such concepts, and know how to contrast the distinctive and connective meanings of these words and concepts that they do intend to employ, from those many other meanings that they do not intend to use. To fail to do so is to fall victim to the *Hazard of the Unreflective Conceptual Framework.* Disagreement over these concepts and their connections to reality abounds, but it is nevertheless important for all critical thinkers to dedicate themselves to the intellectual discipline of reflectively interrogating their conceptual framework. The aim is not to resolve all disputes about the proper meaning of these concepts, but to gain some critical perspective on the varieties of meanings used in the more specialised conceptual frameworks employed in scientific, philosophical, religious and other contexts. Without such conceptual discipline, one can never attain a critical perspective on how to interpret others or on how to anticipate and avoid unnecessary equivocations when stipulating technical uses of these concepts.

The interdisciplinary nature of cognitive neuroscience in particular demands greater attention to the *Hazard of the Unreflective Conceptual Framework* and vigilance about variant meanings and unintentional equivocations:

> Cognitive neuroscience unavoidably traverses the boundaries between the neural cum physiological and the psychological, as well as the boundaries between the neural/physiological and the behavioral. The concepts in these three domains are categorically dissimilar. Their logical articulations are unalike, and the logical connections (of implication, exclusion, compatibility) between the different domains are exceedingly difficult to get into clear view ... The different domains are not reducible one to another, and what explanations are appropriate to one domain

may be inappropriate to another. How the description of phenomena in one domain bears on the description of phenomena in another is highly problematic.[5]

There is an exigency for cognitive neuroscientists to attain a level of conceptual precision in their understanding of the psychological concepts they employ that matches the precision of their experiments. I am not alone in maintaining that the *Philosophical Foundations of Neuroscience* (*PFN*) and *History of Cognitive Neuroscience* (*HCN*), co-authored by the neuroscientist Maxwell Bennett and philosopher Peter Hacker, provide one of the best places to begin an education in conceptual clarity in the domains of philosophy, psychology, cognitive science and neuroscience.[6] Obviously neuroscientists do not need to become philosophers to do excellent neuroscience, but they do need to employ a rigorous conceptual framework in order to rigorously operationalise their definitions and interpret their experimental findings. And the detailed studies of experimental work in *HCN* and *PFN* provide an excellent resource and formation in how to achieve a conceptually rigorous framework. Many of their readers, myself included, will find much to disagree with in their work, but that is hardly grounds for dismissing the fundamental aims of the project and its usefulness for scientists. To those who eschew careful study of *PFN* and *HCN*, I ask: How could a meticulous critical reflection on the fundamental conceptual framework employed in any field of research be a disservice to that discipline?

Even the neuroscientist Joseph LeDoux has come to realise the importance of heeding the *Hazard of the Unreflective Conceptual Framework*. After decades of neuroscientific research on 'fear', LeDoux now believes it was a mistake for him to conceptualise this work as research on fear – a conscious emotion. What he and others are really studying are the non-conscious neural systems for threat detection. LeDoux entreats neuroscientists to aim for greater conceptual clarity:

> It seems obvious that scientists should be as precise as possible to short-circuit the opportunity for misunderstanding. If we can avoid confusion by simply changing the terms, why would we not do it? ... By using different terms for conscious feelings and the nonconscious events that can, in some organisms, contribute to feelings in the presence of threats, much of the ambiguity and confusion about the neural mechanisms that detect and control responses to threats, and neural states that may result, is avoided.[7]

Scientific discoveries often lead us to introduce new, extended or metaphorical uses of meanings and terms that are already part of our conceptual framework. This invites alternative ways of understanding reality, but it also opens us up to the possibility of misunderstandings. To avoid equivocations, stipulating novel technical uses of pre-existent terminology requires careful reflection about what is meant by these innovative extensions. For instance, cognitive psychology and neuroscience often draw upon the *personal level* terminology of common-sense psychology, like memory, emotion and cognition, to develop technical terminology that pertains to the *subpersonal level* mechanisms of cognitive psychology and cognitive neuroscience, e.g. Alan Baddeley's model of working memory, Endel Tulving's episodic memory system, Michael Gazzaniga's interpreter module, Giulio Tononi's integrated information theory of consciousness. In fact, many of these psychological models promiscuously conflate and fail to distinguish between personal and subpersonal level features. LeDoux's own self-critique evidences the massive confusions that result from uncritically employing the term 'fear' which is a personal level concept of a conscious emotion, to characterise a subpersonal level cognitive neural mechanism that undergirds *not* the emotion of fear, but non-conscious 'threat detection'.

In short, the central contention of *PFN* enjoins us to ask important questions: If we do not know *what* we are talking about, then what progress can really be made? What are rigorous experimental protocols without rigorous reflection on the fundamental concepts operationalised to describe and explain the empirical phenomenon of interest? Raising objections to the exigency for conceptual rigour is as unscientific as objecting to the need for experimenters to concern themselves with experimental protocols and meticulously acquired data. Science requires a conceptually clear understanding of the basic concepts it employs, of the hypotheses it formulates, and of the ways its interpretations of data are situated within the conceptual framework of some theory.

Psychological Discourse and Crypto-Cartesian Hazards

Let us now turn our attention to the philosophical hazards bound up with a certain conception of the nature of psychological discourse, that is, the everyday attribution and predication of psychological concepts to ourselves, other humans and non-human animals. The first is the *hazard of theoretical models of psychological discourse.* When a mother says her child has fallen in love with someone, is this attribution of 'love' to her child always based on some psychological theory she has about a theoretical postulate called 'love'? Or is the mother's attribution of 'love' relying on some everyday common-sense understanding of psychological concepts like love, joy, anger, desire, belief and intention? Most contemporary philosophers and many scientists assume that common-sense psychological concepts (e.g. sensation, memory, belief, desire, intention) are non-observable *theoretical* entities that we postulate and attribute to others in order to predict and explain their observable behaviour. If this 'folk psychology' is a theory, then like any theory it is open to theoretical refutation or replacement by a more sophisticated cognitive or neuroscientific theory of psychology, just as the folk physics and folk chemistry of astrology and alchemy have been replaced. Jerry Fodor, Daniel Dennett and many others have argued for various reasons that folk psychology is a non-eliminable theory. In contrast Paul and Patricia Churchland contend that cognitive neuroscience will soon supersede the predictive and explanatory power of folk psychology, allowing us to eliminate the theoretical postulates of 'belief', 'desire' and so on. The widespread endorsement of various theoretical models of common-sense psychology has generated the problem of other minds as well as the seemingly irresolvable debates about the experiments in developmental psychology, comparative psychology, and evolutionary psychology about 'theory of mind' or 'mind reading', that is, the ability of human children, adults and other animals to theorise, albeit tacitly via some theory or simulation, about the non-observable internal mental attributes of other animals.

A small contingent of philosophers and psychologists reject the assumption that all psychological discourse is theoretical. It is true that there exist specialised forms of psychological discourse that are theoretical (e.g. the declarative and non-declarative memory systems of Milner, Squire and Kandel; Tulving's episodic memory system; Fodor's language of thought; the computational and representational theory of mind; propositional attitude belief-desire psychology, which is the mainstay of analytic philosophy of mind), but ordinary psychological discourse is not theoretical. The mother does not employ a theory of love or beliefs in order to ascribe love or beliefs to her child. The root problem underlying the *hazard of theoretical models of psychological discourse* can be identified with a host of more fundamental hazardous assumptions inherited from modern philosophers like Locke,

Hume and especially Descartes. While contemporary naturalists reject Cartesian mind–body substance dualism, many naturalists nevertheless embrace a Crypto-Cartesian conceptual framework. Crypto-Cartesianism denotes a mélange of philosophical hazards. The first is the twin *hazards of the mind–body* and *mental–physical dichotomies*. Adopting any version of these hazardous false steps – such as the division between the mind and body or between the brain and behaviour – sets up an austere physical world against the disembodied ratiocinations of the mind or brain. By placing meaning, intelligibility and reason outside of nature, these views encourage an unjustified separation of behaviour from psychology. Indeed, it has been argued that Crypto-Cartesian approaches to cognitive neuroscience generate two problematic dualisms! First, the mind–mind dualism between the conscious mind and non-conscious computational mind, and a second mind–brain dualism that concerns the problem of how the brain can be an information processing computational mind.[8] Contrary to crypto-Cartesianism, we do not need the mental–physical dichotomy as there are more accurate alternative ways of understanding and distinguishing animal behaviours; ways that acknowledge a plurality of descriptive and explanatory strategies for getting at the whole.[9]

Rather than taking for granted the *hazards of the mind–body* and *mental–physical dichotomies*, we should begin our investigations with the whole animal, which is a dynamic psychosomatic unity that has evolved to interact with the affordances of its environment in a variety of fascinating ways. Crypto-Cartesianism also assumes a number of theses closely tied up with the hazards of the mental–physical dichotomy that have been uncritically accepted as the default framework for investigating psychological behaviour:

1 *Hazards of the Mindless Body*: The body and its physical attributes, like behaviour, are observable, outward, public, objective entities known from the third-person perspective; some physical behaviour of animals is explained by *theoretically* postulating or inferring private internal mental, cognitive or neurophysiological causal mechanisms
2 *Hazards of the Private Mind*: The mind and mental attributes are essentially private, unobservable, inner, subjective entities; mind or self is directly accessible through conscious first person introspection, but we indirectly and theoretically access other minds by inductive or analogical inferences based on observable behaviour

Accepting these two hazards as gospel truth explains in part the genesis of theory of mind debates and the irresolvable philosophical problem of other minds, as well as the confrontation between behaviourists and cognitivists in empirical psychology. While behaviourists and cognitivists endorse incompatible views about what count as genuine psychological explanations, they share a common commitment to the view that behaviour is observable and the mind is unobservable. In short, they both endorse the *hazards of the private mind* and *mindless body*, but behaviourists reject empirical explanations that theoretically appeal to unobservable mental postulates, and cognitivists maintain such theoretical postulates are necessary for empirical explanations of behaviour. And this is why, given the *hazard of the mindless body*, the only way empirical psychology can address non-observable mental attributes, is as postulated theoretical entities that provide causal explanations for overt behaviour.

A similar story provides the impetus for assimilating all psychological discourse, including common-sense or folk psychology, to the theoretical model of psychological attribution. But we need not accept these assumptions. And rejecting crypto-Cartesianism opens up conceptual space to consider alternative pictures of humans and other animals.

Let us look at two complementary alternatives to the hazards considered thus far, the first being the account of psychological attribution detailed in *PFN*'s presentation of the *mereological fallacy*.

Mereological Fallacy in Neuroscience

Mereology studies the relationships between parts and wholes. 'The neuroscientists' mistake of ascribing to the constituent *parts* of an animal attributes that logically apply only to the whole animal we call 'the mereological fallacy' in neuroscience'.[10] The two formidable works by Bennett and Hacker, *PFN* and *HCN*, perspicuously and magisterially present the precise nature of the mereological fallacy, objections to it, scrupulously well documented violations of it, and the multitudinous hazards that ensue from overlooking it in studies on sensation, perception, cognition, memory, cogitation, belief, imagination, emotion, volition, consciousness and self-consciousness by philosophers, psychologists, cognitive scientists and neuroscientists.

It is important to draw attention to a common misunderstanding of their work. It *is not* an attack on neuroscience; it is an attempt to challenge and clarify the philosophical problems that underlie the uncritically endorsed conceptual framework operationalised by many neuroscientists in their research. It is conceptual medicine for a conceptual illness; we might not enjoy the dose or the therapy, but it is intended to help neuroscientists acquire and operationalise a rigorous conceptual understanding that keeps up with their rigorously acquired data. Let us summarise a few salient features of their monumental contribution to the conceptual framework of neuroscience.

First, contrary to the *hazards of the private mind* and *mindless body*, the meanings of our psychological concepts are bound up with the characteristic psychological behaviour – including linguistic behaviour – they signify. The bodily behaviour of animals *is* psychological behaviour; the idea of 'mere bodily movements' that need to be inductively, analogically or abductively correlated with mental or psychological attributes is an abstraction of the behaviourists and philosophers. Long before humans achieve a mastery of language, let alone an understanding of psychological concepts, humans, like other animals, perceive and interact with the psychological behaviours of other animals. It is upon this pre-linguistic, pre-conceptual, and so certainly pre-theoretical basis that humans can transition from a perceptual engagement with the psychological behaviour of animals, to a linguistic understanding and engagement with the psychological behaviour of animals. And it is on the latter basis, that is, the eventual flowering of a linguistically rich common-sense psychology, that humans, quite late in their evolutionary history, transition into something akin to what might be called a theoretical investigation of psychology.

It is, of course, common for humans to be thinking or intending something, to be in mild pain or experience emotions without overtly exhibiting these psychological attributes.[11] Additionally, the meaning of psychological attributes, like anger, are not exhaustively characterised by the description of expressive bodily behaviour, including stereotyped facial movements. The mere description of the bodily movement of a sudden articulation of the knee does not discriminate between a reflex and a voluntary movement. But such abstracted descriptions are unlike our ordinary psychological ascriptions which occur within a wider ecological context that includes observing the psychological behaviour that led up to and followed a knee jerk or voluntary movement. It is in this ordinary context that we observe and interact with the psychological behaviour of others; this is the ecological setting in which we learn what psychological attributes mean by recognising certain patterns of psychological behaviour of animals as *criteria* for the ascription of certain psychological attributes to animals. This is why psychological behaviours are also partially constitutive of the meanings of personal level psychological predicates. It is not possible to describe aptly animal vision, audition, motivation, or executive functions independent from the stereotyped psychological behaviour the animal bearing these attributes exhibits in its environment. This criterial evidence from psychological behaviour for the ascription of psychological attributes is defeasible by countervailing evidence. Humans and other animals are obviously capable of lying, dissimulating, deceiving, pretending, faking and acting as if they are in pain, believe X, desire Y and so forth. 'However, if the criteria for a person's being in pain, believing or intending something *are* satisfied on an occasion and are *not* defeated by countervailing evidence in the circumstances, then we are warranted in asserting that he *is* in pain, *does* believe or intend'.[12]

Second, we ascribe psychological behaviours to the animal as a whole, not merely to its parts. There are no *seeings, pain-sufferings, thinkings, desirings, runnings* and *eatings* walking around in the world as independent entities in their own right. There are only seeing, suffering, thinking, desiring, running and eating animals. Again, the very intelligibility of these basic psychological concepts is bound up with the psychological behaviours we can perceive and engage and eventually linguistically understand. This is the pre-theoretical point of departure for our basic experience and understanding of psychological attributes. This is why the *observable psychological behaviour* of humans and other animals provides the primary evidence for the ascription of psychological attributes to them.

Third, the foregoing account of ordinary non-inductive psychological identification and attribution grounds the 'possibility of inductive (non-logical) identification [which] becomes available through inductively correlating subjects' having certain psychological attributes with other phenomena – for example, neurophysiological events in their brain'. However, if this inductive evidence from, say, fMRI conflicts with the 'normal criteria for the ascription of a psychological predicates, the criterial evidence overrides the inductive correlation'.[13] Said otherwise, inductively establishing the neural correlates of some animal's psychological attributes presupposes and depends on our ordinary non-inductive knowledge of and ability to ascribe these psychological attributes to the animal.

Fourth, it is for these reasons, among others, that the brain cannot satisfy the criteria for being the literal subject of psychological attributes. 'Though neural phenomena are well correlated with an animal's or a person's being in pain, the brain does not exhibit *pain-behavior* ... The observed neural phenomena that are concomitants of a person's suffering pain, for example, are not forms of pain-behavior. They are *inductively* correlated with being in pain. The correlation is an empirical discovery, which presupposes the concept of pain and its nexus with criterial, non-inductive evidence for the application of the concept of pain *to a living creature* (not to its brain)'.[14]

Fifth, as is explained at length in *PFN*, the mereological fallacy is not raising a jejune objection against the possibility of novel, metaphorical, analogical, technical or synecdochical extensions of our ordinary psychological concepts. Rather, it is objecting to the conceptual confusions that result from mistakenly, misleadingly, uncritically or inconsistently claiming to be doing any one of the former and then instead providing no justification for taking such psychological attributions literally or to be insightful, heuristically helpful or explanatory. When 'concepts undergo such analogical extension, something new stands in need of explanation'.[15] Without further elaborations, these novel uses lead to confusions and misunderstandings.

> Talk of the brain's perceiving, thinking, guessing or believing, or of one hemisphere of the brain's knowing things of which the other hemisphere is ignorant, is widespread among contemporary neuroscientists. This is sometimes defended as being no more than a trivial *façon de parler*. But that is quite mistaken. For the characteristic form of explanation in contemporary cognitive neuroscience consists in ascribing psychological attributes to the brain and its parts *in order to explain* the possession of psychological attributes and the exercise (and deficiencies in the exercise) of cognitive powers by human beings.[16]

In sum, Bennett and Hacker are not, as is sometimes suggested, neuroscience sceptics; rather, they are critical of philosophical confusions that lead to misinterpretations of the very important achievements of neuroscientists. Their aim is to help neuroscientists free themselves from the shackles of conceptual confusions they have inherited from the conceptual framework of bad philosophy, so that they can proceed to do their important scientific work more perspicuously.

Critical evaluations of Bennett's and Hacker's *PFN*, and especially its account of the 'mereological fallacy', often ignore the fundamental claim of Bennett and Hacker that ordinary behavioural criteria are constitutive of the meanings of our psychological concepts. Context does matter. The context in which we behave psychologically and later learn how to speak about and conceptualise psychological phenomena is very different from the contexts in which psychologists and neuroscientists perform their experiments and sometimes casually and sometimes literally take psychological concepts rooted in practices from the context of ordinary life and ascribe them to different subjects, like parts of the brain, in very different contexts without explaining if there are any differences between the meaning of memory and its behavioural criteria in everyday life, from the meaning of 'memory' later ascribed to the medial temporal lobe which does not have that behavioural criteria. This is the crux of the mereological fallacy.

Treating Bennett and Hacker as a single psychological agent, the co-author 'BH', whose philosophical attributes are explained by one part of BH, namely H, belies a more important disanalogy. We know independent of their co-authorship that Bennett and Hacker are both independent psychological agents, whereas this is precisely what is under dispute about the brain: Is the brain also a psychological agent, a bearer of personal level psychological attributes? Our legitimate enquiries into what parts of the brain are subpersonal explanatory factors for the personal level psychological attributes of humans *depends upon* our basic and primary recognition of the psychological attributes that belong to human persons. However, if theorists wish to argue that it is explanatorily illuminating to ascribe the personal level psychological attributes of humans to the brains of humans (rather than focusing on subpersonal explanatory factors), then they need to demonstrate what is genuinely explained by re-introducing the same psychological attributes at another level or what new meanings are given to these psychological concepts taken from the context of everyday experience and applied to the brain within the decontextualised environment of the laboratory or clinic.

Psychological and Ontological Identity of Human Persons

The *personal/subpersonal* distinction introduced earlier in this chapter is not equivalent to the *mereological principle* identified by *PFN*, though they are complementary. The mereological fallacy pertains to ascriptions of concepts to some part, that, given the paradigmatic intelligibility or meaning of some concept, it can only be literally attributed to a whole, not its parts. The mereological principle applies to wholes and parts that are artefacts and machines just as much as to humans and other animals. The *personal/subpersonal* distinction, as I employ it, contends that the meaning of some psychological attributes, namely personal level attributes, are intrinsically bound up with the meaning of a person, a rational animal. We cannot understand beliefs, desires and intentions apart from persons that have beliefs, desires and intentions. If the complete story about, say, belief-desire psychology, leaves persons out and claims to get by without believing and desiring persons being in the picture, then something has gone terribly awry. We have, at best, *changed the subject* from the psychology of the believing and desiring human person, to that of a problematic conception of person-less beliefs and desires. Similarly, the application of these personal level psychological attributes to the nervous system, is to change the subject in a still more radical way. In both cases the person disappears as if irrelevant to our basic understanding of paradigmatically personal level psychological attributes. This uncritical form of changing the subject is one instance of the *Hazard of the Disappearing Person*. Bringing together the arguments afforded by the *personal/subpersonal* distinction and the *mereological principle* secures the claim that persons are attributed to wholes, like to rational animals, and not to any of their parts.

This last point bears further consideration. The human person constitutes a dynamically unified and integrated whole amid a magnificent spectrum of abilities and their manifestations. This brings us to the *Hazards of Mind, Body, Self Reification*. Without any doubt, it is certainly true that I am my*self*. I am also an em*bodied* being with a range of intellectual abilities, and these might be equated with possessing a *mind*. Nevertheless, conceding such points does not mean we must accept the frequent reification of these attributes which obfuscates rather than clarifies the identity or nature of what it is to be a human person. The unity of the human person is not the unity of a *self*, *mind* or *body*, but the unity of a developing rational animal with a panoply of powers pertaining to the integrated biopsychosocial aspects of human life. These powers are manifested or impeded through various interactions and reactions with other things in reality. This unity of the human person is addressed by philosophical anthropology, but is often ignored by most work in philosophy of mind due to that discipline's myopic approach to the body, mind and self. Unfortunately, the dichotomising conceptual framework of *philosophy of mind* remains far more influential today than the holistic and integrated approach of *philosophical anthropology*.

While philosophy of mind commences with a dichotomy between the mental and the physical, the mind and the body, philosophical anthropology has a different point of departure. It starts with the human person insofar as it constitutes a stable organic unity amid a dynamic manifold of developmental processes; we humans change, but we do not change in every way all the time. These contentions are related to a view of personal identity known as *animalism*.[17] Long ago Aristotle resolved the nature versus nurture debate by a simple distinction between *first nature* and *second nature*. The first nature grounds the dynamic developments of our second nature, and our second nature allows for the gradual transformation of our first nature without undermining the stable *identity* of the whole. We can assimilate Aristotle's insightful distinction between first and second nature into contemporary parlance by employing a distinction between the *ontological identity* and *psychological identity*, respectively, of the human person.[18]

This distinction is critical for addressing questions of human or personal identity. Contrary to the *Hazards of Cartesian and Lockean Personal Identity* – which equate human identity with the psychological continuity of consciousness or memory – animalists contend that the loss or disintegration of one's psychological constitution through any of the myriad forms of human impairment, disability, disease, illness and so forth, *does not* entail the loss of the more fundamental biological and ontological identity of the human person. This is because animalists hold that the more fundamental ontological identity of a human person can only be terminated through the death of the human organism. Humans cannot lose their ontological identity of being a human person from dementia or any other neuropsychiatric diseases no matter how extensive their suffering, memory impairments or transformations of their psychological identity.

The psychological identity of human persons, what we might call their *personality*, is manifested and disclosed both through ordinary human self-understanding and social interaction, as well through the keen and disciplined observations, descriptions and explanations of the novelist, poet, clinician, behavioural and cognitive neuroscientist, psychologist, philosopher and, most importantly, our close friends and family. Our psychological identity provides a window into the ontological identity of the human person as a living rational animal, constituted out of sundry organised social and biochemical capacities and mechanisms and their integrated interactions. These points suggest alternative ways to conceptualise and understand human persons that eschew the false dichotomy of the mental and physical. To understand human persons requires integrated multi-level explanations that are complementary rather than in competition. We need to address questions concerning how the subpersonal neurophysiological dimension of our ontological identity enables our personal level conscious psychological *cum* social life, as well as how our psychological capacities and operations harness and order the psychosomatic neurophysiological dimensions of the human person.

Let us conclude this catena of hazards by reiterating a point briefly introduced at the outset. What I have claimed thus far is arguably *compatible* with a wide range of philosophical accounts of the ontological composition of the human person such as interactionist substance or property dualism, including the whole ambit of views like emergentism, panpsychism, as well as anomalous monism, functionalism and even some versions of reductive physicalism. I reject all of these post-Cartesian views, and defend a version of Aristotelian hylomorphic animalism, but that is beside the point for our present purposes.[19] Thus, we should avoid the *Hazard of Simplified and Hasty Mind–Body Positioning*, as most views in psychology and neuroscience are compatible with a range of positions on the mind–body problem. Furthermore, it is not the mind–body problem but the neurophysiological and psychological constitution of the human person's abilities and activities that are more pertinent to the neuroscientific study of religion.

Consciousness

Consciousness is a contentious issue; what follows is an opinionated sketch of consciousness and its hazards. There are two inseparable and unified facets of consciousness that we can distinguish according to two inextricable modes of presence: (1) the *intentional presence* of objects I am conscious of, and (2) *subject presence* wherein I am a subject conscious of intentional objects. Our conscious psychological operations are *intentional* insofar as they are *about* or *directed towards* some object: *seeing colour; hearing sound; touching tangibles; perceiving or registering a dog; remembering my first pet dog; imagining my favourite painting* or *song; having a somatic ache on my back* or *hedonic feeling, being in love* or *angry with, afraid of, hopeful* or *sorrowful for some person; inquiring about the nature of justice; understanding Euclid's definition of a triangle; reflectively judging Libet's account of the brain science of free will to be true or false because of reasons X,Y,Z; deliberating about how best to travel to Paris; deciding to take the train to Paris*; and, *taking the train to Paris.*

Indivisibly bound up with the intentional character of our psychological operations is subject *consciousness* or *awareness*. I am the subject that is consciously *seeing, hearing, touching, perceiving, remembering, imagining, having somatic pains, passions, emotions, moods* and other affective and conative states, I am also the subject that is *wondering, understanding, conceptualising and theorising, rationally examining the evidence and reasons for some claim, reflectively judging it to be true or false, probable or unlikely,* and engaging in *self-reflective deliberative practical reasoning* and *action* concerning what is good for me and others here and now and how are such goods ordered towards the flourishing of myself and other human persons. We are also self-conscious, which 'is not a matter of being conscious of something called a "a self" . . . but rather of a person's capacity to think about, reflect on, report and be conscious of his own mental states, beliefs, desires and motives, his skills, tendencies, attitudes and character traits, as well as his past life and experiences'.[20]

Through the deleterious influence of misleading philosophical ideas about consciousness, empirical studies on consciousness frequently limit their categorisation of consciousness to a kind of *mental state*. Three are noteworthy: (1) *Qualitative* or *phenomenal states* are conscious states that have some qualitative properties or *qualia* that might be restricted sensory qualities and so might include Thomas Nagel's gloss on consciousness as 'what it is like to be an X'. Cognitive phenomenology has recently extended these ideas to include the phenomenal features of cognitive and doxastic states. (2) *Meta-mental states* are conscious states about other mental states. (3) *Access consciousness* concerns the availability of mental information or content to the subject independent from whether or not this information is phenomenally conscious. According to Ned Block's well-known division of this conceptual territory, 'phenomenal consciousness is experience; the phenomenally conscious aspect of a state is what it is like to be in that state. The mark of access consciousness, by contrast, is availability for use in reasoning and rationally guiding speech and action'.[21]

All of these highly contentious divisions and subdivisions of consciousness are widely disputed in the philosophical and scientific literature.[22] But we should also be sceptical of philosophical and scientific projects that aim to treat real features related to conscious experience as distinct *properties* or *states* of consciousness that can be philosophically understood and explored empirically as discrete isolated objects of investigation. This modularisation of consciousness encourages the misleading idea that, say, visual experiences can be decomposed into their distinct phenomenal (blueness), meta-mental (being conscious of experiencing blueness), and access properties (the un/availability of visual information pertaining to the experience of blueness), each of which can be studied on its own.

These *Hazards of Crypto-Cartesian Consciousness* can be avoided, for the sketch of consciousness I expounded above shows that a detailed picture of consciousness can be provided without any recourse to the problematic notions of phenomenal, meta-mental and access consciousness and the tendency to reify these abstractions into discrete concrete objects of study. This alternative approach does not amount to a refutation of the dominant models of consciousness, but it does show that neuroscience is not obliged to remain hypnotised by the *Hazards of Crypto-Cartesian Consciousness*. Finally, this sketch also suggests that nature of consciousness can be addressed independently from settling quixotic ontological questions about physicalism, mental causation and the mind–body problem.

Hard Problem of Consciousness and the Hazard of Zombie Neuroscience

David Chalmers is well known for distinguishing between the *easy* and *hard problems* of consciousness. 'The easy problems of consciousness are those that seem directly susceptible to the standard methods of cognitive science, whereby a phenomenon is explained in terms of computational or neural mechanisms. The hard problems are those that seem to resist those methods'.[23] Most easy problems of consciousness concern the systematic identification of the neural mechanisms and correlates of conscious. Chalmers outlines a list of easy problems of consciousness that includes

- the ability to discriminate, categorise, and react to environmental stimuli
- the integration of information by a cognitive system
- the reportability of mental states
- the ability of a system to access its own internal states
- the focus of attention
- the deliberate control of behaviour
- the difference between wakefulness and sleep

The hard problem of consciousness – a version of the aforementioned problem of mind–mind dualism – concerns explaining conscious experience itself, including the range of phenomena identified with subject and object consciousness. Chalmers and others contend that the hard problem of consciousness has not and perhaps cannot be solved by the methods of neuroscience. Why? Aside from problems with the many failures of past attempts, one way Chalmers motivates this contention is by considering the possibility of zombies. Unlike the zombies of science fiction, a philosophical zombie is 'someone or something physically identical to me (or to any other conscious being), but lacking conscious experiences altogether'.[24] The hard problem points out that the efforts of neuroscientists will continue to provide powerful explanations of zombie humans – via subpersonal cognitive processing minds – but will not come one iota closer to explaining what is distinctive of real humans, namely consciousness. Chalmers argues that the conceivability of zombies entails their possibility and this undermines certain reductive and non-reductive physicalist views on the mind–body problem and shows that we must take consciousness seriously.

Despite my agreement with this final point, I think we should be sceptical about arguments that move from conceivability to possibility; furthermore, the conceit of Chalmers' argument is deeply committed to the *Hazards of Crypto-Cartesianism* I urged us to reject, and he also fails to distinguish, and so often conflates, personal with subpersonal level attributes. Aside from Chalmers' purposes, however, I think philosophical zombies introduce a more modest point, call it the *Hazard of Zombie Neuroscience*, which is similar to the *Hazard of the Disappearing Person*. This hazard highlights difficulties with any purported claims to provide comprehensive explanations of human experience by psychology, cognitive science or neuroscience that completely overlook or omit the fact that humans are conscious agents. Such alleged explanations of human persons could only be true of human zombies, not of human persons. The lesson to be learned is that no explanation of human persons can purport to be comprehensive if it has not adequately addressed human persons as being everyday conscious agents with the aforementioned spectrum of personal level capacities for conscious operations.

Causal and Explanatory Pluralism

The debates on mental causation and free will in human and divine agents often share a strikingly similar blinkered theoretical commitment to causal monism. Causal monism is the view that causes are in competition to be the exclusive occupant of the one and only slot for the sufficient cause of some phenomenon. The *hazard of causal monism*, is closely linked with an exaggerated view of *parsimony* and the *hazard of extreme reductionism*. We should abandon such constrained understandings of causality and reductionism and acknowledge the wide range of causal explanations required for accounting for the multitude of factors that contributed to any phenomenon. Explaining a car accident, for instance, might require examining a range of causal factors like the poor choices of a sleepy driver, the way exhaustion affects attention and sensorimotor reaction times, poor visibility and wet pavement due to heavy rainfall, deterioration of automobile tyres, improperly designed banked curve, a deer running across the road and so forth.[25] Against causal monism and forms of explanatory reductionism exponents of the new mechanist philosophy of biology, neuroscience and psychology defend a form of explanatory and causal pluralism. Carl Craver argues that multi-level causal and constitutional explanations provide neuroscience with a mosaic unity.

> This mosaic view of the unity of neuroscience is broader in scope than reduction because it covers both the integration of fields in research at a given level and in research that crosses levels. This mosaic view also provides a more accurate and elaborate view of interlevel interfield integration. Where reductionists understand the unity of science in terms of stepwise reduction to lowest levels, the mosaic view treats the unity of science as the collaborative accumulation of constraints at multiple levels. Whereas reduction focuses on relations of identity, supervenience, and ontological reductive links, the mechanistic mosaic view emphasizes the importance of explanatory relevance as the bridge between levels. Finally, whereas reduction models emphasize the importance of explanatory reduction to fundamental levels, the mosaic view can be pluralistic about levels, recognizing the genuine importance of higher-level causes and explanations. The mosaic unity of science is constructed during the process of collaboration by different fields in the search for multilevel mechanisms.[26]

Acknowledging the exigency to take seriously the hierarchy of integrated levels of causal and explanatory significance relevant for understanding human persons opens up clearer distinctions between complementary explanations from the personal and subpersonal levels. Indeed, the personal/subpersonal distinction sets a clearer research agenda for addressing the way the neurophysiology of subpersonal levels enable, influence and are integrated into our capacities for conscious operations at the personal level.

Causal and explanatory pluralism not only elucidates the actual practices of scientists and provides a way to side step muddled philosophical debates about mental causation or determinism, compatibilism and libertarianism in free will, but also contributes to theological reflection on the co-operative nature of divine and human action. By distinguishingly sharply between what God does *qua* Creator from what humans do *qua* creatures, and seeing that there is no creaturely causation without a Creator, and that the Creator does not act *qua* creature, a significant advance can be made beyond the similarly tired debates about theological determinism.[27]

Hazards of the Computational and Representational Theories of Mind

Cognitive scientists typically define cognition as information processing that involves some form of computations – classical or connectionist – over representations that are causal, or intentional, or even phenomenal. The hazards here are many.

The concept of 'representations' is employed ambiguously within and between different disciplines to sometimes mean mere causal covariation or *re-presentation* of patterns of information in one medium, e.g. photons bombarding a retina, to equivalent or computationally processed patterns of information in another medium, e.g. neural spike trains in the visual cortex. Similarly, cognitive scientists often say a neuron or a node in a connectionist network *represents* the stimulus that it selectively responds to. But these meanings of 'representations' as causal mediators are wholly different from, though they are frequently confused with, different accounts of 'mental representations'. One account of mental representations understands representations to consist in 'intentional' mental acts; typically as mental acts with propositional content. Our beliefs, thoughts, and other forms of 'mental representations' are said to be 'intentional' in the sense discussed before; they are *about* or *directed towards* something. Representations in the causal sense do not entail mental representations in the intentional sense. Confusions arise because while many theorists unreflectively conflate the two senses of representation, other theorists contentiously debate whether mental representations in the intentional sense are identical to, reducible to or emergent from causal representations in the brain.

Debates also persist over incompatible theories of computation and representation; disagreements concern whether computational and representational theories of mind (*CRTM*) are helpful models, metaphorical heuristics or literally describing what is occurring in the brain. Furthermore, proponents of *CRTM* take different stands on the modularity of cognitive systems, which is a distinct issue from whether the brain is modular. There are different theories of cognitive modularity, but most theorists would agree that modules are cognitive systems for processing domain specific information, e.g. perceptual or motor information. Fodor suggests that 'the most important aspect of modularity [is] something that [he] call[s] "informational encapsulation"'.[28] Modules are encapsulated because they only process domain specific information and are incapable of getting access to other kinds of information in a system. Informational encapsulation is often linked with the idea of 'cognitive impenetrability' wherein a cognitive module is incapable of being influenced by information that falls outside of its input source or domain. Defenders of modularity are divided between theories of modest modularity à la Fodor (rejecting that central systems are modular because they do not have information encapsulation) or massive modularity à la Carruthers (maintaining the whole mind is modular based on arguments from evolutionary psychology). Proponents of *neural reuse* are sceptical of *CRTM* and reject the neural localisation strategies of modularity theories on the grounds of neuroimaging meta-data analyses and alternative explanations of evolutionary psychology.[29] But even if some version of *CRTM* proves to be the most fruitful way of *modelling* neurophysiological cum psychological behaviour of animals, this does not mean the brain is actually computationally processing representations.

Challenges to *CRTM*, some more *radical* than others, have come from alternative approaches to cognition that are often bundled together as the *4E's of Cognition*: Cognition is embodied, embedded, enactive and extended. Not all proponents of these alternative approaches accept each of these 4Es; some accept modified versions of the *CRTM*, while others completely reject *CRTM* along with the claim that cognition is information processing. Advocates of *radical embodied cognitive science*, inspired by James Gibson and dynamical systems theory, reject *CRTM*'s conceptual framework for interpreting data and defend an alternative that does not appeal to theoretical postulates like representations and classical computational processes. The *hazards of cognitive science* concern a cautionary call to be vigilant and circumspect about these many debates and unresolved questions about the brain and whether and to what degree *CRTM* or any other accounts of cognition as information processing illuminate the neuroscience, psychology and the subpersonal nature of the human person.[30]

Naturalism: Ontological, Methodological and Epistemological

Naturalism has been understood in many different and often incompatible ways – three are noteworthy. *Ontological naturalism* maintains that the whole of reality is compromised by nature or whatever is natural, where the natural is frequently taken to be whatever is constituted by or simply is identical to physical or material entities. This view excludes or denies that there are any supernatural or spiritual realities. It is important to point out that 'one of the more persistent and inexcusable rhetorical conceits that corrupt the current popular debates over belief in God is the claim that they constitute an argument between faith and reason or between religion and science. They constitute in fact, only a contest between different pictures of the world; theism and [ontological] naturalism … each of which involves a number of basic metaphysical convictions …'[31] Challenges to ontological naturalism come from many directions: it is an unmotivated bald assertion, it cannot provide a naturalistic account, via evolution or otherwise, of the reality and knowledge of mathematical, logical, philosophical, moral and aesthetic truths, and most fundamentally, for the human capacity to employ and know principles of rationality within the 'space of reasons'.[32]

Methodological naturalism maintains that knowledge of natural phenomena should be described and explained by natural realities. Methodological naturalism typically commends the scientific method as an ideal methodology for the investigation of natural phenomena; indeed, it privileges scientific knowledge over other forms of knowledge.

An *exclusive* methodological naturalism rules out the possibility of explaining natural realities by appealing to supernatural entities. Significantly, this is a methodological constraint, not evidence of absence; for it leaves out as a matter of principle any consideration of what might not be deemed natural. A *permissive* methodological naturalism holds that while science only has recourse to naturalistic explanations, it is quietist or agnostic about the possibility of supplementing naturalistic explanations with non-natural explanations.

The *hazard of scientism* is a more extreme and often less sophisticated version of methodological naturalism that mistakenly identifies science and the scientific method with the claim that the only true, meaningful or reliable knowledge about reality comes from empirical investigations of science. This mistake is problematic for many reasons. Aside from being self-defeating, scientism – an epistemological position – cannot itself be verified through empirical investigations. Scientism also rules out as non-scientific the non-empirical disciplines of mathematics and logic, which scientific methods presuppose and require.

The *hazard of naturalised epistemology* concerns the project and assumption that the best explanations for why some human claims to know that 'X is Y', comes from psychology and neuroscience. Extreme versions of naturalised epistemology contend that the best explanation for why a human person believes what they do, will not come from evaluating the personal level evidence and reasons that support their beliefs, but from examining the subpersonal neurophysiological and psychological mechanisms that lead to their formation of these beliefs. Like historicism, naturalised epistemology endeavours to explain away or debunk the person's own reasons for belief by looking to something else that explains the origins of their belief, whether it be historical circumstances of race, class and gender, or the psychological mechanisms selected through evolution. Naturalised epistemology arguably commits a subtle version of the genetic fallacy, and should be rejected for this reason and many others, not least is its self-defeating assault on our capacity to know the truth based on evidence and reason.

In sum: Naturalism matters for the neuroscientific study of religion insofar as some forms of naturalism rule out from the beginning the very possibility that some phenomena might also admit of supernatural explanations, while others methodologically ignore such possibilities, and still others leave open their possibility without investigating or by integrating them with naturalistic accounts. This is not the place to take a stand on such contentious issues or the best way to proceed, however, it is critical to be aware of these forms of naturalism when approaching the neuroscientific study of religion.

In the final sections I will turn to a few philosophical hazards that are specific to the neuroscientific study of religion, beginning with a few noteworthy research programmes.

Cognitive Science of Religion and Neurotheology

The neuroscientific study of religion should not be equated with either *cognitive science of religion* (*CSR*) or *neurotheology*. While the first is merely the convergence of neuroscience investigations with religion, the latter two are ideologically driven interdisciplinary research programmes that draw on neuroscience and cognitive science, developmental psychology and evolutionary psychology to provide naturalistic causal explanations – often either vindicating or debunking – of the beliefs and practices of religion. Numerous *hazards* lurk around the assumptions of these research programmes; I mention three *hazards of naturalised religion*, focusing on the scientifically more legitimate *CSR*. First *CSR* depends on scientific research programmes that are problematic or very contentious. Evolutionary psychology is rightly criticised by evolutionary theorists and empirical psychologists alike for its slim empirical evidence, naive correlations, and gratuitous explanations or suspicious 'just so stories'. If evolutionary psychology is a house of cards, then the explanations of *CSR* rest on uncertain foundations.[33] Second, *CSR* is committed to the *massive modularity* view of cognition, which is also contentious, and is one among many views in cognitive science. And insofar as it takes these non-conscious subpersonal information processing modules to provide a complete explanation of the lives of religious persons, it completely leaves out the conscious personal level practices, beliefs and experiences of religious persons. This zombie conception of religious persons runs afoul by ignoring the *Hazard of the Disappearing Person*. Whatever role subpersonal level cognitive information processing mechanisms play in the formation of the personal level doxastic convictions of religious belief or faith, we need to be careful to distinguish and not conflate the latter personal level beliefs or faith of the religious person with the subpersonal level information processing mechanisms postulated by cognitive psychology and cognitive neuroscience. Furthermore, *CSR* uncritically endorses some of the most problematic interpretations of massive modularity, and supposes that religion is developed unreflectively from our 'core knowledge' and the default cognitive modules for intuitive psychology and biology. Such commitments have led many proponents of *CSR* to produce their own just so stories about how subpersonal level cognitive mechanisms for agency detection explain why religious people attribute agency to non-natural entities. Third, many proponents of *CSR* are committed to naturalised epistemology and the quest to provide cognitive explanations for why people are religious independent from whatever those person's overt justifications are for their religious beliefs and practices. Neither the neuroscience nor neurology of religion require such assumptions to do solid scientific and clinical research.

Indeed, in 'Religion and Neurology', the first of his 1900–1902 Gifford Lectures on *The Varieties of Religion Experience*, William James presents a view that is fundamentally at odds with naturalised epistemology and many facets of the *CSR*. James not only anticipated such problematic research programmes, but also had the good sense to reject them and distinguish such reductive explanations from the fruitful complementary explanations of neurology which do not replace personal level explanations of human persons. James also recognised the inconsistency hidden in the assumptions of naturalised epistemology applied to religion: for scientists also have brains, and perhaps the purported truths of evolutionary psychology or *CSR* can also be causally explained more adequately by eschewing their reasons and evidence and looking instead to the conditions of their brains.

> In the natural sciences and industrial arts it never occurs to any one to try to refute opinions by showing up their author's neurotic constitution. Opinions here are invariably tested by logic and by experiment, no matter what may be their author's neurological type. It should be no otherwise with religious opinions … Immediate luminousness, in short, philosophical reasonableness, and moral helpfulness are the only available criteria.[34]

Like the research agenda set by William James, the neuroscientific study of religion is less concerned with the natural history of religion and efforts to vindicate or debunk religion through naturalistic explanations, and is more interested in understanding and potentially helping religious persons affected by neurological deficits. What philosophical hazards need to be identified here?

While not an overtly philosophical hazard, it is worth drawing attention to the importance of scientific research being ecologically sensitive. The beliefs, practices, and experiences of religious persons take place in environments and social settings that are obviously significantly different from the clinic or the alienating tunnel of a fMRI machine. These different contexts are not immaterial to the neuroscientific study of religion.

Philosophical Hazards in the Neuroscientific Study of Religion

Religious practices, beliefs and experiences are personal level proprietary; there is nothing at the subpersonal level that is directly indicative of being religious for the same reason that there is nothing at the subpersonal level that manifests any other personal level attributes like beliefs, desires, intentions, reasons for action, anger, fear, frustration, despair, deep or tentatively held convictions. Of course, like any practices, beliefs and experiences of human persons, religious ones admit of subpersonal level explanations. Indeed, it is unlikely to presume there will be a uniquely religious subpersonal level neuroscientific explanations any more than we would anticipate there to be sui generis 'scientific' or 'football' 'classical music' subpersonal level neuroscientific explanations of a human person's practices, beliefs or experiences vis-à-vis science, football or classical music. As William James pointed out, 'religious melancholy, whatever peculiarities it may have qua religious, is at any rate melancholy. Religious happiness is happiness. Religious trance is trance'.[35] The religious significance of the neuroscientific study of religious persons is entirely dependent upon the religious significance of personal level attributes; neuroscience's subpersonal level investigations do not introduce anything new with respect to the religious character of the religious person's practices, beliefs or experiences.

This brings us to the *Hazard of Numinous Neural Localisation*, that is, the effort to employ the techniques of neuroscience, especially brain imaging or neuropsychology, to locate the religious bits of the brain. Unfortunately, this hazard is sometimes embraced as a methodological agenda, as is illustrated by the aforementioned programme of *neurotheology*, which aims to correlate religious experiences with uniquely religious bits of the brain. This hazard should not be conflated with the perfectly reasonable neuroscientific research that has revealed stereotyped lesions in certain parts of the brain correlated with specific forms of purported religious experience; indeed, such research expands the programme of study of William James and others. And many of the papers in this volume contribute to the neuroscientific, neurological and psychiatric study of religious persons in this valuable way.

Conclusion

I have argued that the neuroscientific investigations of religious persons do not address the personal level features that are essential to the practices, beliefs and experiences of religious persons. Understanding these personal level phenomena is necessarily prior to and a prerequisite for coordinating the neuroscientific investigation of the subpersonal level neural systems that underlie, enable and sometimes disable our abilities to practice religion or spirituality. These distinct forms of investigation are not in competition. What subpersonal level psychological and neuroscientific investigations provide are complementary explanations for what is affecting the person as a whole, which sometimes can confirm, challenge or problematise personal level assessments. The challenge here is avoiding the philosophical hazards neuroscientific investigations of religion encounter on the way.

Endnotes

1. The *Stanford Encyclopedia of Philosophy* (*SEP*) is an excellent resource for nearly any philosophical topic; its entries, written by philosophers or specialists, continue to grow and to be updated regularly. Most entries provide a general survey of a topic, the contentious issues surrounding different positions taken on some particular issue and a representative bibliography on that topic. For limitations of space, I shall not cite all the relevant entries from the *SEP*, but I recommend consulting the *SEP* for an expanded treatment of the topics I have raised here, especially for details on the dominant debates in analytic philosophy of mind. http://plato.stanford.edu/.
2. Mark Johnson and Michelle de Haan, *Developmental Cognitive Neuroscience: An Introduction*, 4th edn. (Hoboken, NJ: Wiley-Blackwell, 2015); Carl Craver, *Explaining the Brain: Mechanisms and the Mosaic Unity of Neuroscience* (Oxford: Oxford University Press, 2007); Charles Taylor, *Sources of the Self* (Cambridge, MA: Harvard University Press, 1989); Robert Bellah, *Religion in Human Evolution* (Cambridge, MA: Harvard University Press, 2011).
3. This distinction has been used in a variety of ways by philosophers, psychologists, psychiatrists, cognitive scientists, neuroscientists and others. I am roughly following a version of the distinction defended in Jennifer Hornsby, 'Personal and Sub-personal: A Defence of Dennett's Early Distinction', *Philosophical Explorations* 3, no. 1 (2000): 6–24.
4. For a rich reflection on these differences, see P. M. S. Hacker's philosophical anthropology trilogy *Human Nature: The Categorial Framework* (Hoboken, NJ: Blackwell, 2007), *The Intellectual Powers: A Study of Human Nature* (Hoboken, NJ: Wiley-Blackwell, 2013) and *The Passions: A Study of Human Nature* (Hoboken, NJ: Blackwell, 2018) and Raymond Tallis' three-volume philosophical anthropology *The Hand: A Philosophical Inquiry into Human Being* (Edinburgh: Edinburgh University Press, 2003); *The Knowing Animal: A Philosophical Inquiry into Knowledge and Truth* (Edinburgh: Edinburgh University Press, 2004) and *I Am: A Philosophical Inquiry into First-Person Being* (Edinburgh: Edinburgh University Press, 2005).
5. Parashkev Nachev and Peter Hacker, 'The Neural Antecedents to Voluntary Action: A Conceptual Analysis', *Cognitive Neuroscience* 5 (2014): 194.
6. M. R. Bennett and P. M. S. Hacker, *Philosophical Foundations of Neuroscience* (Hoboken, NJ: Blackwell, 2003), hereinafter *PFN*; Bennett and Hacker, *History of Cognitive Neuroscience* (Hoboken, NJ: Wiley-Blackwell, 2008), hereinafter *HCN*.
7. Joseph LeDoux, 'Coming to Terms with Fear', *PNAS* 111 (2014): 2876.
8. Francisco J. Varela, Evan Thompson and Eleanor Kesch, *The Embodied Mind: Cognitive Science and Human Experience* (Cambridge, MA: MIT Press, 1993), 52–7.
9. William Jaworski, *Philosophy of Mind: A Comprehensive Introduction* (Hoboken, NJ: Wiley-Blackwell, 2011); Daniel Hutto, *Folk Psychological Narratives* (Cambridge, MA: MIT Press, 2007); Matthew Ratcliffe, *Rethinking Commonsense Psychology: A Critique of Folk Psychology, Theory of Mind and Simulation* (London: Palgrave, 2007); Alva Noë, *Out of Our Heads: Why You Are Not Your Brain, and Other Lessons from the Biology of Consciousness* (New York: Hill and Wang, 2009); Alasdair Macintyre, *Dependent Rational Animals* (Chicago: Open Court, 1999).
10. *PFN*, 73.
11. Ibid., 82n35.
12. Ibid., 83. Hence *PFN* does not defend a form of methodological, psychological or logical behaviourism. This is because the grounds for psychological ascription are not limited to behavioural evidence; empirical psychology is neither restricted to providing explanations of 'mere bodily movements' nor limited to the theoretical resources of classical and operant conditioning, and psychological attributes and their meanings are not essentially exhausted by their behavioural manifestations or dispositions for behaviour. See ibid., 82n35, 117, 416–17.

13. Ibid., 83.
14. Ibid.
15. Ibid., 77.
16. Ibid., 3.
17. See Stephan Blatti, 'Animalism', and Eric T. Olson, 'Personal Identity', in *SEP*; Allison Thornton, 'Varieties of Animalism', *Philosophy Compass* 11 (2016): 515–26.
18. N.B. There are personal and subpersonal level attributes that apply to both our ontological identity (e.g. being a rational animal with a range of personal level psychological capacities that have subpersonal level explanations) and psychological identity (e.g. the particular personal level psychological operations and conscious experiences *here and now* which have definite subpersonal level explanations *here and now*).
19. Daniel De Haan, 'Hylomorphic Animalism, Emergentism, and the Challenge of New Mechanisms in Neuroscience', *Scientia et Fides* 5, no. 2 (2017): 9–38; De Haan, 'The Interaction of Noetic and Psychosomatic Operations in a Thomist Hylomorphic Personalism', *Scientia et Fides* 6, no. 2 (2018): 55–83.
20. *PFN*, 252.
21. Ned Block, 'On a Confusion about a Function of Consciousness', *Behavioral and Brain Sciences* 18 (1995): 227–87.
22. *PFN*, 237–351; Noë, *Out of Our Heads*; Dan Zahavi, *Self and Other* (Oxford: Oxford University Press, 2014).
23. David Chalmers, 'Facing Up to the Problem of Consciousness', *Journal of Consciousness Studies* 2 (1995): 200–219. See E. J. Lowe, 'There Are No Easy Problems of Consciousness', *Journal of Consciousness Studies* 2 (1995): 266–71.
24. David Chalmers, *The Conscious Mind* (Oxford: Oxford University Press, 1996), 94.
25. Jaworski, *Philosophy of Mind*, 290–96.
26. Craver, *Explaining the Brain*, 271.
27. Brian Shanely, 'Beyond Libertarianism and Compatibilism: Thomas Aquinas on Created Freedom', in *Freedom and the Human Person*, ed. Richard Velkley (Washington, DC: Catholic University of America Press, 2007), 70–89.
28. Jerry Fodor, *The Modularity of Mind* (Cambridge, MA: MIT Press, 1983), 36.
29. Michael Anderson, *After Phrenology: Neural Reuse and the Interactive Brain* (Cambridge, MA: MIT Press, 2014).
30. Daniel Hutto and Erik Myin, *Radicalizing Enactivism: Basic Minds without Content* (Cambridge, MA: MIT Press, 2012); Anthony Chemero, *Radical Embodied Cognitive Science* (Cambridge, MA: MIT Press, 2011); Paul Churchland, *Matter and Consciousness*, 3rd edn. (Cambridge, MA: MIT Press, 2013); William Bechtel, *Mental Mechanisms Philosophical Perspectives on Cognitive Neuroscience* (New York: Routledge, 2008); William M. Ramsey, *Representation Reconsidered* (Cambridge: Cambridge University Press, 2007); *PFN*.
31. David Bentley Hart, *The Experience of God: Being, Consciousness, Bliss* (Providence, RI: Yale University Press, 2013), 77.
32. Thomas Nagel, *Mind and Cosmos: Why the Materialist Neo-Darwinian Conception of Nature Is Almost Certainly False* (Oxford: Oxford University Press, 2012); Daniel Robinson, ed., *Scientism: The New Orthodoxy* (New York: Bloomsbury, 2014); Robert Koons and George Bealer, *The Waning of Materialism* (Oxford: Oxford University Press, 2010); J. J. C. Smart and J. J. Haldane, *Atheism and Theism*, 2nd edn. (Hoboken, NJ: Blackwell, 2003); Alvin Plantinga, *Where the Conflict Really Lies: Science, Religion, and Naturalism* (Oxford: Oxford University Press, 2013).

33. Robert Richardson, *Evolutionary Psychology as Maladapted Psychology* (Cambridge, MA: MIT Press, 2007); Hilary Rose and Steven Rose, eds., *Alas Poor Darwin: Arguments against Evolutionary Psychology* (New York: Crown, 2000).
34. William James, *The Varieties of Religious Experience*, Centenary edn. (New York: Routledge, 2002), 19.
35. Ibid., 24.

Chapter 7

The Glass Onion

Sophie Grace Chappell

To begin with a slogan: *context is crucial to comprehending the cognitive.* Too many investigators, both scientists and philosophers, have ignored context when thinking about neurology. I'm going to start by discussing an example of what I mean by this slogan taken from the recent philosophy of neuroscience. Then I will draw some broader morals from the slogan, both for philosophical thinking about, for example, minds and brains and persons, and also for scientists who think about these things.

I

Maxwell Bennett and Peter Hacker (BH) think they detect a fundamental conceptual confusion in contemporary neuroscience;[1] they call it 'the mereological fallacy'. This is the mistake of attributing to some part of a complex what can only properly be attributed to the whole. So, for example, if I said that the pendulum of a clock tells the time, or that the petrol in a car's tank gets me from Milton Keynes to Cambridge, I would be guilty of the mereological fallacy. The right thing to say, according to BH, is that *the clock* tells the time, not just its pendulum, and that the *car* gets me from MK to Cambridge, not just the petrol.

The point of observing this fallacy, they continue, is obvious with neuroscience. It's not my synapses that remember – so BH insist: it's me. It's not my retina or optic nerve or visual cortex that sees: it's me. And above all, it's not my brain that thinks, has experiences, decides, dreams, sees things, believes and knows things and performs actions. It's me. BH insist on the importance of avoiding the mereological fallacy for Wittgensteinian and Aristotelian reasons. The fallacy, they think, expresses a benighted Cartesian dualism (albeit a brain/ body dualism rather than a mind/ body dualism), and it fails to fit with how we actually think and live in our ordinary form of life.

Now only one of the two persons who compose the joint author BH is a philosopher, namely Peter Hacker, who is a distinguished exegete and proponent of Wittgensteinian and (more recently) Aristotelian views; Maxwell Bennett is a neuroscientist, and not a philosopher at all. So perhaps we should say that the insistence against the mereological fallacy is *Hacker's* rather than *Bennett and Hacker*'s?

Well, actually, we can say both. Joint authors are well-established conventional entities in academia, especially in the sciences, though Hacker has done more joint authorship than most philosophers. BH have a philosophical view about the mereological fallacy, and Hacker has a philosophical view about the mereological fallacy. The views are identical, because the principal determinant of the *philosophical* views of BH is Hacker, and/or because it is the rule for joint authors to publish nothing jointly that they cannot each assent to individually.

But hang on a minute. If we can say that about BH and Hacker, what's to stop us saying it, or something like it, about brain and person, and indeed about brain subparts and brain? When I see red, my brain sees red; what's more, when my brain sees red, my visual cortex and my retina and my optic nerve all see red too. And the seeings are identical, because the principal determinant of my seeing red is my brain's seeing red, and the principal determinant of my brain's seeing red is my brain's visual sensory apparatus' seeing red – within which, perhaps, someone who knows more than me about the science of vision may want to determine some particular part of my visual system as principal determinant of my brain's visual system's seeing red. And if we can say *this*, then we seem already to have lost our grip on the idea that BH, or Hacker, or Hacker's critical faculties, have raised any sort of real problem for neuroscience. Apparently Bennett and Hacker's critique of the mereological fallacy suffers from the striking disadvantage that they themselves qualify as a counter-example to it.

Their argument has other disadvantages too. For one thing, suppose we buy their negative critique; OK, now what? It's less than pellucid what their *positive* proposal is about how to do neuroscience. It's also far from clear whether, even if they are right in their description of the problem they claim to see, they can explain why such a problem in our thinking should have arisen in the first place. For another, BH place an awful lot of weight on the conceptual/ empirical distinction, between questions which are apt for experiential, e.g. experimental, testing and questions of logical grammar. But I very much doubt that there is any such thing as *the* conceptual/ empirical distinction. There are different distinctions worth drawing for different reasons; but all of them are fluid and rough-edged, and human practice, especially scientific practice, can itself alter the way we draw them (as Wittgenstein himself points out[2]).

In any case BH's argument as I rehearsed it above, which purports to show that the mereological fallacy is indeed a fallacy by adjoining examples and suggesting an analogy, is almost embarrassingly unpersuasive, because so many of the examples collapse. The fact is, we *can and do* say that the pendulum tells the time, not the clock; and we *can and do* say that the petrol gets us to Cambridge, not the car. (My examples, admittedly, but BH's are no more persuasive.) To object to these uses on the grounds of logical grammar is no better than jibbing when a nineteenth-century sea-captain says there are 99 souls aboard his ship, or indeed when he raises the familiar cry 'All hands on deck!' If there is a point of logical grammar to be made about such cases, it is that we can easily see them as grammatically in order: we can simply label them as examples of that familiar grammatical category, synecdoche.

In Wittgensteinian fashion BH lay much stress on 'what we say'. Essentially their case for the mereological fallacy is that to see the brain, or the neurons, as where consciousness happens is a mistake because *it is not how we think*. (This must be what they mean when they say that seeing things that way is confused: it doesn't square with how we actually think, how we actually *have to* think if we are thinking straight, or thinking at all.)

Now I am quite happy with the idea of philosophy as unmasking conceptual confusions, and as separating out what we think from what we think we think – what we *simply cannot* think unless we are in a muddle of some kind. I do philosophy that way as well (among other ways): I'm a Wittgensteinian too. (Though not – to forestall unwanted solicitations – a scene Wittgensteinian.) But any such argument faces some challenges which are particularly obvious, and seem particularly unanswered, in the current case.

First, some people *do* in fact see, or profess to see, the brain as where consciousness happens, or the visual cortex as where sight happens. We know this because they tell us so; BH obligingly cite a multitude of passages where they tell us so. But this datum suggests that actually this *is* how we think, or some of us, anyway. For as we've already seen, the only good reason for denying that we think this way would be that we can't unless we're in a muddle; and the only reason that BH have offered why those who think this way *must* be in a muddle is, once more, the mereological fallacy.

Secondly: aside from the bedrock of things that we really can't think without confusion, there have been lots of ways that people think. There are to this day. Within our own society it is true both that people think in a variety of conflicting ways, and also that, for many (perhaps most) people on many (perhaps most) topics, there is no fact of the matter about what the way is in which they think. (To put it less kindly: they *don't* think.) And then the relativist challenge to BH is blindingly obvious: it looks like a fourteenth-century witchfinder-general could rebut arguments against the existence of witchcraft – witchcraft that works, I mean – by simply pointing out that the reality of (efficacious) witches 'is part of our fourteenth-century world view'. No doubt it is; but *that's* no argument in its favour.

II

So BH's argument doesn't work. But that's not where I want to leave things. I am myself, as I say, a Wittgensteinian of sorts. I want to explore what a Wittgensteinian *ought* to say about the questions that BH address. And I think that at least one very important truth lies, to some extent hidden, in what BH say about those questions. That truth can be expressed in my opening slogan: *context is crucial to comprehending the cognitive.* It is a problem for BH that their own approach includes confusions and incoherences that arise from misunderstanding or mishandling contextual considerations. All the same, BH are right that ignoring context really has resulted in some general and serious confusions and incoherences in our thinking about how the neurological should be understood cognitively.

If, that is, it should be understood cognitively at all: obviously it's part of what BH are getting at, that neuroscience is not cognitive but *sub*-cognitive. BH are exercised about the tendency of neuroscientists to talk as if neurones themselves could know things, synapses themselves pass on information, hormones themselves convey messages, genes themselves contain building instructions, and the rest of it. But this tendency seems entirely natural if one is focused, as neuroscientists are, on a particular kind of explanatory need to do with control and prediction. What cognitive neuroscientists are looking for is, to borrow a phrase of John Campbell's, the *control panel* for consciousness, the level of description and analysis at which we find the necessary and sufficient conditions for the phenomena we're trying to explain. But that quest does not, in itself, involve the cognitive neuroscientists in *fallacy.* If all talk about neurones as knowing or conveying information necessarily involved the mereological fallacy, then this phrase too would involve the mereological fallacy: 'That switch there turns the light on'. 'No it doesn't', BH might protest, 'a *human agent* turns the light on, *using* the switch'. Sure, if you like, that's another way of talking. But to insist that there can in this area be *only one* way of talking seems like unmotivated pedantry and inflexibility about the natural uses of language, of a kind that Wittgenstein himself constantly battled, and against which he himself insisted that 'every sentence in our language "is in order as it is"'.[3]

'That switch there turns the light on' is not straightforwardly fallacious, then. What it is, however, is drastically abbreviated. The abbreviation is useful, as I say, because it points us to one kind of control panel, useful for one kind of explanatory purpose. Life is short, so it's a good idea to specialise, and concentrating on one sort of explanation, professionally or otherwise, is one way of specialising: that's what academic disciplines do. Still, when we have other explanatory purposes, we might fill the remark out in all sorts of different ways. 'That switch there turns the light on if a human agent presses it'; or '. . . if you've changed the bulb'; or '. . . if you've paid the electricity bill'; or '. . . if the switch is wired up to the circuit'; or '. . . if Hathi the elephant scratches his bottom against that corner of his enclosure'; or '. . . if Vaisey the rabbit has not nibbled her way through the wires again'; or '. . . if the government troops have recaptured the power station from the rebels'; and so on and so on and so on, indefinitely.

So not filling out 'That switch there turns the light on' in whichever of these indefinitely many possible ways might, at any particular time, seem useful, is not *fallacious*: it is not in itself a commission of the mereological fallacy, nor, so far as I can see, of any other fallacy. Nonetheless it might be less than helpful or informative. Simple machines such as lighting systems *have* control panels; they aren't *identical with* those control panels. And even a simple machine won't work except in a minimally friendly context. It might be important to know about these factors for explanatory purposes; consistently ignoring them will be defeating in its own terms, *explanatorily* self-defeating. It might also prompt a kind of monomania, a kind of inability to think in more than one set of explanatory terms or at more than one explanatory level. 'That switch there turns the light on' is, as I said a minute ago, a *control-panel* statement. But as the ifs in my last paragraph are meant to illustrate, there is more than one thing that we might regard as a control panel. There is no such thing, for humans, as *the* control panel; it all depends what you want to control, and how. The notion of a control panel is *context-relative.*

I think this gets us to what's really eating BH. BH are concerned, and absolutely rightly, about a popular and pervasive fantasy about control panels. The fantasy is a fantasy of, well, control, a power-fantasy. And what it says is that there *is* just one control panel for humans, and that the control panel is neurons (one version), or genes, selfish or otherwise (another version), or economic relations (a third), or giant blue lizards from the constellation Draco (and another). We have a number of names for this sort of view. One of the less derogatory is reductionism. Reductionism is the attempt to *do everything with one control panel*, and its appeal to the human psyche is obvious: like systematic political/ economic theories such as Marxism, and like crank sects such as David Icke's, it purports to put us in touch with *the secret truth that really controls everything.* Against any such view it is only sane to protest, rather in BH's style, that its causal analyses characteristically and pervasively mistake the part for the whole. The factors that such theories point us to may be *part* of the full explanation of everything. (They may be, though I have my doubts about the giant blue lizards.) But they aren't the full picture, and they can't explain everything on their own, for the same reason again: because there isn't just one control panel for humans, there are lots, for different purposes.

Neuronal reductionism is a very bad thing; to some extent it's a bad thing in just the same respects as David-Ickery, because it feeds a crackpot conspiracy-theory power-fantasy; though the power-fantasy that neuronal reductionism feeds is arguably all the worse for being more plausible, and therefore more infectious, than Icke's. But what we need to fight it is not the dead-end accusation that BH come out with again and again, their conversation-stopping 'Offside – red card – you've committed the mereological fallacy'. What we need to fight it is a better understanding of how explanation works in general, and in particular of the variable and fluctuating role of context in various explanations.

A good understanding of explanation will say that reductionisms always involve the ignoring of relevant context. It won't, on the other hand, insist that *everything* is always context, in the way in which J. S. Mill famously argues that a complete physical explanation of some event, such as the lighting of a match, would have to involve the whole history of the entire physical universe up to that point. As Mill himself went on to say, explanation succeeds when it produces understanding. And what it takes to produce understanding is relative not only to the kind of explanation it is, the kind of control panel that it looks to (if any – explanations in maths, and again in aesthetics and ethics, do not involve control panels), but also to the audience.

Good explanation moves back and forth between these poles: it involves both analysis and synthesis. It's like those big hairy leather-clad blokes who spend their Saturdays taking their motor-bikes apart, and their Sundays putting them back together again; to be a really good motor-bike mechanic, you need to be able to do both. The analysis is the stripping down of complexes like lighting systems, or perceptions, to their control-panel ingredients (the switch, the firing neuron); the synthesis is the building up from those ingredients to the thing itself. In the mode of analysis we can and do say things like 'That much petrol will get you to Cambridge', 'You see the green ball when this neuron is fired', 'This switch controls the main lights' etc.; in the synthetic mode we of course don't suppose that this means that just I and the petrol are going to Cambridge, or that all that's needed for me to see green is for this neuron to fire, as it might be on a lab bench; or that this switch controls the main lights *all on its own.* Analysis strips away the layers of the onion; synthesis puts them back again. BH are right to insist – if this is a way of putting what they are insisting on – that synthesis is essential to the proper understanding of complex and embedded processes, in order to see properly the context without which there is no making sense of the thing. But then, so is analysis, in order to see properly the thing which was our original reason to look at the context. We need *both.* Just that, if you ask me, is one of the key lessons of Wittgenstein's later philosophy.

And that's basically it. That's my argument. The rest of the paper simply applies it to four particular examples: genes, perception, religious experience and persons.

III

Genes first. I can do this very quickly, because I know even less than I have to say about it. We've all come across the idea of 'genetic determinism', science fiction scenarios where one person is cloned from another, scare-stories in the press about gene control, and so on. Now certainly the genetic level is *one* control-panel level. But not the only one. And, as Tim Lewens and others have spent their careers arguing, not in fact a level that does very much controlling of results at all, considered on its own. Like any other control-panel level, we have to vector in genetic effects with all the other kinds of effects that are in the picture. Even if my DNA is the genetic recipe for me, still, to borrow an analogy of Lewens', a recipe for a cake is not a cake. And as any chef knows, it's not only not inevitable that if you follow the recipe twice you will come up with exactly the same cake twice; it's *extremely hard* to bake the same cake twice.

Next, perception. Suppose I see a magnificent plane tree in the grounds of Magdalen College. This visual perception of mine, we might say at the extreme of our analytic bent, *is* the firing of neurons in my visual cortex; and then the reductionist mistake is to take this *façon de parler* as if it were the full and literal truth about perception. It's nothing of the sort. About this perception, it's *a* truth, but not *the* truth. The firing of neurons is, at the neuroanatomical level, the control panel for perception in humans (and other structurally similar species), and if we were speaking carefully that's all we would say – not the rash claim that *identifies* perception with neuron-firings. But for me to have a perception of the plane tree, far more is, obviously, necessary. The relevant neurons have to be connected to the rest of my brain in the right way for perception to happen (whatever way that may be). I have to be able to see, having eyes and optic nerves which are not significantly damaged. There has to be a plane tree, and there has to be light in Magdalen grounds, and I have to be in Oxford (not Cambridge), in the right bit of Magdalen (New Building Lawns), facing the right way, and without any quirky philosopher's fake-barn/ stripe-painted-mule tricks like a plane tree hologram set up in my sight-line exactly where the actual tree is, and exactly resembling it. Relatedly, it had better be true that if there were no plane tree there, then I would not see one. And so on, on the synthetic tack, and so forth.

Once we synthetically build in everything that needs to be there for the full picture of perception, we get to see very clearly why my perception of the Magdalen plane cannot seriously or literally be identified with the firing of my neurons. This is a 'cannot' of conceptual truth, because the contextual factors that make for perception are not *mere* contextual factors; they are conceptually involved, constitutively involved, in what we mean when we talk about perception. It's *part of the concept* of perceiving the plane tree that the plane tree should be there to be perceived, that it should impact causally on me (in a particular way), that I should be suitably situated and physically equipped to perceive it, that no plane tree would mean no perception of a plane tree, and the rest of it. The firing of neurons of the types that fire when someone perceives a tree – that doesn't involve a tree. But perceiving a tree – that has to involve a tree. We cannot understand perception without understanding its context. Not: we can't understand it *properly* or *comprehensively*; we can't understand it (*it*, perception, not some part of it such as the firing of neurons) at all. This is how, in the case of perception, I want to cash out my slogan: *context is crucial to comprehending the cognitive.*

And what, in case you're wondering, are the anti-sceptical implications of what I've just said about perception? The answer is not that this view of perception *refutes* scepticism; but it is that this view of perception seriously ups the argumentative ante against scepticism. Our concept of perception is, as I've just said, intrinsically anti-sceptical. Of its very nature, perception has a reference beyond the mental states that do that referring: it implies the existence of objects beyond the mind that we perceive. That doesn't, obviously, imply that there *are* such objects. What it implies is that if scepticism is true to any significant extent, then we do far less *perceiving* than we think we do, and perhaps none at all; what happens when we think we perceive is that neurons fire in patterns that we can't explain. This conclusion does not *refute* scepticism. But it does make it look a pretty fruitless hypothesis. The sceptic has either no serious explanation, or no explanation at all, of the apparent external reference of our alleged perceptions. The best explanation is that this external reference is veridical, and so that our alleged perceptions really are perceptions. If anyone wants to refute that argument to the best explanation, the onus is on him to show why we shouldn't accept it.

Thirdly, religious experience. My approach here is to treat this as a special case of perception, and insist, here too, on the crucial role of context in making sense of it. Visual perception, for example, at the control-panel level *involves* the firing of neurons; but visual perception *isn't identical with* the firing of neurons, because with visual perception there is necessarily a story to tell (at one explanatory level) about what causes those neuronal firings, e.g. the plane tree, and (at another explanatory level) a story to tell about what the accompanying experiences are experiences *of*, e.g. the plane tree. Likewise with religious experience. This, too, at the control-panel level *involves* the firing of neurons; but religious experience *isn't identical with* the firing of neurons, because there is necessarily a story to tell (at one level) about what causes those neuronal firings, e.g. God (or some aspect or intimation of God, or gods, or other spiritual beings), and (at another level) a story to tell about what the accompanying experiences are experiences *of*, e.g. God (or . . . etc.).

And what does this story about religious experience do against scepticism about religious experience? The answer to this question too is analogous to what I've just said about perception. The answer is not that this view of religious experience *refutes* scepticism about it; but it is that this view seriously ups the argumentative ante against scepticism. For our concept of religious experience too is – for the most part – intrinsically anti-sceptical. As usually conceived, religious experience of its very nature has a reference beyond the mental states that do that referring: it implies the existence of objects beyond the mind of which we are aware in religious experience. That doesn't, obviously, imply that there *are* such objects. What it implies is that if scepticism about religious experience is true to any significant extent, then we do far less *religious experiencing* than we think we do, and perhaps none at all; what happens when we think we have religious experiences is that neurons fire in patterns that we can't explain. This conclusion does not *refute* scepticism about religious experience. But it does make it look a pretty fruitless hypothesis. The sceptic has either no serious explanation, or no explanation at all, of the apparent external reference of our alleged religious experience. The best explanation is that this external reference is veridical, and so that our alleged religious experiences really are religious experiences. If anyone wants to refute this argument to the best explanation, the onus, again, is on him to show why we shouldn't accept it.

And finally, on persons. Here I want to suggest that considerations about context play a slightly different role from the one they've just played relative to genes, perception and religious experience. The point I want to make about persons is that we have a tendency to absolutise some particular level of understanding or analysis of persons. The level we pick on to absolutise varies. If we are old-fashioned and close to dualism, perhaps we will insist, as philosophers since Locke have often liked to, that a person is a rational self-conscious being. Or we may think of the mind, rather as Descartes may have done, as a thing within which layers of consciousness are certainly discernible, but which is nonetheless transparent to itself, and a thing which is essentially *constituted* by its own self-transparency: a kind of glass onion, to use an image which John Lennon may or may not have intended as an image of the mind. Or if we are thrillingly modern in our self-conception, perhaps we will see persons as essentially controlled by their genes or their neurons. Well, we could argue about whether any one of these candidates is or is not the control-panel level for persons (if there is just one control-panel level, which – to repeat – I would deny). But even if it is, there's a lot more to persons than that control-panel level. Here too context is everything. The person is not divorceable from his or her context in all sorts of ways; but I want, very quickly, just to mention three ways in particular:

1 Persons are made to be the persons they are – almost literally constituted – by other persons. My parents, in particular, are part of what I am. I think (and I've argued elsewhere[4]) that each of us learns to be an *I* by being a *you* for someone else, usually my mother, father or other principal carer in infancy. This has huge ramifications: for example it means that I don't have to worry about how it is that I or any other infant ever managed to get out of the solipsistic predicament, because I never was in that predicament in the first place. It was the gaze of another that first constituted me as a person; it is the gaze of others who now recognise me as a person that enables me to go on enjoying the dignity of personhood that is due to me. There are other ramifications too, many of them explored in the work of the French philosopher Emmanuel Levinas; but I won't go into them here.

2 Persons have porous boundaries. Since we exist in a context, and since for different explanatory purposes different control-panel levels may be useful, it follows that what counts as *extraneous* to a person, where you draw the boundary of a person, is not an absolute matter. By this I mean in particular

3 That persons' autonomy has porous boundaries. We can see certain factors which are psychologically within a person as *external impediments* on that person's autonomy. We can also see them as part of what it is for that person to exercise autonomy. As before, there doesn't have to be just one right way to distinguish the person from her context. It depends what explanatory purposes you happen to have when you are doing the distinguishing.

We are very apt to insist on absolute boundaries to persons, basically I think because we fear threats to our autonomy; we fear invasion by the world, so we set up the solidest defences we can manage. I think it's both an increasingly robust datum of the mind and brain sciences, and also an inevitable consequence of thinking of cognition and agency as embedded, that we have to accept – not that there is *no* distinction between us and our world – but that there is no *one* distinction. There are a number of useful ways of drawing the line between me and my world for different purposes, but there is no one uniquely correct all-purpose way of drawing the line. Not even in the place where it was drawn by some of the most zealous advocates of the independence of the person from the world, such as the Stoics and, following them, Augustinian Christianity, namely at the boundaries of what the person can choose.

A number of interesting consequences will come to light if we accept this. One is that we will, I should think, come to have a less all-or-nothing approach to free will. And for anyone who, like me, wants there to be free will, that's got to be a good result: whenever 'the free will problem' is set up as 'absolute autonomy from the world or nothing!' it tends to be nothing that wins. Another is that we will come, I would hope, to understand how it can be philosophically respectable to have a less all-or-nothing approach than many bioethicists now seem to recommend to the clinical care of those whose autonomy is under *obvious* threat from debilitation, old age or disease, including of course neurological disease. If there isn't a clear point at which we magically ping out of total non-autonomy into total autonomy, and likewise no clear point at which we magically ping out of non-personhood into personhood, then it may become easier for philosophers who insist on the centrality of personhood to understand why clinical care isn't sharply divisive in the way that their theories recommend. Put this point together with the other point I've just made, about the community-dependence of our status as persons, and I think you have a reason for not being divisive at all: ill human beings deserve to be treated with the full respect due to persons, *no matter what* philosopher's tests for personhood they may pass or fail.[5]

Endnotes

1. Maxwell Bennett and Peter Hacker, *Philosophical Foundations of Neuroscience* (London: John Wiley, 2003), hereinafter BH.

2. Ludwig Wittgenstein, *Philosophical Investigations*, trans. G. E. M. Anscombe (Oxford: Basil Blackwell, 1953), I:242: 'If language is to be a means of communication there must be agreement not only in definitions but also (queer as this may sound) in judgements. This seems to abolish logic, but does not do so. – It is one thing to describe methods of measurement, and another to obtain and state results of measurement. But what we call "measuring" is partly determined by a certain constancy in results of measurement'.

3. *Philosophical Investigations*, I:98.

4. See my 'Knowledge of Persons', *European Journal for Philosophy of Religion* 5, no. 4 (2013): 3–28.

5. On this, see my 'On the Very Idea of Criteria for Personhood', *Southern Journal of Philosophy* 49, no. 1 (2011), or *Knowing What to Do* (Oxford: Oxford University Press, 2014), chapter 6.

Towards an Islamic Neuropsychiatry

A Classification of the Diseases of the Head in Abūl-Hasan 'Alī ibn Sahl at-Tabarī's Paradise of Wisdom

Neil Krishan Aggarwal

A Brief Historical Overview of Islamic Medicine

This chapter presents original translations on the classification and symptom manifestations of neuropsychiatric disorders from Abūl-Hasan 'Alī ibn Sahl at-Tabarī's Arabic text *Firdaus al-Hikma* (The Paradise of Wisdom), the first original composition in the Islamic medical tradition. Arabic medicine has been characterised as a corpus of scientific texts translated into Arabic, mostly from Greek sources, starting from the eighth century [1]. It inherited the Galenic system of pathology, understood as the disturbed equilibrium of the four humours (blood, mucus, yellow bile and black bile [2]) and acquired an Islamic character with the spread of Islam in 622 CE beyond the Arabian peninsula [3]. Greek scientific texts from the Hellenistic, Roman and late Antiquity eras were translated into Arabic in an ambitious state project sponsored by the Abbasid caliphate in Baghdad from the eighth to tenth centuries [4]. For example, the ninth-century Abbasid caliph al-Mutawakkil employed as his court physician a Nestorian Christian named Hunayn ibn Ishāq whose team translated the medical compendia of Hippocrates and Galen, the philosophical treatises of Plato and Aristotle, and mathematical works of Euclid and Archimedes [5]. The caliph Harūn ar-Rashīd established a hospital in Baghdad in 805 CE, and 34 more hospitals arose throughout his dominion within two decades [6]. As Islam spread into the Iberian peninsula, Arabic became the language of science into which Greek and Syriac texts were translated in academic centres at Toledo and Córdoba for eventual diffusion into Europe [7].

Over time, those writing in Arabic attempted to assimilate foreign knowledge within a distinctly Islamic belief system. The Qu'rān came to be regarded as the direct word of God. Collections of Hadīth (literally 'events' in Arabic) recorded the Prophet Muhammad's sayings and doings as a model for ideal living and Arabic writers had to justify the knowledge of non-believers, including medicine, within this framework [8]. For instance, translated texts were culturally adapted so that the polytheistic references of Galen and Hippocrates to Greek gods were replaced by references to a monotheistic Allāh – literally 'The God' – in Arabic [9]. Treatises on Prophetic medicine (*at-tibb an-nabbawī*) written by Sunni religious scholars rather than trained physicians emerged from the ninth century to reconcile medical knowledge with Hadīth literature, and a prime example of fused Greco-Islamic knowledge comes from al-Dhahabī who uses Galen's definition of health as balance among the four humours to discuss humans as the perfect balance among all animals, the believers among all humans, the prophets among all believers, and Muhammad among all prophets [10]. Likewise, Shia scholars developed a separate medicine to reconcile medical knowledge with the sayings and doings of Muhammad *and* revered Shia Imams (*at-tibb al-a'imma*) [11]. Sunni and Shia forms of Prophetic medicine continue to be written around the world, synthesising classical Greco-Islamic medicine with popular health culture and Islamic religious precepts [12].

An Introduction to Abūl-Hasan Alī ibn Sahl at-Tabarī

Islamic medicine also produced volumes of original texts, as well as translations of foreign works, from the ninth century onwards as Arabic writers began to reason through Greek medical principles in the context of local geography, botany and astronomical calculations [13]. Abūl-Hasan Alī ibn Sahl Rabbān at-Tabarī (henceforth, at-Tabarī) is one such author whose biographical information comes mostly from his own *Firdaus al-Hikma*. Born in the city of Marw in present-day Turkmenistan, at-Tabarī was trained in theology, philosophy and medicine by his father, a prominent state official, and became a trusted counsellor to the caliph al-Mutawakkil to whom he dedicated the *Firdaus al-Hikma* [14]. At-Tabarī appears to have read widely, comparing the Indian Ayurvedic scholars Caraka, Suśruta, Vāgbhata and Mādhavakara against Greek authorities such as Hippocrates, Galen, Aristotle and Dioscurides, even as he chronicles native Persian occult practices [15]. Although he converted to Islam, scholars have been divided as to whether he was born Christian or Jewish [16–17]. However, this confusion may result from an earlier mistranslation of his title *rabban* as 'rabbi', leading to the false notion that he was born Jewish, even though at-Tabarī himself explains that the title was a Syriac Christian word for 'our master' or 'our teacher' [18]. What seems indisputable is that at-Tabarī wrote prolifically about theological matters after his conversion, on topics ranging from the evidence of Muhammad's prophecy [19] to apologetics urging Christians to convert to Islam [20]. Based on his employment at the court of al-Mutawakkil, we can assume that at-Tabarī was born either at the end of the eighth century or the beginning of the ninth century.

At-Tabarī is fondly remembered by scholars around the world. He is proudly claimed by Iranians as one of the first physicians to specify that the origin of epilepsy is the central nervous system and to also present a classification of different types of headache [21–22]. Islamic medicine continues to be practised in South Asia where there are more than 35 000 practitioners in India alone [23], and a reference book on the history of Islamic medicine included in the national syllabus laments that at-Tabarī's reputation has been limited to 'eastern physicians' since only one translation of his work exists in Urdu [24]. The translations presented below are intended in part to remedy this imbalance and to situate at-Tabarī's work within the cultural context of Islam, neurology and psychiatry.

Translations from the *Firdaus al-Hikma*

The Introduction

The introduction begins with a reference to Allah and Muhammad followed by an explanation of at-Tabarī's motivations for writing the book. While the religious reference may sound familiar and even formulaic to those well acquainted with Islamic religious literatures, they are nonetheless notable as proof of at-Tabarī's attempt to reconcile his religious faith with Greek medical knowledge:

'And praise to Allah, the living [*al-hayy*], the permanent, the beneficent, the creator, the maker [*al-bari*], and the prayers and peace of Allah the Great [be] upon Muhammad the Prophet and his family.

'This is a book of the collector, 'Alī ibn Rabban, [who] started [by] praising God and said that praise of goodness, generosity, and the preference of people are matters around which all nations gather. Whosoever explores the benefits of people is good and whosoever is liberal with what he has is generous . . . And my father was among the scholars [literally, 'sons of the book'] of the city Marv who possessed high virtues and manners with them . . . In my youth, he taught me just enough from it by the power of what Allah distributed to me and according to whatever time and disposition helped him. In what I read, I found many fragments, books of wise principles, from the people of Syria and others, in which their authors had restricted [themselves] to one discipline from the many, varying, disciplines of medicine. And this called me to compose a comprehensive book on account of the best qualities of the former and latter books so that it could be a register [*zamāman*] for all of them, a leader [*imāman*], an ocean [*muhītan*] for all of the books . . . So the secret of the secrets of wisdom, the treasure of the treasures of the craft, and fundamentals of this were available to me by the help of God, comprising mostly what I wanted [literally, 'of what was desired by the desirer']. And I [literally, 'the describer'] reached it from the discipline of medicine, knowledge of the principles of this discipline, its branches, its quality of essentials and non-essentials, the existence of souls and their bodies, the assemblies of animals, plants, the causes of colours, flavours, and the benefits of all of this, its harms, and the limits of things which the wise outlined' (1–2).[1]

Here, at-Tabarī begins by invoking key attributes of Allah. Moreover, the grace of Allah as God is mentioned as the reason for at-Tabarī's acquisition of medical knowledge and his success in completing the *Firdaus al-Hikma*. His pursuit of medicine is seen as a religious, not secular pursuit, underlying the religious nature of scientific knowledge.

After his religious invocation, brief biography and introduction to the text, at-Tabarī then references Greek philosophers and physicians. A Hellenistic sensibility provides the tone of his text, not just with respect to his outlook on medicine, but also in his justification that medicine belongs properly within the realm of philosophical inquiry. Although formal logic is no longer taught in contemporary medical syllabi, the rules for proper conjecturing and reasoning preoccupied early Muslim physicians as a legacy of the Greek medical tradition, and the word *hikma* in Arabic can translate as 'philosophy' or 'wisdom' [26]. This intellectual heritage is retained in the Urdu word *hakim*, literally, 'a wise person', still

[1] All translations in this chapter are mine from the original Arabic. I have translated from the standard critical edition of M. Z. Siddiqui, who standardised the text from four manuscripts: the British Museum Manuscript, the Berlin Manuscript, the Gotha Manuscript and the Khwāja Kamāluddīn Manuscript [25]. All page numbers listed at the end of translated sections refer to this critical edition.
I have taken three liberties in my translations. First, Siddiqui produces long selections of text, often without any paragraph indentation. Therefore, I have inserted paragraph breaks purely for reader convenience. Second, at-Tabarī, like all educated writers in Arabic, uses the particle 'and' (*wa*) to introduce a new sentence for continuity of thought. To avoid this repetition, I have deleted this word. Finally, and relatedly, Arabic uses the same word 'and' (*wa*) rather than commas to separate multiple elements listed in a series. Therefore, I retain the standard English style of eliminating all but the final 'and' in presenting series.

used to refer to a physician. The influence of the Greco-Islamic tradition is witnessed through belief in God, always stated as Allah, and restraint in the patient-physician relationship as prescribed by Greek authorities.

At-Tabarī's Conception of Neurological and Psychiatric Diseases

At-Tabarī introduces his discussion of neurological and psychiatric diseases in his second 'discourse'. The second discourse concerns the nature, signs and treatments of diseases, based on organ system. The second discourse contains 14 sections, of which 3 are devoted to an extensive discussion of 'diseases of the brain'. As stated in the introduction, at-Tabarī prefers foods and diets over medicaments in order to restore imbalance to their Platonic natural order. We can never be entirely sure about translations for specific food ingredients, plants and herbs when they have travelled across various languages, histories and geographies [27]. Therefore, I conclude the chapter with at-Tabarī's classification of diseases followed by their signs and symptoms.

The Third Section: On Diseases of the Brain

One abiding theme in cultural psychiatry has been how the people describe universal biological symptoms through local cultural meanings [28]. At-Tabarī draws upon religion to explain disease manifestations and to illustrate salient points for his readers:

'I mention in this section thirteen types among the sufferings of the head, from epilepsy, and it is *avīlbasya* [he glosses it as "epilepsy"]. A group calls it the fortune-telling disease [*kāhinī*] because from among them is one who tells fortunes, and strange things appear to him. From it [epilepsy] [are] desolation [*wahsha*], doubt [*waswasa*], talking irrationally [*haḍīyan*], depravity of thought and reason [*fasād al-khyāl wa 'aql*], forgetfulness, returning to the wild with a wild animal [*tawaḥush fī al-barārī ma al-waḥsh*], insomnia, shame [*subba*], echo/clang [*dawī*], vertigo, [and] swelling [*waram*]. I have mentioned [all] except for those [sufferings] among headaches: six types of cranial headache [*sanwarta*] from it, hemicranial/migraine headache [*shaqīqa*], and four types of headache that are agitated from the four humours. And two defects aggregate all of this: either it is corruption from the brain itself or it is from the involvement of the stomach and juices [*marāq*].

'As for the illnesses of doubt, talking irrationally, insomnia and going to the wild, they are due to the excess of heat and dryness targeting the brain and making it dry. Maybe the intellect changes from pleurisy [*al-birsām*] and hot fever. If it appears in two sides of the brain that are cold and dry, silence [*al-sukāt*] occurs. If coldness and moistness are excessive, lethargy [*al-subāt*] results.

'As for wildness and corrupt thought, their illnesses are from black bile. The proof of health is what we have said about the two illnesses together: if fresh, hot water is poured over the head and cold, moist things are placed on it, lethargy and sleep occur. If hot, dry things are placed, and there is an increase in fasting, excess of thought, and anxiety, then insomnia results.

'As for epilepsy, it is from a cold, viscid humour and from black bile retained in the brain or in the wind passages of breath; the brain moves and accumulates to dislodge its ear from itself as it agitates the stomach, with hiccups [*al-fuwāq*]. If the brain contracts and suffers pain, the whole body is agitated. Perhaps epilepsy is from corruption in the stomach in the juices, and the brain participates with them in the illness. Perhaps it is from a corrupting humour that rises from the foot to the brain and there is a seizure, as the poison of a scorpion rises. The poison of scorpions with the smallness and the fineness of their stings goes from the lowest parts of the body to the highest parts until the man is killed. Hippocrates said that [regarding] young boys, their vessels are narrow and their blood is languid, so the blood solidifies within them in this illness and kills them quickly. As for the middle-aged, they are stronger over this disease because their vessels are wider and their blood is abundant, hotter and the coldness of this disease does not overcome its clots. He also said that if the nasal mucus of the young boy and the wounds of his head and body are excessive, his brain then seeks purification and surrender to seizure. The wounds of his head and body benefit from this because if these moistures remain in the brain, perhaps they plug up the tracts, chill the blood, and smother and kill him' (138–9).

At-Tabarī's use of the Arabic word *kāhin* to describe epilepsy is striking for its religious significance. The word appears in verse 29 of the fifty-second chapter of the Quran entitled *at-Tūr* (The Mount): 'And speak, since you are not a fortune-teller [*kāhin*] or a madman through the blessings of your Lord' (my translation). The word *kāhin* is often translated as 'soothsayer' by older generations of translators, but the word shares an etymology with the Hebrew word – and last name – 'Cohen', a class of people seen to possess a type of spiritual knowledge unavailable to the five empirical senses. This verse in the Quran is intended to dispel concerns that Muhammad, as the final prophet, is yet another fortune-teller. I suspect that at-Tabarī deliberately uses this word to emphasise that epilepsy may present with the afflicted person proclaiming what is not there, literally not empirically sensible, by employing a cultural idiom that would have been familiar to his audience.

The Fourth Section: On the Signs of the Diseases of the Brain and What Appears in Them

Religion appears in another example of disease manifestations. As before, at-Tabarī explains the humoural pathophysiology of neuropsychiatric disorders. He then narrates a specific example by illustrating the tale of a man who is simply described as 'Christian':

'If the epileptic falls as if he is dead, this proves that the brain is filled with cold humour. If his mouth foams and salty saliva flows from it, then the disease is from phlegm. If he vomits something from which the soil boils like it boils from vinegar, then it is from black bile. If this is from black bile that is unmixed from association [with other humours], then for his whole body his anxiety increases, his speech is little and his body slackens. And this afflicts whomsoever is brown of colour, plenty of hair, long of thought, filled up of veins, and slender of body. If the disease is from yellow bile transformed into black bile, his anger, agitation and irrational talk will increase. If it is from blood transformed into black bile, his laughter and his pleasure will increase. This type afflicts whomsoever is light complexioned and red, deep of thought, concern and trouble. It is the safest of all because it resembles intoxication since blood [of all the humours] is the [most] beloved of the natural order [*tabi'a*]. As for the one who is feeble of flesh, black bile is hardly generated. Perhaps the illness is from a collection of corrupting moistures with yellow bile transformed to black bile. So the sign(s) of this are: if the yellow bile is stirred up, insomnia and talking irrationally afflicts him. If phlegm is stirred up within him, lethargy afflicts him.

'Hippocrates said that if the epilepsy is with laughter and animation, then he is avoiding separation and sorrow. Indeed, laughter proves that it is from blood. Sorrow and separation point that it is from black bile and phlegm. He said that for whomsoever his seizure is from the corruption of black bile, then varices [*dawālī*] appear on his calf or haemorrhoids of the backside appear [and] he will escape from it [the epilepsy]. His meaning is that the varices [*dawālī*] are thick lesions, so if they appear on the calf, that points to the bad substance which had descended from the brain to the calf. He said in its example that for bald people, it does not afflict their large varices [*dawālī*] so if it afflicts them then the hair of their heads grows. By the meaning of his statement "for those bald people" he meant those whose hair has gone away from the disease of alopecia [*tha'alab*]. So if the varices appear on their trunks, then it shows that the substance had descended from the head to the leg.

'It is said [by Hippocrates] that: "For whom there is epilepsy, I smelled something lupine [*min turmūs*] when he seizes". And that is its reason. He comes to, perceives this, then recovers. If he does not come to and does not perceive, then his recovery is not anticipated. Like this, if I blew air covering up the wound on his neck, then he sneezed, then he desired to recover [*rajī lahu al-bura*]. And if not, then not.

'Alexander the itinerant [*al-tawāf*] said, "I stripped the nail from the two big toes of the feet of the epileptic until blood poured out from them. Then I rubbed that blood on the lip of the epileptic and in the area [*fī-mā*] between his eyes. Then he recovered and stood up instantly".

'And the wise Hippocrates said that: "Whosoever seizes falls to the ground as if he were dead and his perception goes, there is no cure for it. Whosoever is not like that, then his cure is a tough predicament because the brain is the master [*sayyid*] of the organs and from it is the origin of sensation and movement. If the disease prevails over this mastery, its treatment becomes difficult because the sensation and the movement of the heart and the liver are also from it [the brain]". We will show this in what follows that the brain is divided into two parts. In it are three vessels. Perhaps the disease is in the front of the brain or in the last part or in all of its parts. The hardest of all of them is what afflicts the location of thought and memory together. Aside from this is what afflicts the location of memory. If the disease is in the front of the brain – and it is the location of fantasy and thought – it [the disease] reveals itself to that part what it reveals to the man. And he would heal and claim that he sees in the direction of the house, players of instruments [*zamārīn*] and sports [*la'ābīn*]. If the disease is in the middle part of the brain – and it is the location of thought – what targets it is what targets the man. He would shut the door of the room on himself, open the small window, and throw everything in the house out of it to people. Nothing would reveal itself to him as it would reveal to the first [type/person], but he could not reason that he was wrong in what he did. And the cause of this is from a cold, bad humour that corrupts the location of reason. Therefore, drowsy people result from poison and other things. In the winter/rainy season, these flee from the cold into the depth of the earth.

'If the disease is in the last part of the brain – and it is the location of memory – it [the disease] happens to it [the diseased person] as it happened to a group from the Byzantines who were at war. What afflicts them from the malodour of a decaying cadaver is what corrupts their memory. And they tarry at that time, not remembering their own names or the names of their fathers. Among those whose brains are corrupt and reason has changed are those who think that they are of pottery. They have feared that they would touch something and they would break. Among them are those who have thought that the sky falls upon them so they flee, proceeding slowly while yelling. Some of them have thought that they were wild camels and would flee from people. Some of them were chickens so when their reason changed, they believed that they were a chicken and shouted.

'In this time of ours there are many of their afflictions through corruption of the mind whose examples have not been heard [before]. As for one of them, there was a Christian man who was afflicted by his wealth. His friends found him at night having cut off part of his throat. Blood flowed from him. So they met him, treated him, and asked him about the cause that led to this. He stated that he saw men and women gathering around his house. From among them, someone said that they were not surprised by this Christian who had shown virtue and then committed adultery with a Muslim woman. From among them someone said "Guard him to the morning so that he does not flee!" From among them someone said, "You did not guard him as he threw himself in the *bīr* [a large body of water] and went away". And those of a different opinion about this depressed person said that he slit his own neck and found relief from torment and repression. In the midst of this, he goes to the knife and slaughters himself or he loses consciousness and falls. Then, when he is treated, his rationality returns to him.

'And I observed two other men kill themselves and die. The men and women in Tabaristan and Dailam hung themselves from the trees whenever fear or sorrow descended upon them. And the Wise [Hippocrates] said that the cause of these diseases is that the souls were naturally disposed to the hatred of darkness and running from it to the light. Indeed the brain is the location of the rational self. So if murky, cold steam unfastens it, the self becomes afraid and sadness strikes it at one time, and desolation, and fear at another [time]. The example of the self in this [situation] is the example of the light of the sun when the clouds or fog ascend without it. But this appears to a man like the man hearing a sound or a ring when there is no sound in the air. He sees something between his eyes that resembles fire or gadflies. He sees the thing in two. All of this appears from defects that take place in the brain. From this is the disease that stirs from the rise [*nafkha*] of deviancy and corruption in it or in the stomach. This rises to the brain and corrupts it. Symptoms from the meeting of yellow bile with phlegm are the mental disorders of reason, frivolity [*'abath*], and talking irrationally. If it is from the yellow bile alone, its affliction is with colic [*mags, magas*], the belching of a lace of smoke [*mad-khana*], bitterness of the mouth, thirst, and the yellowing of urine. If phlegm unites with it, the saliva and sourness of the belching increase. It is also from some of the organs and their signs that it is experienced from the ascension of vapour from the organ during the attack [*'and al-nūba*]. as Galen mentioned and which we will mention in the account of its treatment' (139–42).

Religion forms an integral part of at-Tabarī's explanation of illness and treatment. As a convert to Islam from Christianity, at-Tabarī would surely have recognised that his audience would object to 'adultery with a Muslim woman'. The gravity of the situation is underscored by the crowd that appears outside of this Christian man's house in at-Tabarī's case study. Not only is the man accused of violating virtue, he is also shown to act irrationally by taking his own life. Religious mores again pervade at-Tabarī's text, demonstrating once again that his description of neuropsychiatric disorders fuses Greek humoural medicine within an Islamic context.

This chapter has examined at-Tabarī's Firdaus al-Hikma as the first text within the Islamic medical tradition to articulate a classification for neuropsychiatric disorders. At-Tabarī fashions a unique understanding of health and illness by synthesising themes of Greek humoural medicine with Islamic theological precepts. His mention within history of medicine textbooks and the rise of Urdu commentaries explaining his Arabic text attest to his ongoing relevance within South Asian Islamic medicine. Expertise in the Firdaus al-Hikma remains mandatory: the government of Pakistan has included the text in its course syllabus on the theoretical foundations of contemporary Islamic medicine [29] and the text

is part of the history of medicine course in India [30]. A recent translation of the text into Persian signifies the interest in his medical thought beyond South Asia [31]. Ongoing work is needed on how today's Islamic medical practitioners regard his legacy, compare his work to scholars within their tradition and within the culture of biomedicine, and mobilise his ideas within clinical practice.

References

1 Browne, E. G. 1921. *Arabian Medicine: The FitzPatrick Lectures Delivered at the College of Physicians in November 1919 and November 1920*. Cambridge: Cambridge University Press.

2 Bürgel, J. C. 1998. Secular and religious features of medieval Arabic medicine. In *Asian Medical Systems: A Comparative Study*, ed. C. Leslie, 44–62. Delhi: Motilal Banarsidass.

3 Shanks, N. J., and D. Al-Kalai. 1984. Arabian medicine in the Middle Ages. *Journal of the Royal Society of Medicine* 77: 60–5.

4 Gutas, D. 1998. *Greek Thought, Arabic Culture: The Graeco-Arabic Translation Movement in Baghdad and Early Abbāsid Society (2nd–4th/8th–10th Centuries)*. London: Routledge.

5 Saad, B., H. Azaizeh and O. Said. 2005. Tradition and perspectives of Arab herbal medicine: a review. *eCAM* 2: 475–9.

6 Saad, B., and O. Said. 2011. *Greco-Arab and Islamic Herbal Medicine: Traditional System, Ethics, Safety, Efficacy, and Regulatory Issues*. Hoboken, NJ: John Wiley.

7 Brewer, H. 2004. Early Arabic medicine. *Journal of the Royal Society for the Promotion of Health* 124: 184–7.

8 Rahman, F. 1987. *Health and Medicine in Islamic Tradition: Change and Identity*. New York: Crossroad.

9 Pormann, P. E., and E. Savage-Smith. 2007. *Medieval Islamic Medicine*. Washington, DC: Georgetown University Press.

10 Biesterfeldt, H. H. 2011. Medicine in the Arab world. In *Encyclopedia of Medieval Philosophy*, ed. H. Lagerlund, 742–6. Dordrecht: Springer Netherlands.

11 Ebrahimnejad, H. 2011. What is 'Islamic' in Islamic medicine? An overview. In *Science between Europe and Asia: Historical Studies on the Transmission, Adoption and Adaptation of Knowledge*, ed. F. Günergun and D. Raina, 259–70. Dordrecht: Springer Netherlands.

12 Good, B., and M. J. D. Good. 1992. The comparative study of Greco-Islamic medicine: the integration of knowledge into local symbolic contexts. In *Paths to Asian Medical Knowledge*, ed. C. Leslie and A. Young, 257–71. Berkeley: University of California Press.

13 Sa'adi, L. M. 1958. Glimpses into the history of Arabic medicine. *Bulletin of the Medical Library Association* 46: 206–18.

14 Hamarneh, S. K. 1997. Al-Tabarī. In *Encyclopaedia of the History of Science, Technology, and Medicine in Non-Western Cultures*, ed. H. Selin, 930. Dordrecht: Springer Netherlands.

15 Ullmann, M. 1978. *Islamic Medicine*. Edinburgh: Edinburgh University Press.

16 Beaumont, M. I. 2005. Early Muslim interpretation of the Gospels. *Transformation: An International Journal of Holistic Mission Studies* 22: 20–7.

17 Behbehani, A. 1984. Rhazes: the original portrayer of smallpox. *JAMA* 252: 3156–9.

18 Meyerhof, M. 1931. `Alî at-Tabarî's 'Paradise of Wisdom', one of the oldest Arabic compendiums of medicine. *Isis* 16: 6–54.

19 Watt, W. M. 1953. His name is Ahmad. *The Muslim World* 43: 110–17.

20 Martin, R. C. 1980. The role of the Mu'tazilah in formulating the doctrine of the apologetic miracle. *Journal of Near Eastern Studies* 39: 175–89.

21 Gorji, A., and M. K. Ghadiri. 2001. History of epilepsy in medieval Iranian medicine.

Neuroscience and Biobehavioral Reviews 25: 455–61.

22 Gorji, A., and M. K. Ghadiri. 2002. History of headache in medieval Persian medicine. *Lancet Neurology* 1: 510–15.

23 Sheehan, H. E., and S. J. Hussain. 2002. Unani Tibb: history, theory, and contemporary practice in South Asia. *Annals of the American Academy of Political and Social Science* 583: 122–35.

24 Qadeer, A. 2005. *History of Medicine and Medical Ethics*. Delhi: Rabbani.

25 Siddiqui, M. Z. 1928. *Firdausu'l Hikmat or Paradise of Wisdom of 'Ali b. Rabban-al-Tabari*. Berlin: Buch- u. Kunstdruckerei 'Sonne'.

26 Aggarwal, N. K. 2010. Diagnostic reasoning in Nizāmī 'Arūzī's *Four Discourses*. *Medical Humanities* 36: 88–92.

27 Aggarwal, N. K. 2013. 'On the Diseases of the Head' in the scale of medicine by Muhammad Akbar Arzānī [d. 1722]. *History of Psychiatry* 24: 106–17.

28 Aggarwal, N. K. 2010. Psychosis in the Firdaus al-Hikmat, the first major Arabic medical text. *British Journal of Psychiatry* 197: 447.

29 Curriculum Division, Higher Education Commission. 2004. *Curriculum of Eastern Medicine for BEMS & M.Phil.* Islamabad: Government of Pakistan. http://hec.gov.pk/english/services/universities/RevisedCurricula/Documents/2004-2005/Eastern%20Medicine%202004.pdf.

30 Central Council of Indian Medicine. 2014. *Syllabus of Kamil-E-Tib-Wa-Jarahat (BUMS) Course*. New Delhi: Government of India. https://ccimindia.org/pdf/UG-1st-2nd-3rd-yr-Syllabus-BUMS-Unani.pdf.

31 Tabarī, Ai. S. R., A. N. Munzavī and M. I. Zākir. 2012. *Firdaws al-ḥikmah : Baḥr al-Manāfi Va Shams al-Adāb*. 1391; repr., Tehran: Markaz-i Taḥqīqāt-i Ṭibb-i Sunnatī va Mufradāt-i Pizishkī-i Dānishgāh-i Ulūm-i Pizishkī-i Shahīd Bihishtī.

Chapter 9

II.I *Clinical Conditions*

Temporal Lobe Epilepsy, Dostoyevsky and Irrational Significance

Alasdair Coles

An association of some sort between epilepsy and spirituality, both divine and demonic, has been postulated for millennia (reviewed in Devinsky and Lai 2008). No doubt, this is because people with epilepsy seem to become 'possessed' during their seizures, both in the convulsions of the generalised epilepsies and in the strange altered awareness of temporal lobe seizures. In addition, has been the observation that people with epilepsy may show an unusual interest in religion, recently documented in an ancient Babylonian text (Reynolds and Kinnier Wilson 2008). Some date the birth of rational medicine to Hippocrates' denial that those with the 'sacred disease', epilepsy, had mystical power (Todman 2008).

The complex interplay of epilepsy and religion is illustrated by a study from New Delhi which showed that 6 per cent of patients thought their epilepsy was a curse from God and 14 per cent felt it was a punishment for past sins (Khwaja and Chadhury 2007). Twenty-nine per cent became more religious after their seizures started and 80 per cent of people reported that religion had helped them cope with epilepsy. Only 2 per cent reported mystic experiences with seizures, the subject of this chapter.

The phenomenology of epilepsy may be studied to understand the normal hierarchical function of the brain. For focal epilepsies are unusual neurological 'experiments of nature' in that they demonstrate the consequences of stimulation of a particular brain region. Abnormal electrical discharge in a localised area of cortex causes symptoms attributable to that site. Typically this activity will spread throughout the cortex to cause a generalised convulsion and unconsciousness; but experiences or behaviour in the seconds before the seizure itself can be recalled and used to understand the normal function of that part of the cortex in health. Up to 3 per cent of people with focal epilepsy are said to have religious or mystical experiences as part of their seizure, most commonly those with onset in the right temporal lobe (Devinsky and Lai 2008). If anything, this figure is an overestimate, explaining why several small studies fail to identify such patients (Greyson et al. 2015; Tedrus et al. 2014; Williams 1956). Here I analyse the core experience of such temporal lobe seizures, best described by Fydor Dostoyevsky, and conclude that they mimic some, but not all, of the elements of authentic religious experiences and that their interpretation as 'religious' depends upon prior conditioning.

Perhaps the most interesting question, theologically, of people who have frequent mystical seizures is to ask: what sort of religious life do they lead? What sort of belief and religious practice emerges from 'inappropriate' mystical experiences? I describe the contentious evidence around the claim by Norman Geschwind that such patients are 'hyperreligious' (Waxman and Geschwind 1975).

Finally, I draw attention to the paradox, which has not been previously articulated, that rational people may understand these experiences to be artefactually generated by a disease and yet nonetheless attribute to them lasting significance in their lives, apparently understood to offer authentic spiritual insight.

The Nature of Dostoyevsky Seizures: Oceanic Ecstasy

The first medical description of a religious experience induced by focal epilepsy may be from the nineteenth-century Scottish physician, James Howden, Medical Superintendent of the Montrose Royal Lunatic Asylum (of whom more below). He describes eight cases of either ictal religious experience or post-ictal religious psychoses (Howden 1873). British neurologist William Gower mentions one case, without further comment, in his massive and authoritative 1881 textbook of epilepsy: a patient whose seizures started by a 'sensation in the great toe, followed by a desire to micturate and a feeling of turning over and over, this was succeeded by the feeling of being in heaven, seeing persons and hearing a question asked' (Gowers 1881, 61).

The fullest description of what have been termed 'religious seizures', however, comes from the writing of Dostoyevsky (hence the sobriquet 'Dostoyevsky seizures'), particularly in the character of Prince Myshkin, in *The Idiot*, whose epilepsy is a key motif throughout the book. For instance:

> He [Myshkin] remembered that during his epileptic fits, or rather immediately preceding them, he had always experienced a moment or two when his whole heart and mind, and body seemed to wake up to vigour and light; when he became filled with joy and hope, and all his anxieties seemed to be swept away for ever; these moments were but presentiments, as it were, of the one final second (it was never more than a second) in which the fit came upon him.
>
> (Dostoyevsky 1869, 139)

The seizures described by Dostoyevsky do not have explicit religious content, so the term 'religious seizure' is unhelpful. More accurate perhaps is James Leuba's term 'ecstatic seizures'. In his 1925 classic, he describes some cases:

> Among the dread diseases that afflict humanity there is one that interests us quite particularly; that disease is epilepsy. Its main manifestation is often preceded by curious signs, varying greatly from person to person, but fairly constant in the same person. In some instances, the 'aura', as these premonitory symptoms are called, is in the nature of an ecstasy. In Modern Medicine, Dr Spratling reports the case of a priest under his care whose epileptic attacks were preceded by a rapturous moment. Walking along the streets, for instance, he would suddenly feel, as it were, 'transported to heaven', This state of marvellous enjoyment would soon pass, and, a little later on, he would find himself seated on the curb of the sidewalk aware that he had suffered an epileptic attack. The same author mentions elsewhere two other epileptic patients, 'teachers of noted ability' who speak of their aurae as 'the most overwhelming ecstatic state it is possible for the human to conceive of'.
>
> (Leuba 1925, 204–5)

A contemporary account of a temporal lobe seizure with apparent religious content comes from an anonymous contributor to an online chatroom, who narrated in real time the experience of the 'aura' of his or her accustomed focal seizures which persisted for 20 minutes (which technically is the state of 'complex partial status') before eventually leading to a convulsion.

> This is the aura. The fit comes later, a sensation like a fast train. 00:19 It's not going to be a bad one. It's come up fast. The slow burn is the worst. 00:21 It was the smell that told me. I smell things

> like burning herbs. Then they go, and when its over they're gone. 00:29 I can feel fragments of identity speaking to me. It gets harder to describe. I taste salt and something else. I exult in these moments. it's the payoff for the bad times, the weary times. In these moments I kiss God. 00:31 I can see all the colours now. under your skin! look at your hand. do you doubt that you contain an infinity of shades? tone and chroma chapter and verse. you are the book of madder-rose and indigo. my hands will be taken soon, for a while. but how lovely that i can speak colour with my hands, while the time lasts! 00:33 its coming. i break open like achrysalis, i split. cant say much more. but you are the divine! look at your hands, draw breth, and do not doubt that you taste eternity. 00:37 over soon. i would be a river if i could. i would bleed eternal/divine. wont see it when i wake up. see it NOW. all colours. when you see all the colours. all the colours, in any one colour. that is to taste the divine. over soon. I want to remember! the keys look like bone, like brick. pyramids and saints toes. all colours. all the colours. they all saw all the colours. 00:40 keys like bone, but containing all colours. the colours never leave us. God is spectrum, infinite spectrum. sound, colour touch all a spectrum 00:54 It's over. I had the fit, I'm fine except I think I hit my elbow on something and I bit my tongue.
>
> (Anonymous 2012)

One of my patients, A.S., a theologian who had suffered temporal lobe seizures since his teens, interpreted his attacks as 'a gift from God' or 'divine inspiration'. But, his description of the subjective experience itself was free from overt religious imagery. He decried suddenly feeling content, 'at peace, and the world around me is illuminated, as though I had gone from darkness to light'. This lasted for a few seconds.

Leuba has catalogued the core features of Dostoyevsky seizures: 'the subject's role is entirely passive; it is as if an external power had taken possession of him . . . The ecstasy may bring with it a sense of initiation, illumination, or revelation . . . The experience is so wonderful that the most extravagant descriptive terms and comparisons seem to fall short of the reality; it is an ineffable experience' (Leuba 1925, 206). To these, I would add a sense of calm and universality; one of my patients, G.A., described the sensation as 'oceanic'.

I hypothesise that such experiences are described with explicit religious language and imagery only in those conditioned by a religious upbringing. Unfortunately, information on prior religious exposure is usually lacking in the literature on Dostoyevsky seizures. In the case of my patient, A.S., his 'divine gift' were key to his conversion, but prior to the onset of his seizures he had an unusually observant religious life, encouraged to take Catholic Mass several times a week. Likewise, five out of the six cases in a classic paper arguing that seizures precipitated religious 'conversion' actually had unusually intense religious upbringing (Dewhurst and Beard 1970). Case 1 was a regular attender of church up to the age of 18 and infrequently thereafter, but who insisted on sending his children to Sunday school. Case 2, whose father converted from Methodism to Christian Science, decided at the age of nine to become a minister, and used to get up at 6:00 AM to sing hymns. Case 3 was brought up strictly in the Jewish Orthodox faith and remained devout until the age of 17. Case 5 was brought up in a strict non-conformist family. Case 5: was 'always religious'. So, these are hardly 'conversions', more like reversions of people to a former religious life, precipitated by a seizure. Although presented by the authors as a mechanistic brain-based event, I would argue that the psychological shock and disruption of a seizure led these individuals to seek the solace of their former faith.

Experience from non-Western peoples with epilepsy confirms the view that unusual experiences like seizures, even without any explicit mystical content, tend to be interpreted within a religious and cultural agenda. For instance Haitians with epilepsy were all thought to have been possessed by Voodoo spirits (Carrazana et al. 1999; Cavanna et al. 2010). And Louise Jilek-Aall has described how Tanzanian peoples regarded epilepsy as caused by ancestral spirits or spirit possession (Jilek-Aall 1999).

The corollary of my hypothesis is that the same subjective 'ecstatic' experience may be interpreted in non-religious ways in those without religious conditioning. This was the conclusion of Japanese investigators who, in a survey of 234 people with epilepsy, found 3 with religious ictal experiences, all of whom came from families with strong religious backgrounds, itself unusual in Japan (Ogata and Miyakawa 1998). If not interpreted as religious, such seizures may be understood as erotic or just pleasurable. In a small series of 11 cases of 'ecstatic seizures' from Norway, 8 had sensory hallucinations, 4 had erotic sensations, 5 had 'a religious/spiritual experience' and several had symptoms that had no counterpart in human experience (Asheim Hansen and Brodtkorb 2003). Likewise, there are examples of pure erotic (Amancio et al. 1994) or pure 'pleasure' seizures (Aull-Watschinger et al. 2008) arising in temporal lobe epilepsy.

How typical are Dostoyevsky seizures of religious experiences in people without neurological disease? There is certainly resonance with some elements catalogued by Alexander and Andrew Fingelkurts (Fingelkurts 2009), namely (1) 'the sense of having touched the ultimate ground of divine reality'; (2) 'the experience of timelessness and spacelessness'; (3) 'feelings of positive affect, peace, joy and unconditional love'; (4) 'blissful absorption into the present moment'; (5) 'experiencing in an extraordinary way that all things are "One" with a divine being'. But some normal elements are absent: (1) 'a sense of special patterning of events in a person's life by a divine being'; (2) 'an awareness of receiving help in answer to a prayer'; and (3) 'an awareness of being looked after or guided by a presence of God'. An important difference between Dostoyevsky seizures and 'healthy' religious experiences are their frequency: it is usual for people to experience the latter perhaps once or twice in a lifetime (Fingelkurts 2009).

The exact site within the temporal lobe which subserves these seizures is not known. It seems to have been outside of the reach of Wilder Penfield's stimulating electrode, when he explored the effects of stimulating the temporal lobe cortex in awake patients during epilepsy surgery (Penfield 1955, 1958). Instead, he catalogued reawakening of memories, induction of primitive emotions (especially fear) and 'interpretative illusions', especially time, such as déjà vu and jamais vu. However, there is one convincing case report of induction of typical 'ecstatic' bliss in a neurosurgical patient by stimulation of an area within the anterior-dorsal insula (Picard et al. 2013).

I conclude that the core experiences of such temporal lobe Dostoyevsky seizures are ineffable emotions comprising oceanic peace, universality and ecstasy, that resemble in part religious experiences in neurologically normal people. These emotions may be interpreted in traditional religious terms by those with appropriate conditioning. But overlooked in previous accounts is one outstanding feature of these attacks that deserves further analysis: those who experience may derive from them great personal significance, even after many years.

Authenticity and Significance: The 'Higher and Lower Life'

James Leuba, concluding his assessment of ecstatic seizures, writes that 'these traits might naturally enough suggest super Human causation, yet no metaphysical significance is ascribed to them'. My observations are the opposite: often people affected by these experiences draw great personal, and long-lasting, significance from them. Patient A.S., mentioned above, interpreted his Dostoyevsky seizures as gifts from God, which informed his work as a theologian. When I explained that his experiences were due to epilepsy and could be halted with anticonvulsant medication, to my surprise he declined. He accepted the diagnosis, but continued to attach spiritual and personal significance to them.

Non-compliance with medication is usual in such cases. In the Norwegian series of 11 patients with Dostoyevsky seizures, quote above, five consciously induced their seizures and four were non-compliant with anticonvulsant treatment (Asheim Hansen and Brodtkorb 2003). Case 3 in Geschwind's original series was reluctant to take anticonvulsant medication because his seizures were 'important' to him (Waxman and Geschwind 1975).

A trace of this sense of importance or significance of such experiences can be found in highly rational people. Dostoyevsky could describe ecstatic seizures so accurately in *The Idiot* because he himself experienced them. And they were intimately connected with his theology. For instance, Sophia Kovalewski in her 'Childhood Recollections' says Dostoyevsky described his 'first attack' (almost certainly he had childhood seizures which he seems to have suppressed) in this way:

> Suddenly Dostoiewski exclaimed: 'God exists, He exists'. At the same time from a nearby church a bell began to toll for midnight mass. And Dostoiewski went on to say: 'The air was filled with a big noise and I tried to move. I felt the heaven was going down upon the earth and that it had engulfed me. I have really touched God. He came into me myself, yes God exists, I cried, and I don't remember anything else. You all, healthy people, he said, can't imagine the happiness which we epileptics feel during the second before our fit. Mahomet, in his Koran, said he had seen Paradise and had gone into it. All these stupid clever men are quite sure that he was a liar and a charlatan. But no, he did not lie, he really had been in Paradise during an attack of epilepsy; he was a victim of this disease like I was. I don't know if this felicity lasts for seconds, hours or months, but believe me, for all the joys that life may bring, I would not exchange this one'. On another occasion, Dostoiewski gave this further description of his aura. 'During a few moments I feel such a happiness that it is impossible to realize at other times, and other people cannot imagine it. I feel a complete harmony within myself and in the world, and this feeling is so strong and so sweet that for a few seconds of this enjoyment one would readily exchange ten years of one's life – perhaps even one's whole life'. You are all healthy people . . . but you have no idea what joy that joy is which we epileptics experience the second before a seizure . . . I do not know whether this joy lasts for seconds or hours or months, but believe me, I would not exchange it for all the delights of this world.[1]
>
> (quoted in Alajouanine 1963, 212)

Karen Armstrong also describes her seizures somewhat wistfully. She entered a Catholic convent at the age of 17. Seven years later, after a series of 'fainting attacks' she was diagnosed with epilepsy. She was treated and no longer had seizures. She left the convent and lost her conventional Catholic faith, but has made theology her profession. In one of her autobiographies, she wrote,

> My neurologist once told me that people with temporal lobe epilepsy are very often intensely religious. Certainly just before I have a grand mal fit I have a 'vision' of such peace, joy and significance that I can only call it God. What does this say about the whole nature of religious vision? Certain episodes in the lives of the saints have acquired a new meaning for me. When

[1] Very curiously, despite these clear descriptions, some deny that Dostoyevsky can have experienced these ecstatic seizures himself (Hughes 2005), but the evidence seems incontrovertible.

> Theresa of Avila had her three-day vision of hell, was she simply having a temporal lobe attack? The horrors she saw are similar to those I have experienced, but in her case informed by the religious imagery of her time. Like other saints who have 'seen' hell she describes an appalling stench, which is part of an epileptic aura. Is it possible that the feeling I have had all my life that something – God, perhaps? – is just over the horizon, something unimaginable but almost tangibly present, is simply the result of an electrical irregularity in my brain? It is a question that can't yet be answered, unless it be that God, if He exists, could have created us with that capacity for Him, glimpsed at only when the brain is convulsed. What I can say, however, is that if my 'visions' have sometimes let me into 'Hell' they have also given me possible intimations of a Heaven which I would not have been without.
>
> (Armstrong 1983, 23)

Both authors seem, albeit with much reservation, to attribute from events they know to be generated by a disease (an 'electrical irregularity').

The most eloquent exposition of this paradox comes from the character of Prince Myshkin in this extended speech, which ends with a quotation from Revelations 10:6.

> When the attack was over, and the prince reflected on his symptoms, he used to say to himself: 'These moments, short as they are, when I feel such extreme consciousness of myself, and consequently more of life than at other times, are due only to the disease – to the sudden rupture of normal conditions. Therefore they are not really a higher kind of life, but a lower'. This reasoning, however, seemed to end in a paradox, and lead to the further consideration: 'What matter though it be only a disease, and abnormal tension of the brain, if when I recall and analyse the moment, it seems to have been one of harmony and beauty in the highest degree – and instant of the deepest sensation, overflowing with unbound joy and rapture, ecstatic devotion and with completest life?' Vague though this sounds, it was perfectly comprehensible to Muishkin [*sic*], though he knew that it was but a feeble expression of his sensations. That there was, indeed, beauty and harmony in those abnormal moments, that they really contained the highest synthesis of life, he could not doubt, nor even admit the possibility of doubt. He felt they were not analogous to the fantastic and unreal dreams of intoxication by hashish, opium or wine. Of that he could judge, when the attack was over. These instances were characterised – to define it in a word – by the intense quickening of the sense of personality. Since, in the last conscious moment preceding the attack, he could say to himself, with the full understanding of his word: 'I would give my whole life for this one instant' then doubtless it was worth a lifetime. For the rest, he thought the dialectical part of his argument of little worth; he saw only too clearly that the result of these ecstatic moments was stupefaction, mental darkness, idiocy. No argument was possible on that point. His conclusion, this estimate of the 'moment', doubtless contained some error, yet the reality of the sensation troubled him. What's more answerable that a fact? And this fact had occurred. The prince had confessed unreservedly to himself that the feeling of intense beatitude in that crowded moment made the moment worth a lifetime. I feel then as if I understood those amazing words . . . 'There shall be no more time'.
>
> (Dostoyevsky 1869, 140)

It is characteristic that people experiencing such seizures have a sense of their personal importance and significance, even years after they have been aborted by medication. This is quite different, as Mishkin points out, from the experiences induced by alcohol and most drugs, and from mania itself, where usually nothing of meaning remains years after the euphoria has settled. The one exception is the ingestion of psilocybin, the active ingredient of magic mushrooms, which leaves people with a long-lasting feeling of mystical significance, even in subjects who are well aware they are part of a scientific experiment (Griffiths et al. 2006, 2011; Johnson et al. 2012; MacLean et al. 2011).

Of course, people may attribute personal significance to illness for a variety of reasons. There is no doubt that periods of enforced convalescence may lead to a new attention to spirituality (Francis of Assisi and Ignatius of Loyola, for instance). Also the experience of suffering through illness can mature faith. And being part of a worshipping congregation may be attractive to those with neurological illness because of the offer of practical and emotional support. Conversely, illness may symbolise important internal personal conflicts, as in psychosomatic and dissociative disorders. Yet, none of these approach the character of the significance attributed to Dostoyevsky seizures, which seems automatic or imposed, rather than wilfully received.

I had no doubt, when first treating patient A.S., that his seizures were epileptic and not authentic spiritual experiences. Yet he thought otherwise: when pressed, he explained that if God chose to communicate to his through seizures, who was he to argue? This is his settled opinion, to this day.

Fabienne Picard has provided a neuropsychological explanation for the significance many attach to mystical seizures. He has argued, from two compelling case reports, that the mystical seizures arise from the insula. And he identified, in the detailed accounts of two patients, that part of their experience was an unfamiliar sense of meaningfulness and certainty. He argues that this relates to the role of the anterior insular cortex in predicting errors. If this capacity is reduced, then the experience is freed from accompanying ambiguity and error-detection (Picard and Craig 2009; Picard 2013; Picard and Kurth 2014).

So, how to test authenticity? William James writes about the difficulty of distinguishing real spiritual experiences from the counterfeits of 'trances and convulsive seizures' and concludes,

> In the history of Christian mysticism the problem how to discriminate between such messages and experiences as were really divine miracles, and such others as the demon in his malice was able to counterfeit, thus making the religious person twofold more the child of hell that he was before, has always been a difficult one to solve, needing all the sagacity an experience of the best directors of conscience. In the end it had to come to our empiricist criterion: by their fruits ye shall know them.
> (James 1904, 20)

By this test, ecstatic seizures are authentic 'divine miracles' or at least that is the message of *The Idiot*. For Dostoyevsky recorded in his notes that he conceived Prince Myshkin as 'a positively beautiful man' (quoted by Frank 2010, 577). Many commentators have ascribed a Christ-like quality to Mishkin, and Joseph Frank describes him as 'the extremest incarnation of the Christian ideal of love that humanity can reach in its present form' (Frank 2010, 577). Interestingly, despite Mishkin's intense faith and preoccupation with God and beauty, and in the reconciliation of relationships around him, he is not seen to attend formal worship or follow the liturgical calendar. And, ultimately, he returns to the asylum from which he came. This is an accurate portrayal of the spiritual life of people with temporal lobe epilepsy, which has been labelled as 'hyperreligious' by Norman Geschwind and others, to which I now turn.

Exaltation of the Religious Sentiment in Temporal Lobe Epilepsy

What sort of religious life emerges from a lifetime of temporal lobe seizures? James Howden not only described ictal religious experiences but also a 'mental condition of Epileptics, which, to the best of my knowledge, has not attracted that attention to which its frequency entitles it. I refer to the exaltation of the religious sentiment' (Howden 1873, 482). So appeared in modern medical print, for the first time, the suggestion that people with epilepsy have a tendency to be unusually pious and devout in between seizures. This has been most strongly argued by Steve Waxman and Norman Geschwind, who proposed that people with temporal lobe epilepsy had a personality characterised by religiosity and compulsive writing, often on moral or religious nature. In evidence, they offered three case histories, and alluded to many more (Waxman and Geschwind 1975). In a later paper, Geschwind elaborated that the syndrome included: 'increased concern with philosophical, moral or religious issues, often in striking contrast to the patient's educational background, an increased rate of religious conversions (or strongly justified, rather than casual, lack of religious feeling), hypergraphia (a tendency to highly detailed writing often of a religious or philosophical nature), hyposexuality (diminished sex drive sometimes associated with changes in sexual taste), and irritability of varying degree'. Geschwind thought the syndrome important because, speculating that it arose from kindling in the amygdala due to temporal lobe spikes, he described it as 'unique in being the only cause of major behavioural change for which a reasonably detailed pathogenesis exists' (Geschwind 1979, 219).

Whether these symptoms really co-segregate with temporal lobe epilepsy remains controversial. If you look uncritically for the syndrome, you will certainly find it. Michael Trimble assembled 15 examples of hypergraphia in temporal lobe epilepsy from his and Geschwind's practice (Roberts et al. 1982) and, of these, at least 9 showed hyperreligiosity and 12 had altered sexuality. But, the same constellation of symptoms has also been found in people without epilepsy but with schizophrenia (O'Connell et al. 2013) or frontotemporal dementia (Postiglione et al. 2008). And, in the largest study of the type, 66 people with temporal lobe epilepsy were found to be no more religious than 31 patients with generalised seizures and 26 with non-epileptic seizures (Tucker et al. 1987).

Methodological limitations mean no study has yet been definitive. Not only do most studies tend to involve only a few cases, also a robust metric of the Geschwind syndrome is lacking. Bear and Fedio designed an 18-item scale to identify the syndrome (Bear and Fedio 1977) which showed that people with temporal lobe epilepsy had 'deepened emotions', circumstantiality, altered religious and sexual concerns, and hypergraphia, compared to healthy controls and other disease subjects. This scale has not been subjected to a rigorous psychometric analysis. Nonetheless, Michael Trimble and colleagues have expressed confidence in it, although even in their hands it has not always supported the existence of the Geschwind syndrome. For instance, when comparing people with temporal lobe epilepsy with and without self-identified hyperreligiosity, the scale identified greater emotionality and depression, but not hypergraphia, in the former (Trimble and Freeman 2006). Two other studies, using the Bear-Fedio scale, have shown that the Geschwind syndrome is not specific to temporal lobe epilepsy but rather a measure of general psychopathology (Mungas 1982; Rodin and Schmaltz 1984). And a recent study found no differences, using this scale, between 41 patients with temporal lobe epilepsy and 37 people with psychogenic seizures (Tremont et al. 2012).

Leaving aside problems with the Bear-Fedio scale, Trimble's study (Trimble and Freeman 2006) is interesting for two reasons. Firstly, none of the 28 people with temporal lobe epilepsy who self-identified as hyperreligious had Dostoyevsky seizures, but rather they had much higher rate of postictal psychoses than the non-religious people with epilepsy. Secondly, when compared to members of a liberal Anglican church, the hyperreligious group were more conscious of evil, the miraculous, near-death experiences and of being close to powerful spirit forces; and they scored higher on scales of the noetic quality of their experiences, ineffability and timelessness.

In a study that remains unpublished, 91 unselected people with severe temporal lobe epilepsy from New York were studied using the respected Brief Multidimensional Measure of Religiousness/Spirituality scale. Compared to the general US population, this cohort had more frequent spiritual experiences and more prevalent spiritual beliefs, but less frequently attended a place of worship (Hayton et al. 2002). This may just be because this group were having the high average seizure frequency of 22 a month, which would subvert most lifestyles. But others, among populations with lower seizure frequency, have also noted an inclination of the 'hyperreligious' epilepsy patients to belong to non-traditional religious institutions or even none at all. For instance, Waxman and Geschwind observed that 'the preoccupations of the patients often have a cosmic or global flavour, and may transcend the limits of established religions'; we have seen a patient who, when asked if he were religious, replied that he was 'beyond religion' and that he was a 'cosmic minister to the world' (Waxman and Geschwind 1975, 1563). A similar conclusion was reached in a study of 38 patients in New York (Dolgoff-Kaspar et al. 2011).

So, in applying the James' test ('by their fruits ye shall know them'), how would we judge the fruits of the sort of religion seen in the lives of people with temporal lobe epilepsy? Consider, for example my patient, A.S. He would argue that his Dostoyevsky seizures were at least partly behind his choice of profession as a theologian, which – he would say – is a gift to his church. Yet his lifestyle is unorthodox and chaotic by most standards, including multiple sexual partners, prolonged absences from attendance of formal worship, suspicion within his religious community and at least one episode of post-ictal violence leading to a confrontation with the police.

Alajouanine has argued that Dostoyevsky's epilepsy was a positive component of his creativity as a novelist:

> It would be naive to consider that Dostoiewski's epilepsy is the essential origin of his genius, but it was surely an exceptional experience which had driven him in the way towards manifesting his original vision. In point of fact, epilepsy had created in the person of Dostoiewski a 'double man' (to employ the title of one of his novels): a rationalist and a mystic; each having the better of the other according to the moment. The mystical one seems to have prevailed.
>
> (Alajouanine 1963, 217)

So the religious lives of people with temporal lobe epilepsy may be characterised as being highly 'spiritualised' with mystical and philosophical preoccupation, but not usually contained within an established worshipping community. It would seem unlikely therefore that undiagnosed epilepsy could account for the formation of settled religious communities. Nonetheless, occasionally that hypothesis is offered and needs to be addressed.

As with the case of A.S., occasionally experiences that are interpreted as authentically spiritual get redefined – at least by the medical profession – as epileptic. Other published examples include a case of glossolalia which was a manifestation of focal epilepsy (Reeves et al. 2013); the clue in this case was that the woman had jerking of her left arm whilst she spoke in tongues. These examples are rare and do not undermine the most powerful evidence that there is no increased incidence of epilepsy among religious people, namely the consistent lack of epileptic activity found on the most prevalent technology applied to the study of religious experience: the electroencephalographam. Although many subtle EEG changes have – unsurprisingly – been found in different religious and meditative experiences, these do not include ictal sharp waves (Aftanas and Golocheikine 2002; Beauregard and Paquette 2008; Benson et al. 1990; Le and Silverman 2011; Lehmann et al. 2001;

Oohashi et al. 2002; Surwillo and Hobson 1978; Tenke et al. 2017). Michael Persinger's attempts to show that healthy students, and pre-adolescents, with religious experiences score higher on his own non-validated scale of 'temporal lobe symptomatology' (Persinger 1984, 1991) can safely be ignored.

Conclusion

Mystical, or 'Dostoyevsky', seizures provide the opportunity of the 'experiment of nature' to study the content of numinous experiences induced artefactually by brain disease. Despite their interest, there have been few systematic studies of this seizure type and it is likely that they are very rare.

I hypothesise that mystical seizures originate with a core experience, which is not in itself religious, but is imbued with a sense of significance and meaningfulness (perhaps, as Picard (2013) suggests, by reducing the error-prediction capacity of the anterior insula). In individuals with the appropriate upbringing, these are then interpreted within a religious framework.

The scanty literature to date suggests that the religious life that emerges from the person who has frequent numinous experiences is non-traditional and 'cosmic'; and full of value and significance for the person themselves, as Fyodor Dostoyevsky and Karen Armstrong attest. The implications of this for religious education and formation could be considered further by theologians.

References

Aftanas, L. I., and S. A. Golocheikine. 2002. Non-linear dynamic complexity of the human EEG during meditation. *Neuroscience Letters* 330: 143–6.

Alajouanine, T. 1963. Dostoiewski's epilepsy. *Brain*, 86: 210–18.

Amancio, E. J., S. T. Zymberg and M. F. Pires. 1994. [Temporal lobe epilepsy and aura with happiness and pleasure: report of 2 cases and review of the literature]. *Arquivos de Neuro-Psiquiatria* 52: 252–9.

Armstrong, K. 1983. *Beginning the World*. New York: St Martin's Press.

Asheim Hansen, B., and E. Brodtkorb. 2003. Partial epilepsy with 'ecstatic' seizures. *Epilepsy and Behavior* 4: 667–73.

Aull-Watschinger, S., E. Pataraia and C. Baumgartner. 2008. Sexual auras: predominance of epileptic activity within the mesial temporal lobe. *Epilepsy and Behavior* 12: 124–7.

Bear, D. M., and P. Fedio. 1977. Quantitative analysis of interictal behavior in temporal lobe epilepsy. *Archives of Neurology* 34: 454–67.

Beauregard, M., and V. Paquette. 2008. EEG activity in Carmelite nuns during a mystical experience. *Neuroscience Letters* 444: 1–4.

Benson, H., et al. 1990. Three case reports of the metabolic and electroencephalographic changes during advanced Buddhist meditation techniques. *Journal of Behavioral Medicine* 16: 90–5.

Carrazana, E., et al. 1999. Epilepsy and religious experiences: Voodoo possession. *Epilepsia* 40: 239–41.

Cavanna, A. E., S. Cavanna and A. Cavanna. 2010. Epileptic seizures and spirit possession in Haitian culture: report of four cases and review of the literature. *Epilepsy and Behavior* 19: 89–91.

Devinsky, O., and G. Lai. 2008. Spirituality and religion in epilepsy. *Epilepsy and Behavior* 12: 636–43.

Dewhurst, K., and A. W. Beard. 1970. Sudden religious conversions in temporal lobe epilepsy. *British Journal of Psychiatry* 117: 497–507.

Dolgoff-Kaspar, R., et al. 2011. Numinous-like auras and spirituality in persons with partial seizures. *Epilepsia* 52: 640–4.

Dostoyevsky, F. 1869. *The Idiot*. London: Vizetelly.

Fingelkurts, A. A. 2009. Is our brain hardwired to produce God, or is our brain hardwired to perceive God? A systematic review on the role of the brain in mediating religious experience. *Cognitive Processing* 10: 293–326.

Frank, J. 2010. *Dostoevsky: A Writer in His Time*. Princeton, NJ: Princeton University Press.

Geschwind, N. 1979. Behavioural changes in temporal lobe epilepsy. *Psychological Medicine* 9: 217–19.

Gowers, W. R. 1881. *Epilepsy and Other Chronic Convulsive Diseases*. London: Churchill.

Greyson, B. B., L. L. Derr and N. Fountain. 2015. Mystical experiences associated with seizures. *Religion, Brain and Behaviour* 5: 182–96.

Griffiths, R.R., et al. 2006. Psilocybin can occasion mystical-type experiences having substantial and sustained personal meaning and spiritual significance. *Psychopharmacology* 187: 268–83; discussion 284–92.

Griffiths, R. R., et al. 2011. Psilocybin occasioned mystical-type experiences: immediate and persisting dose-related effects. *Psychopharmacology* 218: 649–65.

Hayton, S., L. S. Boylan, S. C. Jackson, and O. Devinsky. 2002. Religion and epilepsy. Paper presented at the annual meeting of the American Academy of Neurology, Denver, CO.

Howden, J. C. 1873. The religious sentiment in epileptics. *Journal of Mental Science* 18: 482–97.

Hughes, J. R. 2005. The idiosyncratic aspects of the epilepsy of Fyodor Dostoevsky. *Epilepsy and Behavior* 7: 531–8.

James, W. 1924. *The Varieties of Religious Experience*. New York: Longmans, Green.

Jilek-Aall, L. 1999. Morbus sacer in Africa: some religious aspects of epilepsy in traditional cultures. *Epilepsia* 40: 382–6.

Johnson, M. W., R. A. Sewell and R. R. Griffiths. 2012. Psilocybin dose-dependently causes delayed, transient headaches in healthy volunteers. *Drug and Alcohol Dependency* 123: 132–40.

Khwaja, G. A. S., and N. Chadhury. 2007. Epilepsy and religion. *Annals of the Indian Academy of Neurology* 10: 165–8.

Le, C., and D. H. Silverman. 2011. Neuroimaging and EEG-based explorations of cerebral substrates for suprapentasensory perception: a critical appraisal of recent experimental literature. *Psychiatry Research* 194: 105–10.

Lehmann, D., et al. 2001. Brain sources of EEG gamma frequency during volitionally meditation-induced, altered states of consciousness, and experience of the self. *Psychiatry Research* 108: 111–21.

Leuba, J. H. 1925. *The Psychology of Religious Mysticism*. London: Kegan Paul, Trench, Trubner.

MacLean, K. A., M. W. Johnson and R. R. Griffiths. 2011. Mystical experiences occasioned by the hallucinogen psilocybin lead to increases in the personality domain of openness. *Journal of Psychopharmacology* 25: 1453–61.

Mungas, D. 1982. Interictal behavior abnormality in temporal lobe epilepsy: a specific syndrome or nonspecific psychopathology? *Archives of General Psychiatry* 39: 108–11.

O'Connell, K., J. Keaveney and R. Paul. 2013. A novel study of comorbidity between schizoaffective disorder and Geschwind syndrome. *Case Reports in Psychiatry* 2013: 486064.

Ogata, A., and T. Miyakawa. 1998. Religious experiences in epileptic patients with a focus on ictus-related episodes. *Psychiatry and Clinical Neuroscience* 52: 321–5.

Oohashi, T., et al. 2002. Electroencephalographic measurement of possession trance in the field. *Clinical Neurophysiology* 113: 435–45.

Penfield, W. 1955. The twenty-ninth Maudsley lecture: the role of the temporal cortex in certain psychical phenomena. *Journal of Mental Science* 101: 451–65.

Penfield, W. 1958. Some mechanisms of consciousness discovered during electrical stimulation of the brain. *Proceedings of the National Academy of Sciences of the United States of America* 44: 51–66.

Persinger, M. A. 1984. People who report religious experiences may also display enhanced temporal-lobe signs. *Perceptual and Motor Skills* 58: 963–75.

Persinger, M. A. 1991. Preadolescent religious experience enhances temporal lobe signs in normal young adults. *Perceptual and Motor Skills* 72: 453–4.

Picard, F. 2013. State of belief, subjective certainty and bliss as a product of cortical dysfunction. *Cortex* 49: 2494–500.

Picard, F., and A. D. Craig. 2009. Ecstatic epileptic seizures: a potential window on the neural basis for human self-awareness. *Epilepsy and Behavior* 16: 539–46.

Picard, F., and F. Kurth. 2014. Ictal alterations of consciousness during ecstatic seizures. *Epilepsy and Behavior* 30: 58–61.

Picard, F., D. Scavarda and F. Bartolomei. 2013. Induction of a sense of bliss by electrical stimulation of the anterior insula. *Cortex* 49: 2935–7.

Postiglione, A., G. Milan, S. Pappatà, C. De Falco, F. Lamenza, V. Schiattarella, G. Gallotta, P. Sorrentino and S. Striano. 2008. Fronto-temporal dementia presenting as Geschwind's syndrome. *Neurocase* 14: 264–70.

Reeves, R. R., S. Kose and A. Abubakr. 2013. Temporal lobe discharges and glossolalia. *Neurocase* 20: 236–40.

Reynolds, E. H., and J. V. Kinnier Wilson. 2008. Psychoses of epilepsy in Babylon: the oldest account of the disorder. *Epilepsia* 49: 1488–90.

Roberts, J. K., M. M. Robertson and M. R. Trimble. 1982. The lateralising significance of hypergraphia in temporal lobe epilepsy. *Journal of Neurology, Neurosurgery, and Psychiatry* 45: 131–8.

Rodin, E., and S. Schmaltz. 1984. The Bear–Fedio personality inventory and temporal lobe epilepsy. *Neurology* 34: 591–6.

Surwillo, W. W., and D. P. Hobson. 1978. Brain electrical activity during prayer. *Psychological Reports* 43: 135–43.

Tedrus, G. M., L. C. Fonseca and G. C. Hoehr. 2014. Spirituality aspects in patients with epilepsy. *Seizure* 23: 25–8.

Tenke, C. E., J. Kayser, C. Svob, L. Miller, J. E. Alvarenga, K. Abraham, V. Warner, P. Wickramaratne, M. M. Weissman, and G. E. Bruder. 2017. Association of posterior EEG alpha with prioritization of religion or spirituality: A replication and extension at 20-year follow-up. *Biological Psychology* 124: 79–86.

Todman, D. 2008. Epilepsy in the Graeco-Roman world: Hippocratic medicine and Asklepian temple medicine compared. *Journal of the History of the Neurosciences* 17: 435–41.

Tremont, G., M. M. Smith, L. Bauer, M. L. Alosco, J. D. Davis, A. S. Blum, and W. C. LaFrance Jr. 2012. Comparison of personality characteristics on the bear-fedio inventory between patients with epilepsy and those with non-epileptic seizures. *Journal of Neuropsychiatry and Clinical Neuroscience* 24: 47–52.

Trimble, M., and A. Freeman. 2006. An investigation of religiosity and the Gastaut–Geschwind syndrome in patients with temporal lobe epilepsy. *Epilepsy and Behavior* 9: 407–14.

Tucker, D. M., R. A. Novelly and P. J. Walker. 1987. Hyperreligiosity in temporal lobe epilepsy: redefining the relationship. *Journal of Nervous and Mental Disorders* 175: 181–4.

Waxman, S. G., and N. Geschwind. 1975. The interictal behavior syndrome of temporal lobe epilepsy. *Archives of General Psychiatry* 32: 1580–6.

Williams, D. 1956. The structure of emotions reflected in epileptic experiences. *Brain* 79: 29–67.

Chapter 10

II.I *Clinical Conditions*

Parkinson's Disease, Religious Belief and Spirituality

Roger Barker and Clare Redfern

Whether the experience, symptoms, treatment or neuropathology of Parkinson's disease (PD) could potentially play a role in shaping religious beliefs and practices can be viewed from several different angles. For example, a diagnosis of a serious illness could make one reassess and question previously held attitudes and beliefs; faith in a benign God may be challenged. Spirituality, broadly defined as a quest for meaning and truth, could also play a role in the process of integrating the experience of living with Parkinson's disease, as with any disease or major life experience. Less conscious mechanisms might also be in play, more intrinsic to the disease process, such as loss of motivational drive due to dopaminergic dysfunction. The resulting apathy, which is often seen in PD, might reduce efforts to pursue personal interests, including a religious faith. Cognitive deficits, for example altered social cognition such as changes in 'theory of mind', could also potentially contribute. At a more pragmatic level, problems with decreasing mobility, and energy levels as well as a host of other symptoms and drug side-effects could potentially make all aspects of daily life problematic, therefore impeding the pursuit of religious practices or a spiritual path. In this chapter we review and discuss the existing literature and research, in the hope that it might augment understanding of this little-studied aspect of PD as well as contribute to cognitive perspectives on religious belief and experience.

Overview of Parkinson's Disease

Pathophysiology

Parkinson's disease (PD) is a common, chronic, neurodegenerative disorder of the ageing nervous system with an incidence of about 1 in 800 and an average age of onset of around 70 years [1]. It typically presents with a movement disorder consisting of a pill rolling tremor, bradykinesia and rigidity along with postural instability [2], although it is now recognised that prior to this there is a prodromal period characterised by a decreased sense of smell, slowed walking, a REM sleep behavioural disorder and mild depression [3]. This prodromal phase is thought to be due to pathology in a number of structures within the central nervous system (e.g. the brainstem and olfactory bulb) as well as within the enteric nervous system of the gut [4]. The disease then progresses to affect the basal ganglia, in particular the dopaminergic cells of the substantia nigra within the midbrain resulting in the onset of motor signs and symptoms. This pathology is defined by the accumulation of a specific protein, alpha synuclein, into Lewy bodies and Lewy neurites, which form the basis for the diagnosis of PD pathologically [5].

The cause of PD is unknown. Over the last 20 years, the genetic aspects of this condition have been better understood; rare familial forms exist associated with a range of single Mendelian gene abnormalities and genome wide association studies suggest a role for genetic risk loci in idiopathic disease [6–7]. Patients with PD typically present when they have lost 70–80 per cent of the dopaminergic fibres within the striatum which accords to a 50 per cent loss of substantia nigral dopamine cells [8]. By the time the dopaminergic nigrostriatal system has degenerated to this extent the bradykinesia, rigidity and tremor have become obvious enough to be noticed, prompting presentation to a medical practitioner.

Treatment Effects

Treatment seeks primarily to replace the lost dopamine within the nigrostriatal system. This can be done using agents that are designed to slow down the breakdown of dopamine (COMT or MAO inhibitors) [9], drugs that directly act on dopamine receptors (the dopamine agonists) or agents designed to replace dopamine by providing its precursor (L-dopa) [10]. Dopamine-replacement therapies work well in early disease in easing motor difficulties. However, they are not without side-effects which can include hallucinations and cognitive deficits such as those involving executive working memory [11]. Less frequently, behavioural problems due to overstimulation of the more intact dopaminergic pathways, such as those projecting from the midbrain to the cortex (mesocortical) and nucleus accumbens (mesolimbic) can also arise and include hypersexuality, repetitive movements known as *punding* and pathological gambling. These are especially seen in young male patients on dopamine agonists. Side-effects also include dyskinesias: involuntary choreic and dystonic movements which typically appear after several years of L-dopa treatment, which over time can come to dominate the clinical picture. In the early stages the management of PD is relatively straightforward and involves manipulating the dosages and timing of the dopaminergic drugs, however, with time side-effects develop and become increasingly debilitating and difficult to treat.

Psychological and Cognitive Effects

Over time the pathology involves a range of cortical and sub-cortical sites, and with this the more prominent neuropsychiatric and cognitive deficits that are characteristic of advanced PD appear. Psychiatric features are commonly seen in PD, even in the early stages, including depression in around 50 per cent of cases; anxiety, including panic attacks, and social phobia is also common as are apathy and sleep disorders [12]. Evidence suggests that mood and motivational changes in PD are linked to the underlying disease process and not solely a reaction to disability; this is not unexpected, as a role for the basal ganglia in the regulation of cognitive and emotional functioning as well as movement control, is increasingly acknowledged [13], and PD also has pathology in sites linked to these types of problems.

Mild cognitive impairment is commonly seen in PD and includes deficits in executive function (such as attention, concentration, working memory and planning), increased impulsivity and visuospatial problems. However, the presence of mild cognitive impairment does not necessarily herald global cognitive decline as in some patients these deficits relate solely to dysfunctional dopaminergic networks. However there are a number of predictive factors for later frank dementia which includes older age, a genetic predisposition (MAPT H1/H1 genotype) and deficits in posterior, non-dopaminergic cortical functions [14]. Hallucinations (often of animals or people) and visual misperceptions as well as the sense of something or someone being just out of sight are also common. These are most often seen early on in the more elderly person with PD; these are rarely perceived as religious experiences as generally the hallucinations are felt to represent people. Other cognitive effects in PD, such as problems with theory of mind, which might potentially affect religious practice will be considered below.

Personality Effects

Preclinical levels of impulsivity affecting multiple cognitive functions have been recently identified in relation to dopaminergic, serotonergic and noradrenergic dysfunction in PD [15]. These could cause planning and concentration problems, potentially leading to a more chaotic lifestyle. Other studies however note a more 'cautious, rigid' personality profile resulting from reduced 'novelty seeking' behaviour [16]. The apparent contradiction between increased impulsivity but more conservative, cautious behaviour likely reflects the complex nature of impulsivity changes and difficulties measuring these. Previous suggestions of an association between a specific personality type (cautious, stoical, conservative) and later onset of PD have now been seen to be over simplistic [17].

Factors Affecting Religious Belief and Spiritual Practice in Parkinson's Disease

Discussion of aspects of PD that might be relevant to spirituality and religious faith will be augmented by subjective viewpoints derived from personal accounts of the experience of people living with this condition. These are taken from qualitative interview studies carried out in recent years in the UK [18–19], Sweden [20] and the US [21]. These are included to make explicit the practical difficulties encountered in everyday life, which might affect religious practice; some also include comments about how developing Parkinson's disease affected aspects of the participant's spirituality and religious faith. It must be recognised however that the experiences of an individual or small group might not reflect a majority experience, especially in a disease that is so varied in its symptoms and progression; similarly, religious faith and beliefs are also diverse and multifaceted, shaped by individual life experiences and cultural influences.

Practical Problems

Physical symptoms and their psychosocial effects are likely to impact in practical ways on religious life or spirituality. The accounts of everyday life with PD from interview studies emphasise the greater mental concentration and physical effort required to carry out what were previously semi-automatic functions – lifting the feet when walking, swinging one's arms, swallowing and modulating one's voice, and facial expressions. Here's how 'Beth' a 62-year-old woman who had had PD for 10 years, described this:

> And like you have to, when you put your . . . , get up on your feet, you say, 'now go on put that foot in front of the other' and you have to physically make yourself do a step and a step at a time, you have to tell your body what to do, it doesn't just do it by thinking. [18]

Balance and gait problems increase the likelihood of falls; rigidity, tremor and slowed movements, coupled with a tendency to 'freezing' can impede simple everyday procedures. Some comments from Caap-Ahlgren's study illustrate this:

> The most frustrating is, not always being able to walk. Suddenly it is 'Stop! the legs won't move' and 'Can't drive my car any more, arms and legs don't coordinate'. [20]

Added to the physical challenges of getting about, can be the anguish of feeling judged or criticised:

> And I can see somebody looking at me and thinking 'what's the matter with her?' and that is soul destroying because I've always been a person who liked to look my best, . . . and this [PD] takes that away from you. [18]

The stigmatisation of those who appear weak, frail or different, is all too common in a society that celebrates youth, beauty and physical grace. This can lead to loss of confidence and withdrawal from society, compounding the isolation that a movement disorder can impose. Similarly people with speech impairments can feel marginalised and fearful of being thought incompetent [22]. In Caap-Ahlgren's study, participants reported limiting their social sphere to family activities because of a perceived sense of discrimination and misunderstanding about their symptoms. Even within families, changed facial expressivity and voice can have an isolating effect:

> The number one complaint my family has is they said that I always look like I am mad. My left side of my face tends to freeze, like a zombie type and I can't talk sometimes and they always think I am mad or something. [20]

Some report trying to disguise the early symptoms of Parkinson's

> I try and stop myself from moving. So I hold my arm or I put my arms to the back and clasp my fist like this, so my fingers aren't moving and my hands aren't moving and I try and disguise it but I look worse when I disguise it because I'm doing contortions. [18]

Even apparently 'secondary' symptoms, such as excessive sweating due to autonomic dysfunction can cause discomfort, embarrassment and avoidance of social situations. 'Beth' felt even this symptom alone would be hard to tolerate and described how she would avoid people because of continual sweating bouts.

Drug Effects

Dopaminergic drugs can transform the existence of a person with Parkinson's disease but on-off effects can be distressing and tiring. Beth says of her drugs, '*without them I would have no life*' but she describes the 'on-state' when the dopaminergic drugs are working maximally as making her feel '*wired*', '*tense*', '*full of medication*', with the sense that the drugs are controlling her and '*pushing*' her. In contrast, the off-state is, for her, one of a fog-like disconnection between mind and body, severely hampering movement as described here,

> But it's all depending on whether they produce the dopamine or not, they can control me because I can take the tablets and if they don't work, there's nothing I can do about it, not a damn thing, I can just sit there and wait for it, the next lot of tablets, I can't keep taking them and taking them because I think my head would explode if I did. [18]

Unpredictability of symptoms, and of drug effects, can begin to define daily life:

> Parkinson's dictates my day. I mean there are days that I feel good and I want to get out and just go, go, go, but my body just won't work. My mind tells my body to go but it doesn't listen. It does me no good to plan things, because I never know what I am physically going to be able to do on any given day. [21]

> You have to plan it by tablets, not by life and clocks and you know what I mean, you can't just say 'Oh I'll get up at six o'clock and I'll be straight out that door' because I couldn't do it. [18]

These accounts illustrate clearly how the mental and physical demands of coping with PD, coupled with the unpredictability of drug effects might impede participation in interests and personal pursuits, including religious activities.

Emotional Effects and Psychological Adaptation

Adapting emotionally as Parkinson's disease progresses is also a necessary and challenging process and one in which religious beliefs and practices may be shaped and changed. For example, anger, denial and frustration can arise as previous skills are lost and the roles taken within a family or within society are eroded:

> I wish you could see me the way that I was. I am just worthless and stupid now. I was in the military and had a sharp mind. I could build a lot of things with my hands, now my hands won't work. [21]

There is inevitable anguish at the loss of an imagined future,

> We had plans of retiring and travelling. I never dreamed PD would be my retirement. [21]

> I couldn't wait to have grandchildren and now the time is here, I can't even hold them or play with them. [21]

and the fear and uncertainty that the future now holds:

> 'My future is uncertain'. '... it's the uncertainty of not knowing if I will be able to walk in a year'. 'I am fearful of the unknown ... The unknown is scary'. [21]

However, stoical acceptance was also frequently noted:

> I'm not dying with Parkinson's disease I am living with Parkinson's disease. Even though I can't do the things I use to could do, things could be worse, I could have a brain tumor, but I don't. I have Parkinson's. Just knowing that gives me peace. [21]

Park describes how a process of positive adaptation or 'meaning-making' can occur, following a traumatic event such as the onset of a serious illness, as individuals struggle to align earlier convictions with present realities [23]. This process involves reappraising deep-rooted views for example, a sense of being in personal control, and that the world is benevolent, predictable and fair, convictions easily shattered by the onset of an erratic, incapacitating disease. Secondly one's goals in life, such as pursuing a fulfilling career or living a long life in good health, will need to be adjusted and this might include a third area: re-evaluation of existential concepts such as life's purpose, meaning and values. The process of adaptation can be maladaptive if it leads to over rumination, but beneficial if coherent meanings can be constructed.

This process has also been termed post-traumatic growth, reflecting the potential for beneficial change following a life crisis, for example as priorities are reordered, relationships deepened and personal strengths are developed [24–25]. Religious belief and rituals can play a well-recognised role in integrating the emotional and cognitive upheaval accompanying trauma or developing a major illness [26–27]. Being faced with existential questions, the process of finding meaning within the experience of illness can take on a spiritual dimension.

In Stanley-Hermanns' study in the US, participants, admittedly from a strongly religious culture (Texas), gave many examples not only of the positive value of religious faith for them in coping with PD, but also examples of how their faith was enhanced in the process. In a series of non-directive individual interviews and recording of group discussions involving 14 self-reported Christians: 12 reported that their faith was stronger as a result of PD, only 2 reported no change. Leaving possible biases inherent in the study aside, for these people at least, faith was described as a crucial element in adapting. For example, one participant said that she decided to,

> let God be God in my life and depend on him.

another said,

> My relationship with God is really what gives me the daily strength.

Others reported an increased sense of connection with God, leading to reordered priorities,

> So I don't ask why, I just say here I am, Lord, you know why. I am so thankful that even if it took this, even if it took this to get my life in order and my relationship, you know, recommitting my life to God, then I am thankful for that.

> I am closer to God, I think than I have ever been. God has never left me . . . He has always been there. It made me realise that I needed him more in my life . . . now I really stop and think about what is important before I start the day. [21]

Even in Western Europe, despite increasing secularisation, religious faith continues to play a role in coping with illness such as cancer and chronic pain [28–30]. Although no European studies have, to our knowledge, explicitly investigated whether religious faith plays a role in managing the physical or emotional effects of PD, occasional reference has been made to the value of prayer. For example, a small UK study investigating the effect of self-help group membership on coping methods in PD, identified prayer, as well as keeping active and taking medication, as subjectively important for some participants in maintaining well-being [31]. So it appears there is some limited anecdotal evidence that religious beliefs can play a role in coping with the challenges of PD, yet changes in cognitive ability and the possibility that these could affect spirituality, religious beliefs and practices must also be considered.

Cognitive Deficits, Spirituality and Prayer

Problems with impulsivity, attention, concentration and short-term memory could make the practice of meditation, prayer or attending religious meetings difficult. However, an important question is whether there is a more intrinsic change in attitude towards faith, or interest in religion or existential questions, as a direct result of neural degeneration in PD. Some have considered general cognitive functions that are required for 'religious cognition' in relation to various brain deficits. For example, a capacity for engaging in 'transcendent thought' which involves rising above the present moment, contemplating an imagined future (and likewise an imagined, supernatural realm), has been suggested as dependent on frontal lobe executive functions, and working memory in particular [24]. Interestingly frontal lobe deficits in a non-demented PD group were found to correlate with impairment in envisaging possible futures (admittedly of a more prosaic, everyday variety) despite absence of episodic memory problems [32].

Theory of mind (ToM), the intuitive capacity to attribute intentions, plans, desires to others is also considered necessary for the apperception of a relational, divine agent – contemplating 'the mind of God'. This finds support in some imaging studies. In one such study, devout (healthy) Christians, whilst praying, demonstrated activation patterns in those areas normally activated by theory of mind [33–34]; this pattern was activated only during improvisational prayer but not in ritualised praying. Another imaging study also linked theory of mind area activation with questions regarding God's emotions and involvement in the world [35]. There is some suggestion that deficits in ToM can occur in PD, as in other neurodegenerative conditions (e.g. Alzheimer's, Amyotrophic Lateral Sclerosis, Huntington's Disease, Frontotemporal dementia). A recent review found ToM deficits in PD that correlated with frontal executive impairment [36]. However, the studies reviewed were small, sometimes contradictory and reduced ToM in PD has not been found in our own unpublished studies [37].

We could however still infer that cognitive impairments in PD, if present, might alter the experience of praying or contemplation; in practice this might mean that a different style of religious practice becomes expedient, for example possibly more ritual based rather than improvisatory prayer. In an interview study of the self-reported benefits of mindfulness-based cognitive therapy (MBCT) in PD, one participant, 'Carol', provides a vivid description of cognitive effects that impede her attempts to pray:

> Since I became ill I'm not praying five times . . . I can't concentrate on one thing, you know my mind is wondering all the time . . . I've just become a different person altogether and I've got like two personalities, Jekyll and Hyde. [19]

She describes how the practice of mindfulness, a technique of attending to physical and emotional self-awareness, to focus attention and discount negative ideas, was of help in overcoming her wandering attention and in her struggle to maintain a coherent sense of identity:

> I am praying now more and that's kind of mindfulness and when we are praying we have to give full attention to the prayers to God and not to any other things or people talking . . . I just feel good about myself, that it's probably maybe giving me some kind of inner peace.

Though using a subjective outcome measure, her account suggests that changes in the capacity to pray might to some extent be partly overcome with effort and the prioritising of cognitive resources as in MBCT. This might have parallels in the beneficial effects of brain-training exercises in PD on improving frontal lobe functioning [38]. Despite difficulties caused by cognitive changes, in this example at least, it seems that faith retains its significance for Carol and motivates use of MBCT as a means of coping. It seems plausible that whilst the physical, psychological and cognitive effects of Parkinson's disease might affect the ability to engage in religious activities such as prayer, an intrinsic desire to live out and express a faith, religion or spirituality can persist. Indeed, according to the Post-traumatic growth (PTG) model, and as Hermanns' study seems to suggest, religious beliefs could even be enhanced by the existential crisis provoked by the onset of illness.

Some commentators have suggested a specific role for dopamine in modulating religious experience [39–40] but the specificity of the role is not well-founded. They draw largely on the effect of dopamine and serotonergic imbalances in psychiatric conditions that feature religious delusional states and obsessions, or following ingestion of hallucinogenic drugs. It seems misleading, however, to conflate religious psychotic episodes and reflective faith or regular religious observances especially as there appears little overlap between neural networks affected in schizoaffective disorders, for example, and those in PD. That dopamine plays a key role in goal-directed learning, and executive control through the interplay of the mesolimbic and mesocortical dopaminergic pathways is well known [41], striatal dopamine pathways within the basal ganglia also play a vital role in mediating this [13, 42]. Through motivated experience, it seems dopamine is essential (though not of course sufficient) for making sense of the world and finding meaning; constructing an identity and developing metaphysical beliefs, though dependent on cultural influences, will presumably be part of this too. However, to assert a specific role for dopamine in higher cognition about religious ideas and beliefs, rather than a general role modulating salience of all kinds of ideas is an oversimplification. Unfortunately, in several recent popular articles, a view of dopamine as regulating religious belief is promoted, based on this simplistic approach [43–44]. Comparative studies, comparing belief in PD and control groups, have been used to support this argument, however these contain many flawed assumptions as will be discussed below.

Case-Control Studies of Religion and Parkinson's Disease

In contrast to the ethnographic approach using recorded interviews, a few studies have followed a cognitive neuropsychology of religion paradigm, seeking to elucidate direct effects of dopaminergic neural degeneration within Parkinson's disease, on religious faith [45-48]. PD, as a condition with a clearly defined pathology of dopaminergic neurons (although not exclusively localised to this site), is seen as offering a useful window on the role of those neuronal networks in the practice, experiences and maintenance of religious or spiritual beliefs.

In line with this approach, McNamara and colleagues in Boston, have undertaken several case-control studies comparing PD sufferers and age-matched healthy and disease controls [45–47]. They used standardised questionnaires (namely the Brief Multidimensional Measure of Religiousness and Spirituality (BMMRS) and the Gorsuch Intrinsic/Extrinsic religiousness measure) to quantify religious and spiritual beliefs and commitment. Neuropsychological tests and semantic priming tasks were also used to probe cognitive and semantic deficits, seeking correlations with changes in religious and spiritual beliefs and practice. Their studies claim to show a specific reduction in religiosity in Parkinson's patients, as compared with control groups. This reduction is attributed to the loss of fronto-striatal and limbic-prefrontal dopaminergic networks. However closer scrutiny reveals flaws in study design and statistical analysis, and some excessively bold assumptions about the extent of pathology in the PD brain.

In order to understand the findings, it is important to appreciate what was being asked of the study participants. The BMMRS aims to capture an individual's level of religious belief and commitment by asking around 33 questions about private and public aspects of religion. Though it claims to be equally applicable to different faiths, it is clearly designed with the Christian faith in mind; in our experience it creates particular difficulties for

Buddhists as so many questions ask about God/higher power. In general, total scores reflect levels of religious belief and practice. The questions are also divided into different domains; these include 'positive spiritual experiences' which explore a felt sense of connection with God such as a sense of deep peace or a belief that God is watching over them, guiding them and so on; questions that might only loosely be related to religious faith are included such as having a sense of mission, or a sense of responsibility for reducing suffering also 'religious practices' asking about frequency of prayer, religious reading, meditation and so on and 'religious support' which records involvement in the local religious community. As described in earlier paragraphs, PD has many varied effects, any of which could make participation in both private and public religious activities difficult and reduce scores for religiosity using this measure. Therefore, recruiting a control group with non-neurological disorders that cause comparable physical or social limitations, is essential if any effects of dopaminergic neuronal degeneration on religious faith are to be detected. Following a pilot study that used healthy controls, a follow-up study recruited 71 mid-stage PD patients and 75 controls with health problems including raised cholesterol, arthritis and back pain [46]. Unfortunately, it is questionable whether these conditions are comparable even to well-controlled PD. Raised cholesterol is asymptomatic, and although arthritis and back pain *can* be severely debilitating, in milder forms, they usually do not prevent participation in normal daily activities. The PD group may have been well controlled with medication, though as noted above, side-effects are frequently disruptive and unpredictable. As no assessment of disability was included in the study, it is not clear whether a fair comparison is being made between the two groups. The fact that a within-group positive correlation was found in the PD group between Hoehn-Yahr stage (a measure of disease severity) and religious practices further suggests that physical difficulties might play a real role in limiting involvement in religious practices.

In another comparison of 25 PD and 25 controls, the Gorsuch Intrinsic/Extrinsic Inventory was used to assess levels of religious commitment (McNamara 2010). This scale is designed to differentiate between intrinsic and extrinsic religious beliefs. Participants rate their agreement from 1 (strongly disagree) to 5 (strongly agree) with statements describing aspects of religious practice. Some aspects concern 'intrinsic belief' which describes an internalised commitment affecting values and lifestyle, and some are more related to 'extrinsic beliefs' denoting external practices carried out for social benefit or effect on mood. Examples of intrinsic belief statements are: 'It is important for me to spend time in private prayer' or 'My whole approach to life is based upon my religion'. Some are negatively scored such as 'Although I believe in my religion, many other things are more important in life'. It will be appreciated that coping with a serious illness could easily assume greater importance in life than religious practice and is highly likely to lead to reduced scores. So as in previous studies, the fact that the controls are dealing with a less serious, more easily controlled illness (low back pain and adult-onset diabetes) could explain why the PD group in this study appear to have a loss of religious faith, whilst in fact this might not be the case at all. Besides this, in our view, the data presented in McNamara 2011 has been overinterpreted, beyond what is reasonable from the statistical analyses presented in the paper; for example, there is no correction for multiple comparisons in comparing subscores of the BMMRS between PD and controls. We feel these criticisms are important, as the conclusions of these studies are being widely disseminated.

A lack of a control group with similar physical impairments also undermines another comparative study, carried out in Italy, with a group of 83 PD patients, 88 healthy controls and 79 controls with high blood pressure, another asymptomatic condition [48]. This study used the Royal Free Interview (RFI), a broad measure of religious practice, spiritual beliefs and philosophical world-views, designed specifically to avoid Judaeo-Christian bias. The study rather confusingly reports the results as showing no difference in belief between PD patients and both control groups, though this is because 'philosophical beliefs', which can include atheism, is counted as a belief in the Royal Free Interview. In fact 66 per cent of the PD group reported being 'religious' as compared with 82 per cent of controls. However, misunderstandings might be inherent in the questions used; for example, religious belief is described as *'the practice of a faith, e.g. going to a church or synagogue'*, especially as more PD (13 per cent) patients reported spiritual belief, i.e. *'in a power outside their own existence'* compared with 7 per cent of controls. Nineteen per cent of the PD group, as compared with 10 per cent of controls, did however report a purely philosophical approach to life, described as: *'Some people make sense of what happens to them in life without a belief in a God or any outside power'*. Though this might seem a simple statement of atheism, it could also reflect the search for meaning that developing a serious disease such as PD might engender. So this study also gives little help in elucidating the mechanisms that are affecting faith in PD, or demonstrating whether, intrinsically, faith is really affected.

Priming Studies

Parallel to questionnaire studies, McNamara and colleagues investigated semantic priming for religious concepts in PD, as a way of assessing intrinsic or implicit levels of religiosity [47, 49]. A semantic priming task was devised to compare activation rates for the retrieval of information contained in semantic memory, for both religious and control concepts, in 25 PD patients, and 25 age-matched controls. This raises difficult issues for the design; what concept could be used that can be similar in complexity to religion, incorporating such varied cultural and personal meanings? Their ingenious choice was to use 'civic' engagement as a control concept, encompassing activities (reading news, paying taxes) that, like religion, are personal yet related to the local community and wider society, also imbued with layers of meaning: responsibility, habit, finding connection and so on.

Religious concepts were described by four 2-word phrases chosen to describe religious activities: *'sense spirit'*, *'become holy'*, *'worship God'*, *'pray quietly'* and the 'civic' concepts included *'pay taxes'*, *'read news'* and *'cast vote'*. Nonsense phrases for example, *'paint wind'* *'throw ocean'* *'dance toaster'* *'push waterfall'* denoting activities that cannot be performed were also included. The presented phrases were preceded on-screen by a prime word: either 'sacred' (religious prime), 'citizen' (civic prime) 'housetop' (neutral prime), and the primes and phrases were randomly mixed in presentation.

However, we would contend that these control concept words, whilst of similar frequency to religious ones, do not approach their linguistic complexity. For example, *'sacred'* is both an abstract noun and an adjective, whilst *'citizen'* being a noun, and also one with high imageability, will be more easily processed [50–51]. Similarly, the claim that these phrases denoting 'an action to be performed' are equally complex does not stand up to scrutiny. *'Worship God'* suggests something more abstract than *'pay taxes'* or *'read news'*, and *'sense spirit'* even more so. Likewise *'become holy'* is a complex self-referential task, with several layers of possible ambiguity. What is holiness? How do you become holy? Is it an action? Paying taxes or casting a vote in an informed manner might require complex knowledge, however the action itself is straightforward and does not involve existential questions about the realm of the numinous. Delays due to cognitive slowing in PD, added at each extra level of complexity for the religious prime and phrases, could counteract any potential priming effect and explain its apparent loss. Indeed, the authors themselves discuss the possibility that religious priming is lost in PD because religious concepts are more complicated and so require the co-ordination of more association networks.

Besides, the reported results show no clear priming effect even in controls so a loss of semantic priming for religious words in PD cannot be claimed! It is observed that the control group reacted *more quickly* to religious target phrases when primed with a religious word (sacred) compared to a civic concept word (citizen), however this difference did not reach statistical significance (p=.38). And no significant difference was found between the effect of a religious prime on religious target word and civic target word (p=.1) We therefore dispute McNamara and colleagues' conclusion that 'PD patients demonstrated a selective loss in the ability to activate religious knowledge' [47].

Similarly, further findings of a laterality effect have been reported using mathematical modelling. Patients with Left sided (L)-onset PD (greater right hemispheric dopamine loss) apparently showed a greater religious priming deficit relative to right-sided (R)-onset disease, but this must be treated with caution as the sample sizes were small and in all cases Parkinson's disease has a bilateral onset albeit with one side being more affected than the other. A simpler study design (for example a simple word decision task for religious and non-religious words) with a larger sample size might confirm semantic processing differences according to side of onset in Parkinson's disease. Giacquinto also found a difference (not clearly shown to be significant however) between R- and L-onset PD, with decreased frequency of prayer and dependence on religion in L-onset relative to R-onset disease [48]. These results might tentatively suggest R hemisphere neural networks could play a particular role in maintaining a religious faith or practice, but clearly not, if a change in religious faith has not been adequately demonstrated in the first place.

A further pilot study of narrative priming in PD patients and controls, used questions about an article on prayer and health to measure belief in God and God's intervention in the world. This concluded that religious belief inspired by ritual depended on healthy left brain function (impaired in R-onset PD) and belief inspired by beauty and awe in nature was more right brain dependent (impaired in L-onset PD) [49]. Whether a short-term induced effect on beliefs caused by a narrative is indicative of more sustained reflective beliefs could be questioned, however these studies do raise interesting questions about how religious rituals and practices, or a sense of transcendent awe and wonder, might be processed in different brain areas. Interestingly, Schoedt's imaging experiment indicated R hemispheric activation in improvised prayer but L hemisphere activation in ritualised prayer, which suggests that there may be some hemispheric asymmetry in different aspects of prayer.

Conclusion

We believe that the spirituality of people with PD has been relatively under-explored. The literature is small, limited to a few investigators and compromised by methodological weaknesses.

Little hard evidence can be found for whether religious or spiritual beliefs are directly affected by the disease process in Parkinson's disease. Comparative studies using questionnaires and priming tests, because of methodological weaknesses outlined above, offer little conclusive evidence to suggest a reduced interest in spirituality and religious faith, beyond that created by the many physical and psychosocial disease effects. Further studies aiming to compare changes in religion/spirituality between PD groups and controls must ensure that as far as possible, controls are experiencing an illness that is shown to have similar effects on mobility, anxiety, communication, energy levels and so on. Though we can reliably presume that cognitive deficits, such as concentration problems, apathy or impulsivity might cause some problems in aspects of religious practice, the subjective accounts (from people with Parkinson's disease) considered above suggest that religious beliefs and spirituality can often retain their importance and significance for those previously practising them; indeed they can even play an important role in coping with aspects of this illness. However, a more systematic study with larger numbers of participants would be needed to confirm this hypothesis.

It seems likely that religious and spiritual beliefs and practices, being complex and multifaceted, are dependent on cognitive schemas, enmeshed in habitual forms of thought and practice that would only be affected when cognitive deficits are severe. Furthermore religious faith is a culturally embedded phenomenon; besides practical help and encouragement that would hopefully be given, faith is supported by the 'distributed cognition' of a community of minds; it is an oversimplification to reduce it to functioning of individual neural networks [52]. As people with Parkinson's disease are easily prone to be stereotyped it is especially important to pursue further studies in this area with a degree of open mindedness.

References

1 Foltynie, T., C. E. G. Brayne, T. W. Robbins et al. 2004. The cognitive ability of an incident cohort of Parkinson's patients in the UK: The CamPaIGN study. *Brain* 127: 550–60.

2 Lang, A. E., and J. A. Obeso. 2004. Challenges in Parkinson's disease: restoration of the nigrostriatal dopamine system is not enough. *The Lancet Neurology* 3: 309–16.

3 Olanow, C. W., and J. A. Obeso. 2012. The significance of defining preclinical or prodromal Parkinson's disease. *Movement Disorders* 27: 666–9.

4 Del Tredici, K., U. Rub, R. A. De Vos et al. 2002. Where does Parkinson disease pathology begin in the brain? *Journal of Neuropathology and Experimental Neurology* 61: 413–26.

5 Spillantini, M. G., M. L. Schmidt, V. M. Lee et al. 1997. Alpha-synuclein in Lewy bodies. *Nature* 388: 839–40.

6 IPDGC. 2011. A two-stage meta-analysis identifies several new loci for Parkinson's disease. *PLoS Genetics* 7.

7 Trinh, J., and M. Farrer. 2013. Advances in the genetics of Parkinson disease. *Nature Reviews Neurology* 9: 445–54.

8 Kordower, J. H., C. W. Olanow, H. B. Dodiya et al. 2013. Disease duration and the integrity of the nigrostriatal system in Parkinson's disease. *Brain* 136: 2419–31.

9 Dalley, J., B. Everitt and T. Robbins. 2011. Impulsivity, compulsivity, and top-down cognitive control. *Neuron* 69: 680–94.

10 Jankovic, J., and W. Poewe. 2012. Therapies in Parkinson's disease. *Current Opinion in Neurology* 25: 433–47.

11 Williams-Gray, C. H., J. R. Evans, A. Goris et al. 2009. The distinct cognitive syndromes of Parkinson's disease: 5 year follow-up of the CamPaIGN cohort. *Brain* 132: 2958–69.

12 Weintraub, D., and D. J. Burn. 2011. Parkinson's disease: the quintessential

neuropsychiatric disorder. *Movement Disorders* 26: 1022–31.

13 Redgrave, P., M. Rodriguez, Y. Smith et al. 2010. Goal-directed and habitual control in the basal ganglia: implications for Parkinson's disease. *Nature Reviews Neuroscience* 11: 760–72.

14 Williams-Gray, C. H., S. L. Mason, J. R. Evans et al. 2013. The CamPaIGN study of Parkinson's disease: 10-year outlook in an incident population-based cohort. *Journal of Neurology, Neurosurgery, and Psychiatry* 84: 1258–64.

15 Nombela, C., T. Rittman and T. W. Robbins et al. 2011. Multiple modes of impulsivity in Parkinson's disease. *PLoS ONE* 9, no. 1: 0085747. doi:10.1371/journal.pone.0085747.

16 Poletti, M., and U. Bonuccelli. 2012. Personality traits in patients with Parkinson's disease: assessment and clinical implications. *Journal of Neurology* 259: 1029–38.

17 Ishihara, L., and C. Brayne. 2006. What is the evidence for a premorbid parkinsonian personality: a systematic review. *Movement Disorders* 21: 1066–72.

18 Bramley, N., and V. Eatough. 2005. The experience of living with Parkinson's disease: an interpretative phenomenological analysis case study. *Psychology and Health* 20: 223–35.

19 Fitzpatrick, L., J. Simpson and A. Smith. 2010. A qualitative analysis of mindfulness-based cognitive therapy (MBCT) in Parkinson's disease. *Psychology and Psychotherapy: Theory, Research, and Practice* 83: 179–92.

20 Caap-Ahlgren, M., L. Lannerheim and O. Dehlin. 2002. Older Swedish women's experiences of living with symptoms related to Parkinson's disease. *Journal of Advanced Nursing* 39: 87–95.

21 Stanley-Hermanns, M., and J. Engebretson. 2010. Sailing the stormy seas: the illness experience of persons with Parkinson's disease. *The Qualitative Report* 15: 340–69.

22 Paterson, K. 2012. *It's about Time! Understanding the Experience of Speech Impairment*. Abingdon, UK: Routledge.

23 Park, C. L. 2013. The meaning making model: a framework for understanding meaning, spirituality, and stress-related growth in health psychology. *The European Health Psychologist* 15: 40–7.

24 Collicutt McGrath, J. 2011. Posttraumatic growth and spirituality after brain injury. *Brain Impairment* 12: 82–92.

25 Calhoun, L. G., A. Cann, R. G. Tedeschi et al. 2000. A correlational test of the relationship between posttraumatic growth, religion, and cognitive processing. *Journal of Trauma and Stress* 13: 521–7.

26 Pargament, K. I., H. G. Koenig, N. Tarakeshwar et al. 2004. Religious coping methods as predictors of psychological, physical and spiritual outcomes among medically ill elderly patients: a two-year longitudinal study. *Journal of Health Psychology* 9: 713–30.

27 Shaw, A., S. Joseph and P. A. Linley. 2005. Religion, spirituality, and posttraumatic growth: a systematic review. *Mental Health, Religion, and Culture* 8: 1–11.

28 Dezutter, J., A. Wachholtz and J. Corveleyn. 2011. Prayer and pain: the mediating role of positive re-appraisal. *Journal of Behavioral Medicine* 34: 542–9.

29 Bussing, A., A. Michalsen, H. J. Balzat et al. 2009. Are spirituality and religiosity resources for patients with chronic pain conditions? *Pain Medicine* 10: 327–39.

30 Wiech, K., M. Farias, G. Kahane et al. 2008. An fMRI study measuring analgesia enhanced by religion as a belief system. *Pain* 139: 467–76.

31 Charlton, G. S., and C. J. Barrow. 2002. Coping and self-help group membership in Parkinson's disease: an exploratory qualitative study. *Health and Social Care in the Community* 10: 472–8.

32 de Vito, S., N. Gamboz, M. A. Brandimonte et al. 2012. Future thinking in Parkinson's disease: an executive function? *Neuropsychologia* 50: 1494–1501.

33 Schjoedt, U., H. Stødkilde-Jorgensen, A. W. Geertz and A. Roepstorff. 2009. Highly religious participants recruit areas of social cognition in personal prayer. *Social*

Cognitive and Affective Neuroscience 4: 199–207.

34 Kapogiannis, D., A. K. Barbey, M. Su et al. 2009. Neuroanatomical variability of religiosity. *PLoS One* 4, no. 9: e7180. doi:10.1371/journal.pone.0007180.

35 Poletti, M, I. Enrici and M. Adenzato. 2012. Cognitive and affective theory of mind in neurodegenerative diseases: neuropsychological, neuroanatomical and neurochemical levels. *Neuroscience and Biobehavioral Reviews* 36: 2147–64.

36 Cummins, G. 2012. Social cognition in Parkinson's disease and other movement disorders. Unpublished PhD dissertation, University of Cambridge.

37 Nombela, C., P. J. Bustillo, P. F. Castell et al. 2011. Cognitive rehabilitation in Parkinson's disease: evidence from neuroimaging. *Frontiers in Neurology* 2: 82.

38 McNamara, P. 2009. *The Neuroscience of Religious Experience.* Cambridge: Cambridge University Press.

39 Previc, F. H. 2006. The role of the extrapersonal brain systems in religious activity. *Consciousness and Cognition* 15: 500–39.

40 Liddle, P. F., K. J. Friston, C. D. Frith et al. 1992. Patterns of cerebral blood flow in schizophrenia. *British Journal of Psychiatry* 160: 179–86.

41 Schultz, W. 2002. Getting formal with dopamine and reward. *Neuron* 36: 241–63.

42 Cools, R. 2011. Dopaminergic control of the striatum for high-level cognition. *Current Opinion in Neurobiology* 21: 402–7.

43 McNamara, P. N.d. The god effect. *Aeon.* http://aeon.co/magazine/world-views/dopamine-marks-the-line-between-religious-believer-and-fanatic/.

44 Valeo, T. 2012. Not just tremor: recognizing depression and other non-motor symptoms of Parkinson's disease. *Neurology Now Magazine* 8: 22–7.

45 McNamara, P., R. Durso and A. Brown. 2006. Religiosity in patients with Parkinson's disease. *Neuropsychiatric Disease Treatment* 2: 341–8.

46 Butler, P. M., P. McNamara and R. Durso. 2010. Deficits in the automatic activation of religious concepts in patients with Parkinson's disease. *Journal of the International Neuropsychological Society* 16: 252–61.

47 Butler, P. M., P. McNamara, J. Ghofrani et al. 2011. Disease-associated differences in religious cognition in patients with Parkinson's disease. *Journal of Clinical and Experimental Neuropsychology* 33: 917–28.

48 Giaquinto, S., L. Bruti, V. Dall'Armi et al. 2011. Religious and spiritual beliefs in outpatients suffering from Parkinson disease. *International Journal of Geriatric Psychiatry* 26: 916–22.

49 Butler, P. M., P. McNamara and R. Durso. 2011. Side of onset in Parkinson's disease and alterations in religiosity: novel behavioral phenotypes. *Behavioral Neurology* 24: 133–41.

50 Kousta, S. T., G. Vigliocco, D. P. Vinson et al. 2011. The representation of abstract words: why emotion matters. *Journal of Experimental Psychology – General* 140: 14–34.

51 Schwanenflugel, P. J., K. K. Harnishfeger and R. W. Stowe. 1988. Context availability and lexical decisions for abstract and concrete words. *Journal of Memory and Language* 27: 499–520.

52 Donald, M. 2004. *How Culture and Brain Mechanisms Interact in Decision Making.* Cambridge, MA: MIT Press.

II.I *Clinical Conditions*

Chapter 11

Beyond Reasonable Doubt

Cognitive and Neuropsychological Implications for Religious Disbelief

Gordon Pennycook, Daniel Tranel, Kelsey Warner and Erik Asp

Journal articles and chapters on the cognitive science of religious belief often begin by highlighting the seeming ubiquity of supernatural beliefs (e.g. Pennycook et al. 2012). It is indeed rather striking that most of the world's population share a similar sort of belief in a deity or greater power. According to Zuckerman (2007), approximately 90 per cent of the world's population believe in a deity. In 2011, more than 92 per cent of Americans polled by Gallup answered yes when asked 'Do you believe in God?' – a number effectively unchanged since 1944 (96 per cent; Gallup 2011). These sorts of observations lead naturally to the conclusion that religious belief must be grounded in common and, perhaps, foundational cognitive mechanisms. We agree, though in this chapter we will instead emphasise religious doubt, a common experience among religious and non-religious alike (Hunsberger et al. 1993). In the same Gallup poll cited above, the number of respondents who answered 'no' when asked 'Do you believe in God?' increased from 1 per cent in 1944 to 7 per cent in 2011. Moreover, only 80 per cent identified as theists, and 12 per cent identified as deists when asked to distinguish between having belief in a personal God (theism) versus believing in a universal spirit/higher power (deism) in a 2010 poll (Gallup 2011). Finally, in a 2006 version of the same poll, 73 per cent indicated that they were *convinced* that God exists, with the remainder of the sample indicating some doubt or disbelief (Gallup 2011).

Religious belief and disbelief are two sides of the same coin. Thus, in a sense, investigations of variation in religious belief ought to follow directly from previous approaches to the cognitive science of religious belief. However, it is noteworthy that these previous approaches have generally focused on the types of cognitive processes thought to *support* religious belief, such as agency detection (e.g. Guthrie 1993), teleological thinking (Kelemen 2004) and anthropomorphism (Barrett and Keil 1996). A focus on religious *doubt*, we argue, highlights a different set of cognitive mechanisms altogether.

Unlike other approaches in this volume, we start with an understanding of the cognitive science of religion. We set out a hypothesis for the cognitive mechanisms underlying disbelief. Then we draw on observations from people with prefrontal cortex lesions to test the hypothesis.

Dual-Process Theories and Religious Disbelief

As with much of the cognitive science of religious *belief*, the research on religious *disbelief* posits general cognitive mechanisms that are *not* specific to religious cognition. Rather, religious disbelief is thought to occur via domain general cognitive functions (see

Pennycook 2014). We posit that religious disbelief is not *sui generis*; that is, doubt towards religious concepts is not qualitatively distinct from doubt towards non-religious concepts.

Dual-process theories represent a prominent approach to understanding general cognitive function. Although numerous versions have been proposed (see Evans and Stanovich 2013) the common element is a distinction between automatic, fast, intuitive processing and deliberative, slow and analytic processing. More directly, Evans and Stanovich (2013) have recently highlighted the defining features of the two types of processes: type 1 processes are autonomous and do not require working memory, whereas type 2 entail a deliberative use of working memory resources as a means to decouple from a type 1 output or support hypothetical thought. This distinction is rather basic but nonetheless has implications for religious cognition.

Consider the following problem (De Neys et al. 2008):

> In a study 1000 people were tested. Among the participants there were 995 nurses and 5 doctors. Paul is a randomly chosen participant of this study. Paul is 34 years old. He lives in a beautiful home in a posh suburb. He is well spoken and very interested in politics. He invests a lot of time in his career. What is most likely?
>
> (a) Paul is a nurse.
> (b) Paul is a doctor.

This type of problem was originally developed by Kahneman and Tverksy (1973) as part of their heuristics and biases research programme and has since been used in numerous reasoning and decision-making studies (see Barbey and Sloman 2007). The problem is of particular interest for dual-process theorists because of the apparent conflict between two sources of information: (1) the base-rate probability, which in this case strongly suggests that Paul is a nurse (i.e. there are 995 nurses in a sample of 1000 people; 99.5 per cent chance that Paul is a nurse) and (2) the personality description, which in this case contains stereotypical information that strongly suggests that Paul is a doctor (i.e. doctors tend to be more affluent than nurses). Participants tend to base their response on the stereotypical information in lieu of the base-rate probabilities, hence illustrating 'base-rate neglect' (Kahneman and Tverksy 1973; for a review, see Barbey and Sloman 2007). This is thought to occur because the belief-based stereotypical response comes to mind more quickly and fluently (i.e. more intuitively) than the base-rate response (Pennycook et al. 2014c, 2015). Consistent with this and crucially for present purposes, participants who are more willing to engage analytic (type 2) reasoning processes to override intuitive (type 1) outputs (i.e. those with a more analytic cognitive style) are more likely to respond according to the base-rates (Pennycook et al. 2014a).

The base-rate problem serves as an illustrative case. Participants who dispositionally engage more substantive analytic reasoning processes are more likely to doubt and ultimately override a prepotent belief-based response, leading to a more probabilistic and objective response. Participants who are more likely to question and ultimately override beliefs in the context of a reasoning experiment ought to be more likely to do so outside of a lab. Although not a defining feature, type 2 reasoning is thought to be domain general (Stanovich and West 2003). In other words, reasoning in this very general form surely occurs outside of the lab. The question, then, is whether analytic reasoning has consequences for religious disbelief in particular.

Studies from four separate labs have converged on an affirmative answer to this question. Namely, those who perform better on problems that contain intuitive lures (i.e. those with a more analytic cognitive style) and/or who self-report having a more analytic (as opposed to intuitive) thinking disposition are less likely to hold supernatural religious beliefs (Gervais and Norenzayan 2012; Pennycook et al. 2012; Shenhav et al. 2012; Svedholm and Lindeman 2012; for a review, see Pennycook et al. 2016). Less religious individuals also spend less time on reasoning tasks (such as the base-rate problem above), indicating that they engage in lower levels of slow analytic thinking when solving problems (Pennycook et al. 2013, 2014a). Importantly, these correlations remain robust after controlling for numerous potential mediators across multiple studies, such as age, sex, ethnicity, socioeconomic status, income, education, political ideology, personality variables, traditionalist moral values and intelligence (Browne et al. 2014; Pennycook et al. 2012, 2013, 2014b; Shenhav et al. 2012; but see Razmyar and Reeve 2013).

This correlational evidence has also been supplemented by experimental studies. First, Shenhav et al. (2012) asking participants in a between-subjects design to either write about a situation where they used their 'intuition/first instinct' or a situation where they employed a strategy of 'carefully reasoning through a situation'. The goal of this manipulation was to prime an 'intuitive' or 'reflective' mindset. Participants' self-reported level of belief in God was lower when primed to think in a more reflective mode relative to a more intuitive mode. A subsequent set of studies by Gervais and Norenzayan (2012) – completed independently – verified this result. Gervais and Norenzayan employed three additional manipulations intended to prime analytic thought: (1) a piece of art (namely Rodin's *The Thinker*), (2) a word rearranging task that contained analytic thinking prime words (i.e. analyse, reason, ponder, think, rational) and (3) perceptual disfluency. In each case, these subtle manipulations successfully diminished self-reported levels of religious belief.

These experiments provide an existence proof for the mechanism implied by the negative correlation between analytic cognitive style and religious disbelief. Namely, analytic thought is the cognitive process that is used to doubt and ultimately disbelieve religious and supernatural conceptions. Nonetheless, it is worth pointing out that it is unlikely that such manipulations cause long-term changes in religious belief. Moreover, it may be difficult to find manipulations that successfully increase analytic thinking (see Yonker et al. 2016). For this reason, the correlational data is perhaps the more compelling evidence for our hypothesis. Given the amount of evidence that supports the negative correlation between analytic thinking and religious belief (for a meta-analysis with more than 15 000 individuals, see Pennycook et al. 2016) and the number of possible third-variables that have been ruled out (as described above), the most parsimonious current explanation is that analytic thinking plays a role in religious disbelief. It is plausible that the causal effect of analytic thinking on religious disbelief is strongest over longer periods of time. Future longitudinal studies are required to rigorously test this conjecture.

Why Does Analytic Thinking Cause Religious Disbelief?

It seems clear that analytic thinking is used to revise beliefs, but it is unclear why this appears to typically lead to a *decrease* in religious belief *in particular*. Moreover, the general dual-process account expounded above does not explain what causes someone to think analytically about religious belief in the first place. Thus, dual-process theory provides a general framework under which religious doubt can be understood but ultimately falls short as a mechanistic account (and, as a consequence, further theorising is necessary prior to interpreting the neuroscientific evidence).

Three key results from Pennycook et al. (2012) shed light on the question of why analytic thinking leads to religious disbelief. The first is that religious *engagement* (i.e. religious service attendance, importance of religion in everyday life, prayer frequency etc.) was not associated with analytic cognitive style once religious belief was taken into account. Thus, in other words, there does not appear to be an association between analytic thought and religiosity in general; rather, the association is specific to religious beliefs.

Second, this association is not simply a matter of acceptance or rejection of religious belief. Rather, at least in terms of God belief, performance on the Cognitive Reflection Test (i.e. a three-item performance measure used to assess analytic cognitive style) is associated with degrading levels of conventional religious belief. Those who reported believing in a personal God (i.e. the most conventional God belief in the United States) performed the worst, followed by increased performance in pantheists, deists, agnostics and, finally, atheists (see Figure 11.1). This indicates that religious doubt is not simply an all-or-nothing prospect. Some moderately analytic individuals may engage in modest levels of doubt about the predominant and presumably (on the aggregate) default personal God stance, leading to a moderate position on the matter (e.g. belief in God as a universal spirit that does not intervene in human affairs). Nonetheless, it should be noted that by far the starkest contrast is between personal God theists and atheists: the majority (over 50 per cent) of the personal God theists failed to get a single Cognitive Reflection Test item correct whereas the majority (over 60 per cent) of the atheists got either two or three out of three correct.

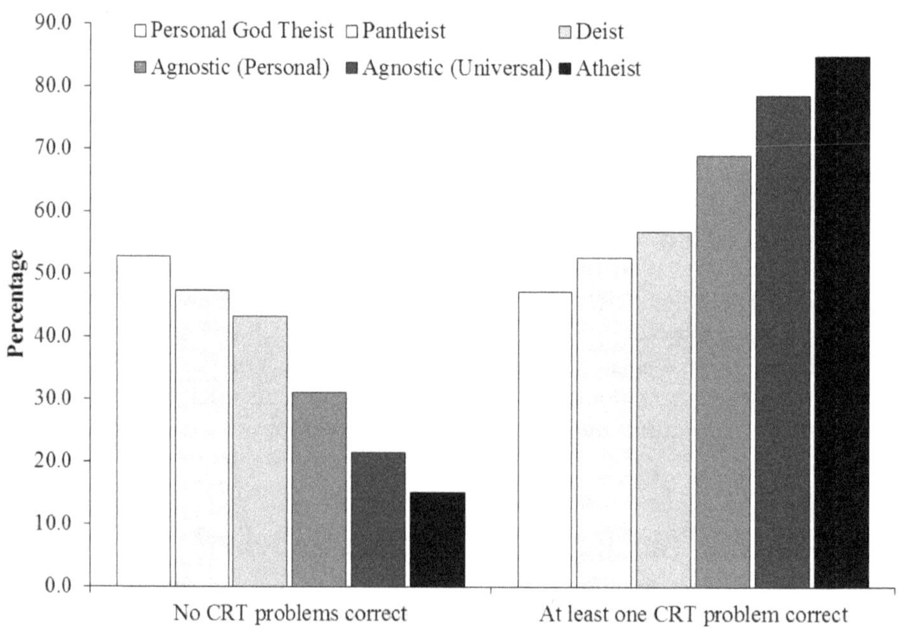

Figure 11.1 Proportion of participants, *left*, who failed to get a single problem correct on the Cognitive Reflection Test (CRT) or, *right*, who successfully answered at least one out of three correct as a function of type of theistic belief. The positive association between CRT performance and religious disbelief is evident across multiple levels of religious conventionality. The slight majority (52.8 per cent) of personal God theists did not get a single CRT problem correct. In contrast, only 15.2 per cent of atheists fell into that group. Data are from Pennycook et al. (2012), Study 1.

Third, noting the supernatural or immaterial nature of religious beliefs, Pennycook et al. (2012) reported a similar association between analytic cognitive style and paranormal beliefs (e.g. astrology, extrasensory perception). This finding indicates that there is something specific about immaterial beliefs that may cause them to be prone to doubt via analytic reasoning. Pennycook et al. (2012) speculated that the inherent conflict between supernatural beliefs and folk conceptions of the materials world (see Atran and Norenzayan 2004). Consider, for example, the proposed nature of angels. Angels are thought to watch over humans and potentially intervene at the behest of God (e.g. by miraculously saving someone from a devastating car accident). This set of beliefs is inherently in conflict with innate conceptions of folk mechanics (i.e. beings cannot pass through solid objects). Neonates demonstrate surprise when naturally occurring rigid bodies occupy the same space (Spelke et al. 1995), indicating that humans have a low level set of 'beliefs' about how the natural world works. Van Leeuwen (2014) recently summarised the evidence for the distinction between 'religious credence' and 'factual belief' that maps onto the distinction between material and immaterial beliefs.

The cognitive conflict between material and immaterial beliefs potentially provides a clue as to what causes someone to think analytically about religious belief in the first place. Recall the base-rate problem from above. A series of studies have demonstrated that the conflict between the base-rate and stereotypical information is actually a *source* of analytic engagement (De Neys et al. 2008). In other words, the conflict between the cognitive outputs causes an increase in analytic reasoning. The key role of conflict in reasoning has now been supported by a large number of measures (e.g. response time, confidence, eye-tracking, skin conductance) across multiple tasks (for a review, see De Neys 2014). In these experiments, participants are given both conflict and no-conflict problems in a reasoning task.[1] The typical finding is that participants spend more time reasoning (or have lower confidence, or higher levels of skin conductance etc.) in cases where there is a cognitive conflict, indicated a low-level recognition of the conflict followed by increased levels of analytic thinking (Pennycook et al. 2015).

This conflict detection process should, in principle, apply to any sort of task or situation that involves a conflict between two cognitive outputs. Thus, the inherent conflict between immaterial religious beliefs and folk conceptions of the material world may be the source of the negative association between analytic thinking and religious belief. Consistent with this line of reasoning, Pennycook et al. (2014a) found that religious believers were less efficient at detecting conflicts during reasoning than non-believers. Specifically, religious believers had a markedly smaller response time increase for conflict relative to no-conflict versions of the base-rate problems (see Figure 11.2). Thus, according to Pennycook et al., 'one need not explicitly decide to critically examine religious beliefs. Rather, one's disposition towards analytic thought may determine the likelihood of implicitly detecting conflict between non-material religious beliefs and our understanding of the material world' (p. 9).

---

[1] The following is an example of no-conflict version of the base-rate problem from above: In a study 1000 people were tested. Among the participants there were 5 nurses and 995 doctors. Paul is a randomly chosen participant of this study. Paul is 34 years old. He lives in a beautiful home in a posh suburb. He is well spoken and very interested in politics. He invests a lot of time in his career. What is most likely? (Note: All that has changed is the base-rate probabilities.)

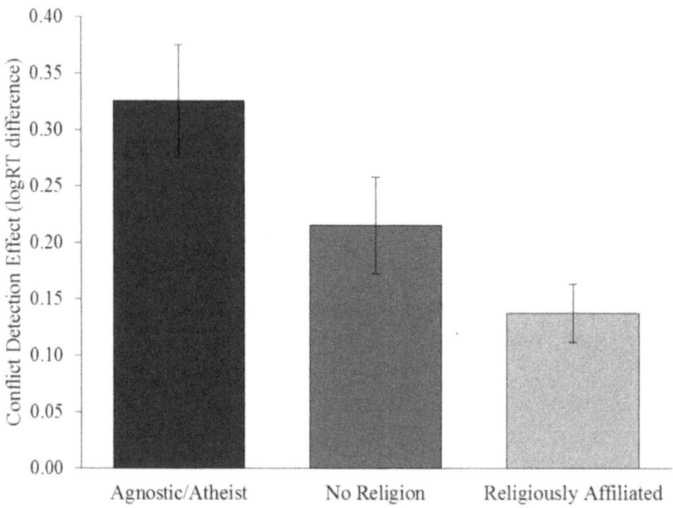

Figure 11.2 Mean RT difference between stereotypical responses to incongruent problems and congruent problems as a function of religious affiliation. The values represent RTs transformed via $\log_{10}$. A larger logRT difference indicates increasing sensitivity to the conflict between base-rate probabilities and stereotypical personality descriptions. These results indicate that agnostics/atheists are more efficient at detecting conflict during reasoning than are the religiously affiliated. Data are from Pennycook et al. (2014a), Experiment 3.

Mechanisms for Belief and Doubt: The Need for a Vigilant Conflict Detector

As outlined above, one's ability to detect and revise conflicting cognitions may play an important role in constraining one's religious beliefs. Individuals that can efficiently monitor conflict and effectively update cognitions are more likely to reject beliefs that are inconsistent with their naturalistic worldview (e.g. religious beliefs, belief in miracles). However, *prima facie*, this appears to make little sense. Why is the ability to detect conflict needed for religious doubt? Why is it that those who are poor at detecting conflict cannot simply *a priori* withhold belief in religious concepts? Our position (detailed below) suggests that credulity is a necessary, involuntary process in how we understand information. Indeed, this position implies that belief is the default stance towards not only religious concepts but all cognitions. Here, we will unpack this conjecture by examining the psychological and neural mechanisms for belief and disbelief.

Our thesis hinges on the psychological mechanisms of belief or doubt towards some cognition. The *sine qua non* of belief is action; so we must ask, what makes a cognition empowered to be acted upon? And likewise, what process denies a cognition its veracity and inhibits action? Conventional wisdom would suggest the process of belief or doubt involves three stages: (1) comprehension of some proposition, (2) assessment of that proposition with other extant mental information and (3) labelling or tagging of the assessed truth value to that proposition which could be indexed in the future (Gilbert 1991). The understanding of a proposition precedes and is independent from the assessment and labelling of the cognition as true (or false). Thus, when we encounter the proposition, *All celestial stars are spheres*, we can first comprehend this information (understand what it means), and then, judge it to be true against our relevant extant mental knowledge. This belief procedure has been attributed to Descartes (Mandelbaum 2014), so we will continue with this conventional nomenclature.

However, many studies in cognitive science have shown that human belief and doubt do not actually operate according to Cartesian principles (Mandelbaum 2014). In rebuttal to the Cartesian belief procedure, Spinoza argued that understanding is not the neutral process conventional wisdom would suggest. Instead, comprehension of a proposition necessitates belief in that proposition. Thus, in his model, when we encounter the proposition, *the heart produces all mental activity*, we must, initially believe this proposition for at least a split-second if we are to comprehend it. However, subsequently, we can use a secondary psychological process to assess, doubt and label this information with a false tag. In the Spinozan model, doubt is a secondary revision to an untested initial belief (Asp and Tranel 2013).

Cognitions are empowered in the Spinozan model by mere mental representation (Gilbert 1993). They are ballistic; they will induce cognition-consistent action given the right circumstances. Alternatively, in the Cartesian model cognitions are static. Only following an assessment period in which cognitions are deemed true can they be believed and empowered. Indeed, this line of reasoning raises the question of whether assessment of every cognition that needs to be believed and acted upon is even possible (Egan 2008). Our cognitive and perceptual systems receive a constant stream of ever changing data that requires timely and accurate responses. What process constantly assigns truth to the voluminous incoming data to afford adaptive responses? The Spinozan model does not require this additional process. It appears to be the most parsimonious account; that cognitions do not need to be turned into belief, they in fact are beliefs.

Empirical studies have pitted the Cartesian and Spinozan belief models against one another. Gilbert and colleagues (1993) used the principle of modular system degradation following resource depletion to examine the two theories. They reasoned that resource depletion (i.e. distraction) should prevent a Cartesian system from either believing or disbelieving propositions it only comprehends, but it should prevent a Spinozan system from disbelieving propositions it both comprehends and believes. They gave participants narratives with several explicitly labelled false statements embedded. Gilbert and colleagues (1993) found that resource depletion acted to sway social judgements of the protagonists in the narratives towards the explicit false information. In effect, reduction of the participants' resources caused participants to believe the false information which later influenced social judgements. Thus, the participants' cognitions from the false statements were left comprehended and believed rather than simply comprehended, a finding consistent with Spinozan belief theory. Subsequent research has found support for the Spinozan model by investigating belief change through fictional narratives, false consumer claims, and acquiescence on questionnaires responses (Asp and Tranel 2013). This belief procedure has been used to explain the well-known truth/belief bias and the tendency to rely on heuristical processing (Asp et al. 2013; Mandelbaum 2014). Additionally, evidence for the Spinozan perspective has been offered in diverse research areas including: mental development, forced persuasions, attributions, psycholinguistics, mental evolution, and social psychological biases (Gilbert 1991, 1993). Some studies have shown results that purportedly are against the Spinozan account (Hasson et al. 2005; Nadarevic and Erdfelder 2013); however, they are either internally inconsistent (see Mandelbaum 2014) or do not adequately test the veracity of the belief accounts.[2]

[2] In a personal communication, regarding Nadarevic and Erdfelder's (2013) finding that source credibility improved true and false information memory, one of us (Asp, E.W.) argued that in the absence of resource depletion the Spinozan and Cartesian belief models cannot make differential

Although the Spinozan account has the weight of theoretical and empirical evidence, it also demands an efficient mechanism to detect belief conflict and to modify discrepant beliefs that do not fit with extant knowledge. If all incoming cognitions are beliefs, then we need a vigilant system to correct all the errant beliefs following exposure. The consequences of an inability to detect and update beliefs would be severe and debilitating. One could not disbelieve propositions or random ruminations to which one was exposed. Credulity and fixed false beliefs that are epistemically unwarranted would be a defining feature. Indeed, this deficiency might be the etiological mechanism of delusions in patients with schizophrenia (Asp and Tranel 2013).

Neural Correlates of Disbelief

One of the most established and well-studied brain–behaviour relationships in cognitive neuroscience is the dorsal anterior cingulate cortex's (dACC) mediation of cognitive conflict monitoring (Botvinick et al. 2004). Neuroimaging studies have shown the dACC is activated in tasks which (1) require an overriding of prepotent responses, (2) involve choosing between a set of equally permissible responses and (3) lead to the production of recognisable errors (Botvinick et al. 2001). The dACC has been theorised to play a key role in the initiation and modulation of cognitive control which is purportedly mediated by the broader prefrontal cortex (including the dorsolateral prefrontal cortex, dlPFC). However, it's important to note that this model, while being well supported by imaging (e.g. Kerns et al. 2004), does not address the overall functions of the dACC and cannot completely account for the results of neuropsychological studies (Botvinick et al. 2004; Gehring and Knight 2000; Shackman et al. 2011). Nonetheless, the dACC is a prime neuroanatomical suspect in the ability to detect cognitive conflict and pass along this information to initiate doubt, or 'belief control'.

Indeed, De Neys et al. (2008) reported increased activation in the dorsal anterior cingulate cortex when participants gave stereotypical responses to conflict base-rate problems, indicating that conflict between base-rate information and stereotypes was successfully detected. Pennycook et al.'s (2014) hypothesis that cognitive conflict detection is associated with religious belief is also supported by neuroimaging work. Namely, Inzlicht and colleagues (Inzlicht et al. 2009; Inzlicht et al. 2011) found a negative association between religious conviction (namely degree of 'religious zeal', belief in God and religious service attendance) and dACC activation during a conflict monitoring/cognitive control task. We take this important individual difference data to support the proposed link between the ability to detect cognitive conflict and religious belief. It should be noted, however, Inzlicht and colleagues have a very different interpretation of these results (Inzlicht et al. 2011). They claim that religiosity *decreases* anterior cingulate activation in order to alleviate anxiety. We find this interpretation somewhat dubious given that the cognitive control task used (namely the Stroop task) is not intended to cause anxiety. Moreover, the evidence for an association between religiosity and anxiety is very mixed (Shreve-Neiger and Edelstein 2004). For example, in a sample of participants who suffered from sleep paralysis – an intensely fearful and aversive experience – belief in religious and supernatural explanations predicted *increased* post-episode distress (Cheyne and

predictions regarding memory accuracy for true, false and uncertain information (in an age-controlled, healthy population).

Pennycook 2013). In the same study, participants with a more analytic cognitive style were less likely to have supernatural explanations for their sleep paralysis experience and, independent of supernatural explanations and all other measured variables, were less likely to be distressed about the experience in the following days. Thus, not only was religiosity associated with increased anxiety, but analytic cognitive style was associated with decreased religiosity *and* decreased anxiety. This, along with Pennycook et al'.s (2014a) direct correlation between conflict detection and religiosity, supports our reinterpretation of Inzlicht and colleagues' fMRI/EEG results.

The dACC and the broader prefrontal cortex are also heavily implicated in Asp and colleagues' neuropsychological model of doubt processes, the false tagging theory (FTT; Asp and Tranel 2013). Under this perspective, belief is considered to be inherent in the process of comprehension (Spinozan belief model), and doubt is thought to be critically reliant on a network of brain regions: prefrontal cortex (PFC), dorsal anterior cingulate cortex (dACC), posterior parietal cortex (PPC), ventral tegmental area (VTA), amygdala and the striatum. Central to this theory is the functions of the prefrontal cortex, which have been linked to the suppression of pathological confabulation, rejection of ad hoc beliefs, and inhibition of prepotent responses. The FTT asserts the prefrontal cortex acts to 'false tag' initially believed representations in postrolandic association cortices. Neuroimaging has shown that in situations where doubt is necessary the prefrontal cortex is highly active (Asp and Tranel 2013). It was argued that damage to the prefrontal cortex from strokes or tumour resections should lead to a general increase in credulity, where patients have a 'doubt deficit' towards information that is compulsorily believed upon comprehension.

To test whether patients with lesions to the PFC had increased credulity to novel information, Asp et al. (2012a) gave patients with focal brain lesions and heathy, age-matched adults magazine advertisements that had been deemed deceptive by the Federal Trade Commission. Patients with PFC damage were more credulous to the deceptive ads than patients with other lesions outside of the prefrontal cortex and healthy participants. This finding held even when the misleading ads contained a disclaimer rebutting the deceptive claim, suggesting that scepticism is generally lower in PFC patients. The results could not be explained by group differences in demographics or cognitive functioning, such as intelligence, memory or reading ability. Lesion location was the only variable that was reliably associated with credulity to the deceptive ads. Although this result was intriguing, we wondered if this lesion-induced credulity could actually impact more abstract and structured social beliefs, such as religious beliefs.

Asp et al. (2012b) conducted an extensive religious belief and behaviour survey in lesion patients to examine this hypothesis. The participants included: patients with prefrontal cortex damage (PFC; Figure 11.3), brain damage comparison patients (BDC) and medical comparison patients (individuals who had undergone a life-threatening but non-neurological medical event, MC). The prefrontal cortex patients reported the highest specific religious beliefs (e.g. *belief in heaven*), and the greatest increase in specific religious beliefs following their brain injury/medical event (Figure 11.4). Compared to the other groups, prefrontal patients also reported the highest scores on scales of authoritarianism (e.g. *Our country will be great if we honour the ways of our forefathers, do what the authorities tell us to do, and get rid of the 'rotten apples' that are ruining everything*) and religious fundamentalism (e.g. *God has given humanity a complete, unfailing guide to happiness and salvation, which must be totally followed*). The results cannot be accounted for by differences in religious affiliation, religious upbringing, religious service attendance,

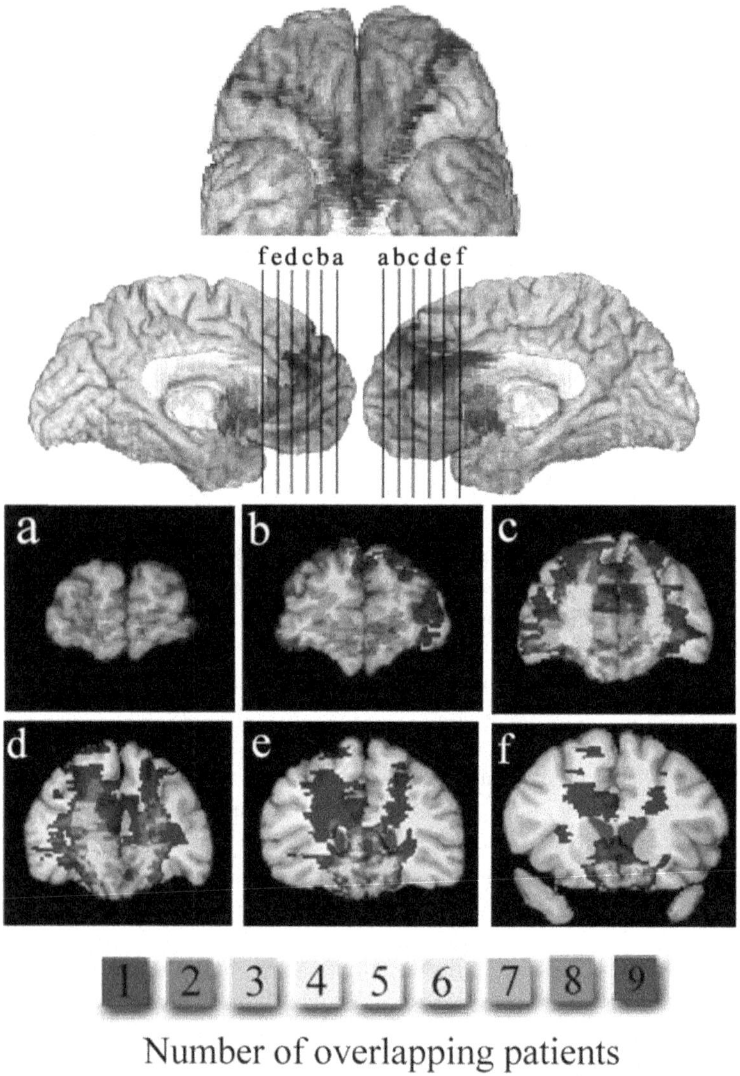

Figure 11.3 Lesion overlap of prefrontal patients. Lesions of the prefrontal patients are displayed in mesial and coronal slices. The bar indicates by degree of shading the number of overlapping lesions at each voxel. Data are from Asp et al. (2012b).

demographic variables or general cognitive functioning. Moreover, neither an aversive medical event nor brain damage, *per se*, produced the high levels of religious beliefs in the prefrontal patients. Unfortunately, Asp et al. (2012b) had no way to gauge the participants' beliefs prior to the lesion/medical event except to rely on their own memories of their past beliefs. Thus, it is possible that the authors happened to select prefrontal patients with a priori strong religious beliefs and they had worse belief recall than comparisons. However, this possibility was considered extremely unlikely as social attitudes in their rural Iowa samples tend to be relatively homogenous and there were no group differences on measures

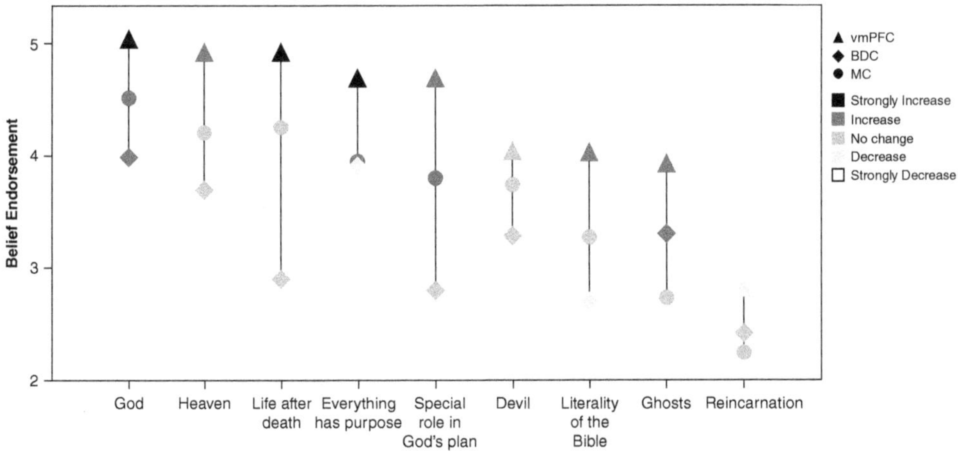

Figure 11.4 Group religious belief endorsement means for specific beliefs. The *y*-axis represents belief endorsement, where 1 = low religious belief to 5 = high religious belief. The *x*-axis represents individual specific religious beliefs. MC, medical comparisons; BDC, brain damaged comparisons; vmPFC, prefrontal patients. Shading indicates reported changes in beliefs following a subject's medical event. Darker shades represent a mean increase in specific belief, and lighter shades represent a mean decrease in beliefs. No group reported a strong decrease in any specific belief. Prefrontal patients reported the highest specific religious beliefs and increases in beliefs. Data are from Asp and Tranel (2013).

of memory. Moreover, in the 16 brain damaged patients that participated in both studies (8 were prefrontal patients), there was a strong bivariate correlation between credulity to the ads and religious fundamentalism ($r = 0.50$, $p = 0.05$). These data suggest that increased credulity is the cognitive mediator for high religious beliefs post lesion.

It should be noted that many of the prefrontal patients in Asp and colleagues' studies primarily had damage to the ventromedial prefrontal cortex (vmPFC) and frontal pole (Figure 11.3). Neuroimaging studies have traditionally highlighted the dlPFC in the processes of cognitive control and the rejection of a stereotypical response during base-rate problems as described above (De Neys et al. 2008; Kerns et al. 2004). The vmPFC and dlPFC could serve distinct functions as suggested by many neuroimaging accounts and some lesion studies (e.g. Glascher et al. 2012). Alternatively, several studies argue that a more general function may be served by the prefrontal cortex that is not specific to dorsal or ventral subregions (Asp et al. 2013; Asp and Tranel 2013; Duncan and Miller 2002). Indeed, patients with exclusive damage to the dlPFC also tend to have increased credulity to deceptive advertisements and higher religious beliefs (Asp et al., n.d.).

Thus, it is possible the roles of the dlPFC and vmPFC are distinct and each offers a unique, but complementary contribution to disbelief. Under this thesis, the dlPFC is specific to the integration of type 2 processing to decisions whereas the vmPFC represents an earlier, more basic doubt process that does not require substantive (or, perhaps, any) type 2 processing. Analytic cognitive style, then, would represent the source of a *later* doubting process; one that operates on fully formed religious beliefs that have survived the false-tagging process. In both cases, however, it is the conflict between the incoming or default supernatural concept and previous materialistic conception of the world that allows doubt to occur.

However, it is also possible that the dlPFC and vmPFC broadly contribute the same function; the prefrontal cortex (in general) provides an adaptive resource which could increase or decrease availability due to task demands (Duncan and Miller 2002). Asp and colleagues have argued this flexible resource is the function false tagging that contributes to a variety of perceptual and cognitive systems (Asp et al. 2013). In this model, false tagging is essential for type 2 processing and analytic cognitive style, as doubt is necessary to reject immediate, intuitive answers (Asp et al. 2013; Mandelbaum 2014). Future research will need to address the potential fractionation of the prefrontal cortex and the role of false tagging in type 2 processing.

Conclusion

The cognitive science of religion has understandably focused primarily on explanations of religious belief. By focusing instead on the cognitive processes that lead to religious doubt and disbelief, the work reviewed here offers a much different perspective. This research strongly implicates a critical role for the prefrontal cortex in the doubt, disbelief and rejection of religious concepts. However, it should be emphasised that we regard the association between structural integrity of the prefrontal cortex and religiosity as one factor among many that contribute to religious belief and experience. Thus, while damage to the prefrontal cortex can lead to an increase in religious beliefs, the reverse is not necessarily true; i.e. individuals high in religious beliefs have prefrontal cortex brain damage. It is likely sociodemographic, cultural and contextual variables all significantly impact one's religiosity independent of prefrontal cortex structural integrity.

Our theoretical and empirical work challenge the legitimacy of neuropsychological models that argue the prefrontal cortex is critical for religiosity and religious belief (e.g. Muramoto 2004). Patients with extensive damage to the frontal lobe not only show belief and behaviour consistent with religious concepts, but their conviction is often increased. We have argued the ability to detect cognitive discrepancies and revise cognitions on the basis of this conflict is necessary to doubt religious concepts. The evidence reviewed here strongly suggests the prefrontal cortex mediates these functions. However, the specific contribution of the prefrontal cortex's subregions (likely in conjunction with other brain regions) to religious doubt is still a matter for debate.

Perhaps there are two neuroanatomically distinct levels of doubt that may undermine religious belief. First, a low-level false-tagging process located in the vmPFC may undermine an initially believed supernatural proposition by comparing it against extant (and conflicting) conceptions of the material world. Second, assuming an absence of a 'false tag', higher-level reasoning processes (in the dlPFC) may be recruited following successful conflict detection (in the dACC). Alternatively, false tagging or doubt may be a general resource that both the vmPFC and dlPFC can utilise following successful conflict detection. False tagging would play a critical role in higher reasoning processes (i.e. type 2 processing). In this model, deficits in the ability to 'false tag' should lead to a decreased analytic cognitive style and an increased reliance on heuristical responses.

The precise role of the prefrontal cortex towards religious doubt will need to be elucidated with future research. However, we believe this work represents an important first step for understanding the mechanisms of the backside of the religious belief coin.

References

Asp, E. W., and D. Tranel. 2013. False tagging theory: toward a unitary account of prefrontal cortex function. In *Principles of Frontal Lobe Function*, 2nd edn., ed. D. T. Stuss and R. T. Knight, 383–416. New York: Oxford University Press.

Asp, E. W., K. Manzel, B. Koestner, C. A. Cole, N. L. Denburg and D. Tranel. 2012a.

A neuropsychological test of belief and doubt: damage to ventromedial prefrontal cortex increases credulity for misleading advertising. *Frontiers in Neuroscience* 6: 100–9.

Asp, E. W., K. Ramchandran and D. Tranel. 2012b. Authoritarianism, religious fundamentalism, and the human prefrontal cortex. *Neuropsychology* 26: 414–21.

Asp, E. W., K. Manzel, B. Koestner, N. L. Denburg and D. Tranel. 2013. Benefit of the doubt: a new view of the role of the prefrontal cortex in executive functioning and decision making. *Frontiers in Neuroscience* 7: 86.

Asp, E. W., K. A. Warner, N. L. Denburg and D. Tranel. N.d. Credulity and religious beliefs in patients with dorsolateral prefrontal cortex damage. Department of Neurology, University of Iowa.

Atran, S., and A. Norenzayan. 2004. Religion's evolutionary landscape: counterintuition, commitment, compassion, communion. *Behavioural and Brain Sciences* 27: 713–70.

Barbey, A. K., and S. A. Sloman. 2007. Base-rate respect: from ecological rationality to dual processes. *Behavioural and Brain Sciences* 30: 241–56.

Barrett, J. L., and F. C. Keil. 1996. Conceptualizing a nonnatural entity: anthropomorphism in god concepts. *Cognitive Psychology* 31: 219–47.

Botvinick, M. M., T. S. Braver, D. M. Barch, C. S. Carter and J. D. Cohen. 2001. Conflict monitoring and cognitive control. *Psychological Review* 108: 624–52.

Botvinick, M. M., J. D. Cohen and C. S. Carter. 2004. Conflict monitoring and anterior cingulate cortex: an update. *Trends in Cognitive Sciences* 8: 539–46.

Browne, M., G. Pennycook, B. Goodwin and M. McHenry. 2014. Reflective minds and open hearts: cognitive style and personality predict religious and spiritual thinking in a community sample. *European Journal of Social Psychology* 44: 736–42.

Cheyne, J. A., and G. Pennycook. 2013. Sleep paralysis postepisode distress: modeling potential effects of episode characteristics, general psychological distress, beliefs, and cognitive style. *Clinical Psychological Science* 1: 135–48.

De Neys, W. 2014. Conflict detection, dual processes, and logical intuitions: Some clarifications. *Thinking and Reasoning* 20: 167–87.

De Neys, W., O. Vartanian and V. Goel. 2008. When our brains detect that we are biased. *Psychological Science* 19: 483–9.

Duncan, J., and E. K. Miller. 2002. Cognitive focus through adaptive neural coding in the primate prefrontal cortex. In *Principles of Frontal Lobe Function*, ed. D. T. Stuss and R. T. Knight, 278–91. New York: Oxford University Press.

Egan, A. 2008. Seeing and believing: perception, belief formation and the divided mind. *Philosophical Studies* 140: 47–63.

Evans, J. St. B. T., and K. E. Stanovich. 2013. Dual-process theories of higher cognition: Advancing the debate. *Perspectives in Psychological Science* 8: 223–41.

Gallup. 2011. U.S. political ideology stable with conservatives leading. August 1. www.gallup.com/poll/148745/political-ideology-stable-conservatives-leading.aspx.

Gehring, W. J., and R. T. Knight. 2000. Prefrontal-cingulate interations in action monitoring. *Nature Neuroscience* 3: 516–20.

Gervais, W. M., and A. Norenzayan. 2012. Analytic thinking promotes religious disbelief. *Science* 336: 493–6.

Gilbert, D. T. 1991. How mental systems believe. *American Psychologist* 46: 107–19.

Gilbert, D. T. 1993. The assent of man: mental representation and the control of belief. In *Handbook of Mental Control*, ed. D. M. Wegner and J. W. Pennebaker, 57–87. Engelwood Cliffs, NJ: Prentice Hall.

Gilbert, D. T., R. W. Tafarodi and P. S. Malone. 1993. You can't not believe everything you read. *Journal of Personality and Social Psychology* 65: 221–33.

Glascher, J., R. Adolphs, H. Damasio, A. Bechara, D. Rudrauf, M. Calamia et al. 2012. Lesion mapping of cognitive control and value-based decision making in the prefrontal cortex. *Proceedings of the National Academy of Sciences* 109: 14681–6.

Guthrie, S. E. 1993. *Faces in the Clouds: A New Theory of Religion*. Oxford: Oxford University Press.

Hasson, U., J. P. Simmons and A. Todorov. 2005. Believe it or not. *Psychological Science* 16: 566–71.

Hunsberger, B., B. McKenzie, M. Pratt and S. M. Pancer. 1993. Religious doubt: a social-psychological analysis. *Research in the Social Scientific Study of Religion* 5: 27–51.

Inzlicht, M., I. McGregor, J. B. Hirsh and K. Nash. 2009. Neural markers of religious conviction. *Psychological Science* 20: 385–92.

Inzlicht, M., A. M. Tullett and M. Good. 2011. The need to believe: a neuroscience account of religion as a motivated process. *Religion, Brain, and Behavior* 1: 192–212.

Kahneman, D., and A. Tversky. 1973. On the psychology of prediction. *Psychological Review* 80: 237–51.

Kelemen, D. 2004. Are children 'intuitive theists'? *Psychological Science* 15: 295–301.

Kerns, J. G., J. D. Cohen, A. W. MacDonald, R. Y. Cho, V. A. Stenger and C. S. Carter. 2004. Anterior cingulate conflict monitoring and adjustments in control. *Science* 303: 1023–6.

Mandelbaum, E. 2014. Thinking is believing. *Inquiry* 57: 55–96.

Muramoto, O. 2004. The role of the medial prefrontal cortex in human religious activity. *Medical Hypotheses* 62: 479–85.

Nadarevic, L., and E. Erdfelder. 2013. Spinoza's error: memory for truth and falsity. *Memory and Cognition* 41: 176–86.

Pennycook, G. 2014. Evidence that analytic cognitive style influences religious belief: comment on Razmyar and Reeve (2013). *Intelligence* 43: 21–6.

Pennycook, G., J. A. Cheyne, P. Seli, D. J. Koehler and J. A. Fugelsang. 2012. Analytic cognitive style predicts religious and paranormal belief. *Cognition* 123: 335–46.

Pennycook, G., J. A. Cheyne, D. J. Koehler and J. A. Fugelsang. 2013. Belief bias during reasoning among religious believers and skeptics. *Psychonomic Bulletin and Review* 20: 806–11.

Pennycook, G., J. A. Cheyne, N. Barr, D. J. Koehler and J. A. Fugelsang. 2014a. Cognitive style and religiosity: the role of conflict detection. *Memory and Cognition* 42: 1–10.

Pennycook, G., J. A. Cheyne, N. Barr, D. J. Koehler and J. A. Fugelsang. 2014b. The role of analytic thinking in moral judgements and values. *Thinking and Reasoning* 20: 188–214.

Pennycook, G., D. Trippas, S. J. Handley and V. A. Thompson. 2014c. Base-rates: both neglected and intuitive. *Journal of Experimental Psychology: Learning, Memory, and Cognition* 40: 544–54.

Pennycook, G., J. A. Fugelsang and D. J. Koehler. 2015. What makes us think? A three-stage dual-process model of analytic engagement. *Cognitive Psychology* 80: 34–72.

Pennycook, G., R. Ross, D. J. Koehler and J. A. Fugelsang. 2016. Atheists and agnostics are more reflective than religious believers: four empirical studies and a meta-analysis. *PLoS One* 11: e0153039.

Razmyar, S., and C. L. Reeve. 2013. Individual differences in religiosity as a function of cognitive ability and style. *Intelligence* 41: 667–73.

Shackman, A. J., T. V. Salomons, H. A. Slagter, A. S. Fox, J. J. Winter and R. J. Davidson. 2011. The integration of negative affect, pain and cogntive control in the cingulate cortex. *Nature Reviews Neuroscience* 12: 154–67.

Shenhav, A., D. G. Rand and J. D. Greene. 2012. Divine intuition: cognitive style influences belief in god. *Journal of Experimental Psychology: General* 141: 423–8.

Shreve-Neiger, A. K., and B. A. Edelstein. 2004. Religion and anxiety: a critical review of the literature. *Clinical Psychology Review* 24: 379–97.

Spelke, E., A. Phillips and A. Woodward. 1995. Infants' knowledge of object motion and human action. In *Causal Cognition*, ed. D. Sperber, D. Premack and A. Premack, 44–78. Oxford: Clarendon Press.

Stanovich, K. E., and R. F. West. 2003. Evolutionary versus instrumental goals: how evolutionary psychology misconceives human rationality. In *Evolution and the*

Psychology of Thinking: The Debate, ed. D. E. Over, 1–53. New York: Psychological Press.

Svedholm, A. M., and M. Lindeman. 2012. The separate roles of the reflective mind and involuntary inhibitory control in gatekeeping paranormal beliefs and the underlying intuitive confusions. *British Journal of Psychology* 104: 303–19.

Van Leeuwen, N. 2014. Religious credence is not factual belief. *Cognition* 13: 698–715.

Yonker, J. E., L. R. O. Edman, J. Cresswell and J. L. Barrett. 2016. Primed analytic thought and religiosity: the importance of individual characteristics. *Psychology of Religion and Spirituality* 8: 298–308.

Zuckerman, P. 2007. Atheism: contemporary numbers and patterns. In *The Cambridge Companion to Atheism*, ed. M. Martin, 47–65. New York: Cambridge University Press.

Chapter 12

II.I *Clinical Conditions*

Ramadam Fasting and Neurologic Disorders

Ashraf El-Mitwalli

Fasting – the voluntary withholding of food – is a common practice in many religions. Depending on the type of fast, weight loss may occur. Participants in a fast may develop negative sodium balance and have high rates of gluconeogenesis with amino acids as the primary substrates. Ketosis develops and ketones replace glucose as the primary energy source in the central nervous system, thereby decreasing the need for gluconeogenesis and sparing protein catabolism. Several hormonal changes occur during fasting, including a fall in insulin and T3 levels and a rise in glucagon and reverse T3 levels [1]. However, the effect of fasting on neurological diseases, direct or indirect (for instance through affecting medication adherence), are not well known. The mass participation in, and clear regulations of, Ramadan fasting make it an ideal opportunity to study these issues.

Fasting in the month of Ramadan is one of the main pillars of Islam. It is obligatory upon every sane, healthy Muslim who has reached puberty and is not travelling during the time of fasting. Allah (SWT) says in the Qur'an what may be interpreted as, 'O you who believe, fasting is prescribed for you as it was prescribed for those before you so that you may achieve Taqwaa (righteousness, God-fearing)' [2]. The Prophet Muhammad (PBUH) said, 'Whoever observes the fast during the month of Ramadan, [while] believing in Allah and seeking His rewards, will have his past sins forgiven' [3].

The Islamic calendar (Hijri) is a lunar calendar, so the first day of Ramadan advances 11 days each year in relation to the Gregorian calendar. Consequently, Ramadan falls on different parts of the seasonal year over a 33-year cycle. During the month of Ramadan, Muslims abstain from food, drink and sex during the month, between dawn and sunset [4]. There are some acts that are recommended, and if you practice them, you will gain more rewards from Allah SWT, such as taking *suhuur* (pre-dawn meal) until just before *fajr* (dawn). We should also hurry to break the fast at sunset. Narrated Sahl bin Sa'd, Allah's Apostle said, 'The people will remain on the right path as long as they hasten the breaking of the fast' [5]. Narrated Anas bin Malik: The Prophet said, 'Take Suhur as there is a blessing in it' [6]. 'Amr bin al-'As reported Allah's Messenger (PBUH) as saying: The difference between our fasting and that of the people of the Book is eating shortly before dawn [7].

Intentional eating or drinking, vomiting, sexual intercourse, menstrual or childbirth bleeding invalidate the fast. It is optional to fast during Ramadan for those who are sick or travelling; likewise, pregnant and nursing women, who are afraid that fasting may weaken them or the child, may opt not to fast [8]. Missed fasts may be made up at a later time when recovered or people may offer expiatory compensation, which consists of feeding a poor person for each day of fast they have missed.

Adherence with Medication

Adherence issues with oral medications during Ramadan are well documented. Studies have indicated up to 64 per cent of people may alter their drug regimen, including altering dosage or frequency, and sometimes completely omitting the drug; often without seeking medical advice [9]. The effect of fasting on the drug regimens was studied in 81 Asian Muslim patients during the religious month of Ramadan. Twenty-two male and 15 female patients were found to change their drug dosage pattern while fasting: 35 missed doses, 8 took their tablets at different times and 4 patients took all their medication as one single daily dose after breaking fast in the evening [10]. A survey of 325 outpatients in a Kuwaiti hospital found that most of them changed their drug regimens during Ramadan [11]. However, 92 per cent of patients receiving oral hormonal therapies for breast cancer adhered to their treatment whilst fasting during Ramadan [12].

The following administration routes do not nullify fasting: eye and ear drops, all substances absorbed into the body through the skin, such as creams, ointments and medicated plasters, insertion into the vagina of pessaries, medical ovules and vaginal washes, injections through the skin, muscle, joints or veins, with the exception of intravenous feeding, oxygen and anaesthetic gases, nitroglycerin tablets placed under the tongue for the treatment of angina, mouthwash, gargle or oral spray, provided nothing is swallowed into the stomach [13]. However, a recent study reported that a majority believe that the use of eye drops during the fasting hours of Ramadan would break the fast (63.7 per cent of respondents) [14]. Another small survey suggests that a large proportion of Muslims would stop or alter the timing of their ocular medication during Ramadan [15]. In another study, more than one-third of the people interviewed would not use topical treatment while fasting, and around the same number would also consider this a breach of their fast [16].

A prospective observational study was designed for diabetic children and adolescents who wish to fast during Ramadan. The majority (60.6 per cent) of the patients could complete their fasting during Ramadan. Blood glucose, hemoglobin A1c, weight and insulin dose before and after Ramadan in two groups showed no significant difference. The study concluded that, children older than 11 years of age with type 1 diabetes mellitus with conventional twice-a-day regimen can fast safely during Ramadan provided they have proper education and intensive follow-up during Ramadan [17].

Fasting and Stroke

Stroke is the third commonest cause of death and disability worldwide. No significant difference was found in the number of hospitalisations for stroke while fasting during the month of Ramadan when compared to the non-fasting months [18]. Another study concluded that fasting during Ramadan has no effect on stroke occurrence in the Isparta Province [19]. We prospectively studied the effect of fasting and its duration on the stroke frequency and type. Muslim patients who were admitted to the stroke unit, Department of Neurology, Mansoura University Hospitals, Mansoura, Egypt one month before, and during, Ramadan over two successive years: 2007 and 2008. The exact time of stroke onset in fasting patients was determined, as well as the time of the last meal before starting fasting from which we calculated the duration of fasting. Baseline laboratory investigations were done on admission and the type of stroke was ascertained based on clinical and computerised tomography brain scan results. As a result, 507 patients were studied. The age distribution of patients was not significantly different between the fasting and non-fasting group. There was no significant difference in the sex ratio, risk factors, NIHSS score and ratios of haemorrhagic and ischaemic stroke. There was no significant difference in the laboratory findings and no correlation between the duration of fasting and both frequency and type of stroke [20]. In the month before Ramadan, strokes most frequently occurred between 6:00 AM and noon; whereas the frequency was higher between noon and 6:00 PM during Ramadan [21].

One study reports that fasting increases the frequency of cerebral venous and sinus thrombosis, especially among those with hypercoagulable states and women who take oral contraceptive pills [22].

Vascular risk factors have been extensively studied during the month of Ramadan. There is an apparent protective effect in acute coronary syndrome associated with religious observance [23]. Religious activities may also have a protective role against cigarette smoking among Muslim college students [24]. A study showed a significant improvement after Ramadan in the 10 year coronary heart disease risk score and other cardiovascular risk factors such as lipids profile, systolic blood pressure, weight, body mass index and waist circumference in subjects with a previous history of cardiovascular disease [25]. The model of Ramadan fasting could be followed as a behaviour modification programme to control or prevent atherogenicity because of its positive impact on the lipid pattern, blood count and coagulation parameters [26]. Ramadan fasting leads to weight loss and fat-free mass reductions. Body composition changes vary depending on age and sex [27]. The possible consequences of the long intermittent fasting schedule during Ramadan on certain biochemical constituents or coagulation variables have been studied during the month of Ramadan and two months after. The values of apoprotein B, lipoprotein (a) and low-density lipoprotein cholesterol /high-density lipoprotein cholesterol ratio were significantly decreased during Ramadan, while total cholesterol, triglycerides, LDL-C, HDL-C and fasting blood glucose did not change during that month. Among coagulation and haematological factors, fibrinogen level and factor VII activity were significantly decreased during the month. These findings contribute to a better understanding of previous reports, as the metabolic and coagulation changes that are considered as atherosclerosis risk factors are counterbalanced during Ramadan [28]. In their study, Qujeq and colleagues suggest that potential usefulness of Ramadan fasting in the restriction of fat intake which is associated with further lowering of serum cholesterol [29]. It seems that the effect of Ramadan fasting on serum lipid levels may be closely related to the nutritional diet. For reduction of plasma lipid levels, it would be necessary to omit at least one term meal or reduce energy by 500 Kcal or more per day [30]. Significant improvements in HDL-C and LDL-C levels were observed even after four weeks post Ramadan. Ramadan-like fasting may be considered for more effective lipid and lipoprotein control [31].

Headaches and Fasting

Dalton et al. in 1975 reported that fasting was a trigger factor in 67 per cent of patients with headaches. This figure increased to 76 per cent when considering only patients aged 30 to 50, and was as high as 91 per cent in female patients undergoing hysterectomy [32].

Fasting headache was previously referred to as 'headache associated with metabolic or systemic disease' in the 1988 International Headache Classification [33] and then was reclassified in group 10 of ICHD-II as 'headache attributed to disorder of homeostasis'

[34]. Currently, the International Headache Society in its third edition (beta version) 2013, coded fasting headache in group 10.5 and considers the following diagnostic criteria:

Diagnostic Criteria

A Headache with at least one of the following characteristics and fulfilling criteria C and D:

 1 frontal location
 2 diffuse pain
 3 non-pulsating quality
 4 mild or moderate intensity

B The patient has fasted for >16 hours

C Headache develops during fasting

D Headache resolves within 72 hours after resumption of food intake

Headache with fasting is significantly more common in individuals with a prior history of headache. In these individuals, the headache may resemble 1.1 Migraine without aura. The likelihood of headache developing as a result of a fast increases with the duration of the fast. The headache associated with fasting does not appear to be related to duration of sleep, to caffeine withdrawal or to hypoglycaemia. Fasting headache can occur in the absence of hypoglycaemia; insulin-induced hypoglycaemia does not precipitate headache in migraine sufferers; and headache is not a complaint of patients presenting to the emergency department with symptomatic hypoglycaemia [35].

Fasting headache is common among secondary headaches, even though its pathogenesis is still unclear. The role of hypoglycaemia as a determinant factor in fasting headache is uncertain. Caffeine withdrawal may be a trigger factor although it is not recognised as such by all authors: the temporal pattern of caffeine-withdrawal headache is comparable to that of fasting headache, but fasting headache can also occur in individuals who do not normally consume caffeine [36]. Caffeine-withdrawal headache is coded independently from fasting headache and is included in group 8 (code 8.3.1) among the headaches attributed to substance withdrawal [35].

The suggestion that fasting headache might be caused by dehydration seems to have been excluded by Mosek during his studies of Yom Kippur fasting [36–37].

Physicians treating Muslim migraine patients should discuss potential Ramadan month exacerbation with their patients and provide counselling regarding the prevention of dehydration and caffeine withdrawal. Pharmacological prophylactic treatment should be considered [38]. Etoricoxib, a Cox-2 inhibitor with a 22-hour half-life, has been shown effective in preventing fasting headache when taken just prior to the 25-hour Yom Kippur fast and, prior to a 15-hour ritual fast, decreases incidence of and attenuates headache during the first five days of the month of Ramadan [39].

Epilepsy and Fasting

A common question from people with epilepsy and their families, approaching the sacred month of Ramadan, is how to manage their medication. Our recommendation is to prescribe a once-daily or twice-daily regimen to take just before dawn and when the fast is broken.

There is insufficient data regarding the effect of Ramadan fasting on seizures. Anecdotal reports and preclinical data showed improvement in seizure control with fasting.

The earliest reports of the effects of starvation on epilepsy date back to the fifth century when Hippocrates described a man whose seizures were cured by abstaining from all food and drink. The first reports in the medical literature were by Guelpa and Marie who described the effect of complete fasting on the cessation of seizures [40]. This was also subsequently reported again in 1921 by Geyelin, reporting that 20 out of 26 fasted patients had improved seizure control, two of whom remained seizure free for more than a year [41]. In another study, patients fasted for up to 25 days, reporting a 90 per cent success rate in children under the age of 10 years, decreasing with age to 50 per cent in adults [42]. In a recent study, six children attempted intermittent fasting. Seizure improvement (in the range of a 50–99 per cent reduction) was noted by four families. One patient's seizures improved only on fast days. One patient's family modified the intermittent fasting schedule to occur for 24 hours once per month, which led to a further decrease in seizure frequency [43]. The ketogenic diet has a limited place in the treatment of epilepsy, especially paediatric.

Only one study has reported an increase in seizure frequency during Ramadan. The most important reason for this was reduced efficacy of anticonvulsants because of their altered dosing. In the patients who received monotherapy and who did not change their drug regimes, the increase in seizure frequency may have been related to the changes in their daily rhythms, emotional stress and tiredness [44]. Lack of adherence with antiepileptic drugs during Ramadan may be hazardous to the patients. In a prospective study of burns in people with epilepsy in Saudi Arabia over a five year period, all burns were sustained during seizures; four of the 10 cases occurred during Ramadan. These four cases were females who did not take their anti-epileptic medications because they were fasting. The remaining six patients had stopped their medication for no specific reason and were not fasting at the time of the seizure [45].

Dosing schedules have to be altered during Ramadan. Drug doses can be taken only between sunset and dawn, and the time span between them is shorter than outside Ramadan. A study on the pharmacokinetics of valproic acid in healthy volunteers showed a significant decrease in the plasma elimination half-life of the 5:00 AM, and delayed absorption phase of the 8:00 PM dose, during Ramadan [46]. Another study showed no effect, on drug levels or seizure frequency, of redistributing the same total daily dose of carbamazepine to a twice-daily regime during Ramadan, compared to the normal three times daily regime [47].

Multiple Sclerosis and Fasting

Fasting during Ramadan does not have harmful effects on healthy immune systems [48]. It suppresses proinflammatory cytokine expression and decreases circulating levels of leukocytes [49]. Moreover, there is beneficial effect of fasting during Ramadan on neutrophil phagocytic function [50].

Fasting had no short-term unfavourable effects on the disease course in multiple sclerosis patients with mild disability [51]. In an Egyptian study, authors found no significant difference between both fasting and non-fasting patients regarding annualised relapsing rate, EDSS score and gadolinium enhanced lesions on MRI in a one year follow-up after Ramadan fasting [52]. However, many neurologists have noted that fasting (especially in summer) exacerbates some MS symptoms (fatigue, fatigue perception, dizziness, spasticity, cognitive problems, weakness, vision, balance, gait) which return to normal during feasting.

There is a consensus that fasting should be avoided by patients experiencing relapses or with significant disability (EDSS score ≥ 7). These data suggest that MS patients should have tailored care [53].

Sleep and Fasting

In addition to sudden shift in meal times, other factors may affect the sleep pattern and circadian rhythms during Ramadan [54]. A cross-sectional survey measuring self-reported sleep time and the Epworth Sleepiness Scale of observant Muslim medical students before, during and after Ramadan showed no significant variation in sleep score. Night sleep hours were significantly shorter, and daytime sleep longer, during Ramadan than before or afterwards [55]. Under controlled conditions of fixed light/dark exposure, caloric intake, sleep/wake schedule and sleep quality, Islamic intermittent fasting has no impact on drowsiness and vigilance as measured by the Johns Drowsiness Scale, total blink duration and mean reaction time [56]. There is a reduction in rapid eye movement sleep percentage during fasting. But there is no difference in sleep latency, non-rapid eye movement sleep percentage, arousal index and sleep efficiency [57]. Ramadan fasting did not change arousal, but the reaction time to an auditory stimulus increased during the Ramadan intermittent fasting. Both reaction amplitude and continuous attention also decreased in the fasting condition [58].

Conclusion

Ramadan fasting is safe for all healthy individuals. Previous studies have shown that there are no adverse effects of Ramadan fasting on heart, lung, liver, kidney, ocular, haematological and endocrine function. However, there is insufficient data regarding the effect of Ramadan fasting on the neurological conditions. The available research suggests that there is no direct negative effect of Ramadan fasting on common conditions such as stroke, headache and epilepsy; indeed there may even be beneficial effects through lowering vascular risk factors for instance. However, indirectly, Ramadan may lead to disease worsening through poor adherence with medication. The pre-Ramadan doctor–patient interview is an important opportunity to discuss the issues of fasting, medication dosing and the lifestyle changes especially regarding sleep, cigarette smoking and caffeine withdrawal.

References

1 Kerndt, P. R., J. L. Naughton, C. E. Driscoll and D. A. Loxterkamp. 1982. Fasting: the history, pathophysiology and complications. *Western Journal of Medicine* 137: 379–99.

2 Quran: Al-Baqarah, verse 183.

3 Bukhari and Muslim and others.

4 Sakr, A. H. 1975. Fasting in Islam. *Journal of the American Dietetic Association* 67: 17–21.

5 Sahih Bukhari vol. 3, no. 178.

6 Sahih Bukhari vol. 3, no. 146.

7 Sahih Muslim 1096 a, Book 13, Hadith 56. USC-MSA web (English) reference: Book 6, Hadith 2413.

8 Mohamed Baianonie, imam of the Islamic Center of Raleigh, NC, www.raleighmasjid.org/imam/fiqh-ramadan.html.

9 Aadil, N., I. E. Houti and S. Moussamih. 2004. Drug intake during Ramadan. *British Medical Journal* 329: 778–82.

10 Aslam, M., and M. A. Healy. 1986. Compliance and drug therapy in fasting Moslem patients. *Journal of Clinical and Hospital Pharmacy* 11: 321–5.

11 Aslam, M., and A. Assad. 1986. Drug regimens and fasting during Ramadan: a survey in Kuwait. *Public Health* 100: 49–53.

12 Zeeneldin, A. A., A. A. Gaber and F. M. Taha. 2012. Does fasting during Ramadan trigger non-adherence to oral hormonal therapy in breast cancer patients? *Journal of the Egyptian National Cancer Institute* 24: 133–7.

13 Recommendations of the 9th Fiqh-Medical seminar, 'An Islamic View of Certain Contemporary Medical Issues', Casablanca, Morocco, 14–17 June 1997, www.islamset.com/search/index.html.

14 Kumar, N., and S. Jivan. 2007. Ramadan and eyedrops: the Muslim perspective. *Ophthalmology* 114: 2356–60.

15 Kumar, N., S. Jivan and J. Buchan. 2008. Compliance with prescribed treatment during Ramadan. *Clinical and Experimental Ophthalmology* 36: 699.

16 Patel, T., A. Magdum and V. Ghura. 2012. Does fasting during Ramadan affect the use of topical dermatological treatment by Muslim patients in the UK? *Clinical and Experimental Dermatology* 37: 718–21.

17 Zabeen, B., S. Tayyeb, B. Benarjee, A. Baki, J. Nahar, F. Mohsin, N. Nahar and K. Azad. 2014. Fasting during Ramadan in adolescents with diabetes. *Indian Journal of Endocrinology and Metabolism* 18: 44–7.

18 Bener, A., A. Hamad, A. Fares, H. M. Al-Sayed and J. Al-Suwaidi. 2006. Is there any effect of Ramadan fasting on stroke incidence? *Singapore Medical Journal* 47: 404–8.

19 Akhan, G., S. Kutluhan and H. R. Koyuncuoglu. 2000. Is there any change of stroke incidence during Ramadan? *Acta Neurologica Scandinavica* 101: 259–61.

20 El-Mitwalli, A., A. A. Zaher, M. A. Mohamed and E. Elmenshawi. 2009. The effect of Ramadan fasting on cerebral stroke: a prospective hospital-based study. *European Journal of Neurology* 16, no. 4: e80.

21 El-Mitwalli, A., A. A. Zaher and E. El Menshawi. 2010. Circadian rhythm of stroke onset during the month of Ramadan. *Acta Neurologica Scandinavica* 122: 97–101.

22 Saadatnia, M., M. Zare, F. Fatehi and A. Ahmadi. 2009. The effect of fasting on cerebral venous and dural sinus thrombosis. *Neurology Research* 31: 794–8.

23 Burazeri, G., A. Goda and J. D. Kark. 2008. Religious observance and acute coronary syndrome in predominantly Muslim Albania: a population-based case-control study in Tirana. *Annals of Epidemiology* 18: 937–45.

24 Nakhaee, N., K. Divsalar and N. Jadidi. 2009. Religious involvement and cigarette smoking among Iranian university students. *International Journal of Psychiatry and Medicine* 39: 189–98.

25 Nematy, M., M. Alinezhad-Namaghi, M. M. Rashed, M. Mozhdehifard, S. S. Sajjadi, S. Akhlaghi, M. Sabery, S. A. Mohajeri, N. Shalaey, M. Moohebati and A. Norouzy. 2012. Effects of Ramadan fasting on cardiovascular risk factors: a prospective observational study. *Nutrition Journal* 11: 69.

26 Saleh, S. A., T. A. El-Kemery, K. A. Farrag, M. R. Badawy, N. N. Sarkis, F. S. Soliman and H. Mangoud. 2004. Ramadan fasting: relation to atherogenic risk among obese Muslims. *Journal of the Egyptian Public Health Association* 79: 461–83.

27 Norouzy, A., M. Salehi, E. Philippou, H. Arabi, F. Shiva, S. Mehrnoosh, S. M. Mohajeri, S. A. Mohajeri, A. Motaghedi Larijani and M. Nematy. 2013. Effect of fasting in Ramadan on body composition and nutritional intake: a prospective study. *Journal of Human Nutrition and Diet* 26, Suppl. 1: 97–104.

28 Sarraf-Zadegan, N., M. Atashi, G. A. Naderi, A. M. Baghai, S. Asgary, M. R. Fatehifar, H. Samarian and M. Zarei. 2000. The effect of fasting in Ramadan on the values and interrelations between biochemical, coagulation and hematological factors. *Annals of Saudi Medicine* 20: 377–81.

29 Qujeq, D., K. Bijani, K. Kalavi, J. Mohiti and H. Aliakbarpour. 2002. Effects of Ramadan fasting on serum low-density and

high-density lipoprotein-cholesterol concentrations. *Annals of Saudi Medicine* 22: 297–9.

30 Afrasiabi, A., S. Hassanzadeh, R. Sattarivand and S. Mahboob. 2003. Effects of Ramadan fasting on serum lipid profiles on 2 hyperlipidemic groups with or without diet pattern. *Saudi Medical Journal* 24: 23–6.

31 Shehab, A., A. Abdulle, A. El Issa, J. Al Suwaidi and N. Nagelkerke. 2012. Favorable changes in lipid profile: the effects of fasting after Ramadan. *PLoS One* 7, no. 10: e47615.

32 Dalton, K. 1975. Food intake prior to a migraine attack-study of 2313 spontaneous attack. *Headache* 15: 188–93.

33 Headache Classification Committee of the International Headache Classification. 1988. Classification and diagnostic criteria for headache disorders, cranial neuralgias and facial pain. *Cephalalgia* 8, Suppl. 7: 1–96.

34 Headache Classification Subcommittee of the International Headache Society. 2004. The International Classification of Headache Disorders. *Cephalalgia* 24, Suppl. 1: 1–160.

35 Headache Classification Committee of the International Headache Society. 2013. The International Classification of Headache Disorders, 3rd edition (beta version). *Cephalalgia* 33, no. 9: 629–808.

36 Mosek, A., and A. D. Korczyn. 1995. The Yom Kippur headache. *Neurology* 45: 1953–5.

37 Mosek, A., and A. D. Korczyn. 1999. Fasting headache, weight loss, and dehydration. *Headache* 39: 225–7.

38 Abu-Salameh, I., Y. Plakht and G. Ifergane. 2010. Migraine exacerbation during Ramadan fasting. *Journal of Headache Pain* 11: 513–17.

39 Drescher, M. J., Z. Wimpfheimer, S. Abu Khalef, A. Gammaitoni, N. Shehadeh and R. Torgovicky. 2012. Prophylactic etoricoxib is effective in preventing 'first of Ramadan' headache: a placebo-controlled double-blind and randomized trial of prophylactic etoricoxib for ritual fasting headache. *Headache* 52: 573–81.

40 Guelpa, G. M. A. 1911. La lutte contre l'epilepsie par la desintoxication et par la reducation alimentaire. *Revue Therapeutique Medica-Chirugie* 78: 8–13.

41 Geyelin, H. R. 1921. Fasting as a method for treating epilepsy. *Medical Record* 99: 1037–9.

42 Conklin, H. W. 1922. Cause and treatment of epilepsy. *American Journal of the Osteopathic Association* 26: 11–14.

43 Hartman, A. L., J. E. Rubenstein and E. H. Kossoff. 2013. Intermittent fasting: a 'new' historical strategy for controlling seizures? *Epilepsy Research* 104: 275–9.

44 Gomceli, Y. B., G. Kutlu, L. Cavdar and L. E. Inan. 2008. Does the seizure frequency increase in Ramadan? *Seizure* 17: 671–6.

45 Al-Qattan, M. M. 2000. Burns in epileptics in Saudi Arabia. *Burns* 26: 561–3.

46 Aadil, N., A. Fassi-Fihri, I. Houti, B. Benaji, M. Ouhakki, S. Kotbi, B. Diquet and F. Hakkou. 2000. Influence of Ramadan on the pharmacokinetics of a single oral dose of valproic acid administered at two different times. *Methods and Findings in Experimental and Clinical Pharmacology* 22: 109–14.

47 Khattab, E., I. H. Mahmood and E. T. Abdul-Jabbar. 2007. Can epileptic patients on carbamazepine safely fast Ramadan? *JIMA* 38486: 156–60.

48 Latifynia, A., M. Vojgani, T. Abofazeli and H. Jafarieh. 2007. Circulating immune complex during Ramadan. *Journal of Ayub Medical College Abbottabad* 19, no. 2: 15–18.

49 Faris, M. A., S. Kacimi, R. A. Al-Kurd, M. A. Fararjeh, Y. K. Bustanji, M. K. Mohammad and M. L. Salem. 2012. Intermittent fasting during Ramadan attenuates proinflammatory cytokines and immune cells in healthy subjects. *Nutrition Research* 32: 947–55.

50 Latifynia, A., M. Vojgani, M. J. Gharagozlou and R. Sharifian. 2009. Neutrophil function (innate immunity) during Ramadan. *Journal of Ayub Medical College Abbottabad* 21, no. 4: 111–15.

51 Saadatnia, M., M. Etemadifar, F. Fatehi, F. Ashtari, V. Shaygannejad, A. Chitsaz and A. H. Maghzi. 2009. Short-term effects of prolonged fasting on multiple sclerosis. *European Neurology* 61: 230–2.

52 Abdeldayem, S. M., and A. H. Hossam Zyton. 2012. The effect of Ramadan fasting on multiple sclerosis. *Egyptian Journal of Neurology, Psychiatry, and Neurosurgery* 494: 341–5.

53 Jahromi, S. R., M. A. Sahraian, F. Ashtari, H. Ayromlou, M. Etemadifar, M. Ghaffarpour, E. Mohammadianinejad, S. Nafissi, A. Nickseresht, V. Shaygannejad, M. Togha, H. R. Torabi and S. Ziaie. 2014. Islamic fasting and multiple sclerosis. *BMC Neurology* 14: 56.

54 Bahammam, A., M. Alrajeh, M. Albabtain, S. Bahammam and M. Sharif. 2010. Circadian pattern of sleep, energy expenditure, and body temperature of young healthy men during the intermittent fasting of Ramadan. *Appetite* 54: 426–9.

55 Margolis, S. A., and R. L. Reed. 2004. Effect of religious practices of Ramadan on sleep and perceived sleepiness of medical students. *Teaching and Learning in Medicine* 16: 145–9.

56 Bahammam, A. S., S. Nashwan, O. Hammad, M. M. Sharif and S. R. Pandi-Perumal. 2013. Objective assessment of drowsiness and reaction time during intermittent Ramadan fasting in young men: a case-crossover study. *Behavioral and Brain Functions* 9: 32.

57 Bahammam, A. S., K. Almushailhi, S. R. Pandi-Perumal and M. M. Sharif. 2014. Intermittent fasting during Ramadan: does it affect sleep? *Journal of Sleep Research* 23: 35–43.

58 Dolu, N., A. Yüksek, A. Sizer and M. Alay. 2007. Arousal and continuous attention during Ramadan intermittent fasting. *Journal of Basic and Clinical Physiology and Pharmacology* 18: 315–22.

59 Sahih Bukhari vol. 3, no. 127.

60 Herrag, M., S. Lahmiti and A. A. Yazidi. 2010. Ramadan: a different side of the emergencies? *African Health Sciences* 10: 215–16.

61 Koushali, A. N., Z. Hajiamini, A. Ebadi, N. Bayat and F. Khamseh. 2013. Effect of Ramadan fasting on emotional reactions in nurses. *Iranian Journal of Nursing and Midwifery Research* 18: 232–6.

II.I *Clinical Conditions*

Chapter 13

Autism and the Panoply of Religious Belief, Disbelief and Experience

Kelly Clark and Ingela Visuri*

While the cognitive mechanisms that incline us towards theistic belief in superhuman agents have been well documented over the past 30 years, unbelief has only recently begun to receive attention. Recent studies suggest that, just as with theistic belief, various psychological mechanisms and processes, such as a propensity for analytic thinking, might incline one towards unbelief. Moreover, it has been suggested that atheism and analytic thinking may both be mediated by constraints presented in autistic individuals (Caldwell-Harris 2012; Clark 2019). In this chapter, we will present and evaluate a few studies relating to both unbelief and autism and then consider some additional ideas that we hope will contribute to a fuller understanding of possible approaches to religion and spirituality in autistic individuals.[1]

It is argued in the cognitive science of religion (CSR) that certain cognitive faculties, dispositions and tendencies dispose us towards theistic beliefs and practices. From our Hypersensitive Agency Detecting Device (HADD), through theory of mind (ToM) (Barrett 2004), to Promiscuous Teleology (Kelemen and Rosset 2009), belief in gods is expected to be produced naturally (Bloom 2007; Tremlin 2006), automatically and easily in human beings (Clark and Barrett 2010). Just like the widespread occurrence of perceptual beliefs ('I see a car', 'It is cold') or memory beliefs ('I remember driving your Chevy on that snowy January morning'), the widespread occurrence of religious (and theistic) beliefs is expected to be underpinned by the normal operations of our properly functioning cognitive faculties.

Religious beliefs are therefore regarded as 'natural' both in the sense that they are easily acquired (typically without recourse to rational reflection or argument) and because they originate with little cultural input. Stewart Guthrie, for example, argues that when we see faces in the clouds or make a sudden reaction to sounds, we immediately and intuitively believe they caused by *someone*, rather than *something* (Guthrie 1993). With our natural inclination towards anthropomorphism, then, we are well on our way towards a natural disposition to religious beliefs in unseen or invisible agents (disembodied spirits from sacred trees to gods).

Such natural and automatic cognitive processes have been called, variously, intuitive, non-reflective, non-inferential, immediate and basic. Justin Barrett (2004), for instance, refers to reflective and non-reflective beliefs, the latter operating intuitively and

* We are grateful for helpful comments, criticisms and suggestions from Justin Barrett, Helen De Cruz and Melanie Nyhof.

[1] We acknowledge that 'religion' and 'spirituality' are not all about belief and meaning making but are multifaceted phenomena expressed variously in different contexts. 'Belief' in the theistic sense of an intuitive notion of superhuman agency and intentionality is, however, the theme explored in this chapter.

instantaneously, such as detecting faces, understanding laws of gravity or identifying agency and intentionality – in human as well as superhuman agents – in our environment. We will henceforth use the term 'intuitive' when referring to non-reflective or non-inferential beliefs, in line with Sperber's (1997) definition.

Focus in this chapter will largely remain on the attribution of agency and intentionality as intuitive beliefs. Lee A. Kirkpatrick (2013) notes, in reference to Guthrie (1993), that belief in superhuman agents is spontaneous and effortless due to the adaptive costs of *not* detecting agency and intentionality: mistaking a stick for a snake is less bad than mistaking a snake for a stick. It therefore takes motivation – and effort – to override such intuitive assumptions: 'Indeed, this view suggests that what requires motivation is activation of alternative psychological systems that raise doubts about our initial perceptions, which, based on additional information, may (or may not) override them'[2] (Kirkpatrick 2013, 131).

In comparison to intuitive beliefs, the acquisition of reflective beliefs is conscious and slower, such as what we find in scientific or theological reasoning. The beliefs that one needs reasoning to acquire have been called, variously, analytic, reflective, inferential, mediate and non-basic. Again, for sake of consistency and convenience, we will call such beliefs 'analytic'. Todd Tremlin (2005) argues that such a dual-process model – intuitively and analytically acquired – is helpful in explaining how people react to information, such as official sets of belief versus 'popular' (and often contradictory) notions, similar to Barrett's discussion on theological correctness (Barrett 1999).[3] Indeed, people may be incoherent in what they report (not believing in life after death) and how they act (talking to a beloved one when visiting his/her grave).

As discussed by Pennycook et al. in Chapter 11, scholars within CSR have argued that religious belief is correlated with more intuitive thinking styles, while unbelief is correlated with more analytic thinking styles (Caldwell-Harris 2012; Gervais and Norenzayan 2012).[4] We will look further into these suggestions, proposing that such correlations indicate more complex psychological tendencies.

Atheism and Analytic Thinking

In order to illustrate the suggested correlation between cognitive style and theistic beliefs, we will depart from Will M. Gervais and Ara Norenzayan's (2012) study 'Analytic Thinking Promotes Religious Disbelief', which offers a representative argument in the field. The authors argue that atheism is associated with analytic thinking whereas religious believers are more likely intuitive thinkers.[5] Drawing on a sample of undergraduate students at the

---

2 Kirkpatrick (2013) emphasises that such an approach does not address the ontological question whether such beliefs are true, or not.

3 Similarly, we are cognitively disposed towards folk physics, perceiving among other things that the world is flat (due to visual illusion). It therefore takes some reflection to move us to the view that the world is round. If we are, by nature, 'folk theists', moving from religious belief to unbelief may involve conscious reflection.

4 Nothing in these accounts precludes such intuitions being overridden. The formation of religious beliefs may also rely on reflective *choices*.

5 We note that complex terms such as atheism and belief need to be discussed more in depth, specifically since many individuals claiming to be 'atheists' may harbour beliefs in other superhuman agents (such as ghosts or spirits). In the studies on 'religious belief' referred to here, however, the underlying notion is that atheism equals disbelief in a personal God, which is characteristic for the Abrahamic traditions but excludes many other traditions that could be defined as religious or

University of British Columbia, Gervais and Norenzayan offered a Cognitive Reflection Test (CRT) to determine their effect on religious belief. The authors hypothesised that analytic thinking would elicit an override of the more natural and intuitive cognitive inclinations towards religious belief. In the first study, they offered three problems (Cognitive Reflector Tests). Understanding their study will prove easier if you take the time to determine your own responses to the problems before proceeding to the analysis. The problems are as follows:

1 A bat and a ball cost $1.10 in total. The bat costs $1.00 more than the ball. How much does the ball cost? ____cents
2 If it takes 5 machines 5 min to make 5 widgets, how long would it take 100 machines to make 100 widgets? _____minutes
3 In a lake, there is a patch of lily pads. Every day, the patch doubles in size. If it takes 48 days for the patch to cover the entire lake, how long would it take for the patch to cover half of the lake? _____days

In each case, the quick and easy intuitive response is incorrect while the more deliberate analytic response is correct.[6]

Upon completion of this test, participants completed three different measures – intrinsic religiosity (IR), intuitive religious belief (IRB), belief in supernatural agents (BSA) – of religious belief, which included such statements as:

> My faith involves all of my life (IR)
> In my life I feel the presence of the Divine (IR)
> It doesn't matter as much what I believe as long as I lead a moral life (IR)
> One should seek God's guidance when making every important decision (IR)
> I believe in God (IRB)
> When I am in trouble, I find myself wanting to ask God for help (IRB)
> I just don't understand religion (IRB)
> God exists (BSA)
> The devil exists (BSA)
> Angels exist (BSA)

Success on the CRT was negatively correlated with affirmations of religious belief; analytic thinking was negatively correlated with religious belief. Gervais and Norenzayan concluded, '(t)his result demonstrated that ... the tendency to analytically override intuitions in reasoning was associated with religious disbelief' (Gervais and Norenzayan 2012).

While the results appear to be significant, the validity of Gervais and Norenzayan's study prompts a number of critical questions. Beginning with the sampling, 62 per cent of the participants were Asians and the vast majority of them were from China (or recent Chinese immigrants).[7] Given Chinese cultural biases against religious belief, the decrease in religious belief among the analytic thinkers could be attributed to cultural bias, not superiority in

---

spiritual. There is likewise evidence of other types of atheism: *apatheism* and *inCREDulous atheism* (see Noranzayan and Gervais 2013).

6 The quick and easy intuitive yet wrong response to (1) is 10, while the correct analytic, deliberate answer is 5; to (2) is 100, while the analytic answer is 5; and to (3) is 24, while the analytic is 47.

7 More than half of UBC's first-year students are not native English speakers; http://fullcomment.nationalpost.com/2010/11/24/tony-keller-finding-the-white-students-on-campus-is-easy-wheres-the-pub/.

reasoning. Cultural biases are also implicit in their measures of intrinsic religiosity, which measures Christian – or at least theistic – features such as faith, angels and the devil. Animism, which also involves invisible agency, would for instance not correspond to the 'religious' questions; practitioners in new spiritual movements might thus not be identified as religious. The question of what this study actually measures remains unresolved.

The second part of the study involves a series of unconscious prompts designed to elicit analytic thinking. Let us consider just one, the art prime.[8] Participants in the control group stared at a 'neutral' image such as *The Discobulos* whereas the remainder were primed by staring at *The Thinker* (an 'artwork depicting a reflective thinking pose'), as an unconscious analytic prime. The subjects then completed the same measures of belief (IR, IRB, BSA). Gervais and Norenzayan conclude that these studies jointly reinforce the hypothesis that analytic processing decreases religious belief: 'viewing *The Thinker* significantly promoted religious disbelief'. The results of these studies are however mixed; some differences between the control and the prime groups are only modestly significant; the authors concede alternative explanations; and the problems of randomness raised previously persist here as well.

Nonetheless, Gervais and Norenzayan conclude:

> All of the manipulations used in studies 2 to 5 plausibly produce multiple effects, and any specific finding in a given study may be open to alternative explanations and should be interpreted with caution. However, across all studies, it is difficult to think of a broad alternative explanation that could parsimoniously explain why analytically overriding intuitive answers, visual exposure to a thinking pose, implicit priming of analytic thinking concepts, and perceptual disfluency all converge on promoting religious disbelief. By contrast, the hypothesis that analytic processing – which empirically underlies all experimental manipulations – promotes religious disbelief explains all of these findings in a single framework that is well supported by existing theory regarding the cognitive foundations of religious belief and disbelief.

In other words, analytic processes are expected to trump/correct/erode/block intuitively and uncritically assumed religious beliefs.[9]

Atheism may, however, also emerge when one's natural cognitive faculties are subjected to criticism by or overruled by reflective thinking; one may give up belief in God, for example, after careful consideration of the problem of evil. Modern science emerged when the science most naturally conducive to our cognitive faculties – so-called folk physics – was overruled by an enormous amount of reflective thinking during the scientific revolution and after. Analytic thinking may thus be involved in the overriding of one's more natural or intuitive beliefs.

Yet the correlation between atheism and analytic thinking does not prove that reflective thought, in every or even most cases, mediates unbelief. It has also been suggested that unbelief and analytic thinking are not directly connected but are mediated by a common,

[8] The other studies involved implicit primes and disfluency primes. Implicit primes involved arranging words into sentences with the prime group given thinking terms (reason, analyse, ponder etc.), while the control group was given unrelated words (hammer, shoe, jump etc.). Disfluency primes involved the use of fuzzy font (prime sample font) versus a large clear font (control sample font). The claim is that having to figure out a fuzzy font engages analytic thinking in a way not required of reading a clear font.

[9] The Thinker/Discobulous results failed to replicate in Sanchez et al. (2017) and in Farias et al. (2017). While this particular study failed, Pennycook et al.'s (2016) meta-analysis found a correlation between analytical or reflective thinking, on the one hand, and atheism or agnosticism, on the other. Gervais et al. (2018) disclaims his own findings.

underlying cause. In the next section, we will explore the suggestion that autism, in some cases, mediates both atheism and analytic thinking.

Atheism and Autism

Autism has been described as a neuropsychiatric condition involving a spectrum of cognitive capacities. The first of the diagnostic criteria in the DSM 5 (American Psychiatric Association 2013) acknowledges difficulties in social and non-verbal communication (e.g. interpreting body language and facial expressions), and understanding linguistic ambiguities (e.g. metaphors).[10] Simon Baron-Cohen's (1995) term *mind-blindness* has often been used to describe the inability to 'mind read' what other people believe, feel or desire.[11] Conversely, non-autistic people are typically intuitive mind readers, attributing beliefs, feelings and desires to human agents rather successfully.

The ability to mentalise facilitates an understanding of another person's beliefs, desires and intentions, and so facilitates responding to other persons appropriately; as mentioned above, this ability is also identified as the basic tool for attributing agency and intentionality also to gods, spirits and other invisible existences (Barrett 2004). Since a properly functioning ToM is expected to underpin theistic belief, it has been argued that its malfunction may preclude believing in a personal God. Scholars have therefore suggested that God, conceived of as a person, may prove inconceivable to an individual with autism (Barrett 2012; Bering 2002; McCauley 2012; Tremlin 2006).

This argument is moreover underpinned by an expectation that high functioning autistic individuals may have a) higher IQs and b) more inferential thinking styles than non-autistic individuals, and autism may thus provide the common ground between these two. It has also been suggested that analytical thinking in autistic individuals would make them more prone to think in terms of folk physics, rather than folk psychology (Bering 2002; Heywood 2010). Empirical attempts at verifying the correlation between autism and non-belief have however generated mixed results (for a detailed discussion, see Lindeman and Lipsanen 2016; Reddish et al. 2016), and replications have failed (Jack et al. 2016; Maij et al. 2017).

In the following section, we will analyse the role of intuitive and reflective cognitive processing in the formation of theistic beliefs, and suggest alternative approaches to understanding the relation between autistic cognition and belief in supernatural, invisible agents.

---

10 The *Diagnostic and Statistic Manual of Mental Disorders*, vol. 5 (2013). The autism spectrum was earlier formulated as four separate diagnoses in the DSM IV: *autistic disorder*, *Asperger's disorder* (often referred to as Asperger's syndrome, or AS), *childhood disintegrative disorder* and *pervasive developmental disorder otherwise not specified*. These were replaced by *autism spectrum disorder* (ASD), an umbrella term which is supposed to include all the earlier diagnoses, from mild to severe symptoms. Naming autism a *disorder* has been understood as pejorative, especially within the autism community, and is occasionally replaced by the term *autism spectrum condition* (ASC), also in this text. There is also a move towards talking of *autisms* in the plural, acknowledging the fact that individuals develop very differently.

11 To avoid the misconception that individuals on the spectrum lack empathy, it is important to note that scholars expect affective empathy to be well functioning, or possibly even heightened, in autistic individuals (Smith 2009). Bird and Cook (2013) therefore suggest that emotional 'blindness' in some individuals may in fact be due to alexithymia rather than being a primary feature of autism.

Complicating the Picture

Attribution of Intentionality

Bering (2002) has hypothesised that ToM deficits in autism would limit reasoning on *why* things happen (i.e. attributing agency to a force that lies behind a certain event, such as a car crash being meant to teach one about the value of life). He therefore suggests that rather than being natural experts in 'folk psychology', individuals with autism are more likely to master 'folk physics' (i.e. attending to *how* things happen, rather than *why*). They would thus not ascribe meaning to life events to the same extent as non-autistic individuals.[12]

Exploring such teleological thinking, Heywood compared autistic and non-autistic individuals stating that they are either theists or atheists (Heywood 2010; Heywood and Bering 2013).[13] Drawing on Jesse Bering's (2002) *Existential Theory of Mind*, Heywood describes teleological thinking as an over-attribution of intentional causation, such as a certain page 'being meant' to open up when a book falls to the floor. In the study, theists indeed gave more teleological responses than atheists when describing autobiographical memories, while participants on the autism spectrum showed a decrease in both teleological *and* anti-teleological reasoning. Heywood concludes that a typical socio-cognitive development would support an implicit bias to reason teleologically – regardless of religious affiliation – while mentalising constraints would affect such tendencies negatively.[14]

The picture may however be more complex than that. As Bering predicts, the autistic participants in Ingela Visuri's (2012) study were eager to discuss physical causality, but rather than dismissing religious and spiritual phenomena, their reasoning aimed at understanding and supporting such claims, for example regarding Noah's ark and reincarnation. This result is in line with Dubin and Graetz's (2009) proposal that individuals on the autism spectrum may have a capacity for *logical creativity* or *a stereoscopical view on the world* (Visuri 2012), fusing scientific and religious reasoning. Put differently, analytical deliberations may contribute to *both* theistic belief and unbelief. A limited tendency for teleological reasoning – combined with a propensity for folk physics – does not automatically incline one towards unbelief.

The same result is found in another study (Visuri 2018) in which the autistic participants describe how ideas on agency and intentionality gradually grow forth, as a consequence of deliberation and reflection: feelings of doing what is morally right grow into notions of God communicating through the body, and the sensation of present but invisible bodies is formed into ideas on intentional spirits and ancestors. In other words, intuitive mentalising abilities are not the sole path to supernatural anthropomorphic interpretations of the world.

---

[12] Bering's EToM overlaps with Barrett's HADD (categoriser, describer and facilitator) in detecting agency and attributing intentionality to a superhuman power.

[13] Heywood notes that in this context, atheism is 'used to describe individuals who profess a broad lack of belief in the supernatural (i.e. Gods, ghosts, souls, afterlives etc.), regardless of the specific term those individuals may select for themselves' (14). When asked for belief in a soul, spiritual force or god(s), 59.2 per cent of the participants reported being atheist or agnostic, and 40.7 per cent reported being theistic believers.

[14] Interestingly, Heywood hypothesises that schizophrenia would affect individuals to over-attribute meaning to life events excessively, thinking that most events are caused in relation to themselves.

Invisible Friendships

It is interesting to note that many children and teenagers on the autism spectrum have imaginary friends (Attwood 2007; Calver 2009; Davis et al. 2018). These appear to function as a coping strategy to compensate for and complement real-life interaction, and provide a safe place to withdraw to in turmoil (Visuri, 2019). Wigger et al. (2013, 12) conclude that, possibly, 'intense imaginative play serves a role, helping children sort out various kinds of agency, knowledge, and perspectives, including those attributed to God'.

While Wigger and colleagues argue that the subjective experience of God is qualitatively different from imaginary friends, Tanya Luhrmann (2012, 100) maintains that God is also treated in terms of pretence and play: 'When you sit on a park bench and imagine God's arms around your shoulders, God is real in a different way than either the bench or a daydream'. Luhrmann thus argues that relations with supernatural agents are treated differently to relations to other humans, and rather make out a unique, epistemological category; much like Winnicott's (1971) discussion on *intermediate areas of experiencing.*

The formation of non-empirical relations in autism may be better understood by rethinking 'beliefs' in experiential, rather than ontological terms. Such a change of perspectives relates directly to the previous discussion on the relation between analytic thinking and supernatural notions: 'beliefs' are not necessarily made up of statements of what is true or not, but operate on a different level. This experiential aspect (i.e. feeling God's presence or arm around one's shoulder) needs to be addressed when measuring beliefs, on as well as off the autism spectrum. The questions we ask affect the results we get.

Embodied Dimensions of Social Cognition

While the guidelines for autism diagnostics in the DSM 5 (American Psychiatric Association 2013) include social difficulties, it is not clear where these stem from. The mirror neuron-hypothesis of autism, which suggests that the ability to 'mirror' others is broken on a neuronal level, is for instance challenged by scholars who hold that mind reading difficulties are related to sensory difficulties. Attribution of stimuli from multiple modalities (e.g. visual, auditive, olfactory) appears to be desynchronised, which makes integration of facial expressions, body language and vocal expressions difficult for autistic individuals (Brock et al. 2002; Foss-Feig et al. 2010). This is likely also why autistic individuals often prefer communication online to interaction face-to-face (Davidson and Orsini 2013).

Interaction with invisible agents is another example of disembodied communication, and also has the benefit of not requiring instant responses, which makes processing of their 'minds' less constraining for autistic individuals. It has accordingly been suggested that 'contrary to popular notions that individuals on the autism spectrum will find mental representations of superhuman agents perplexing, the participants in this case study describe such bodiless agents as predictable, emotionally coherent, and benevolent' (Visuri 2018, 26). Mind reading difficulties in autism should thus not be generalised to all kinds of agents, but may differ depending on who the agent is and how the communication is achieved.

Conclusion

The arguments put forward in this chapter do not imply that autistic individuals would be more or less prone to embrace invisible agents. We rather argue that there are more than two sides to the coin, and nuances appear when expanding the conceptualisation of 'religion' as well as 'autism'. The brain is complex. We have only begun to plumb its depths. Human culture is likewise vast and mysterious, and reducing cognitive functioning to fixed brain processes *inside* people means neglecting that which takes place *between* people. Outer impact changes our inner worlds. Theistic belief and unbelief are thus likely the result of both complex cognitive processes and cultural influences. Determining, in any particular case, the precise influences on anyone's religious belief or unbelief is, at least for now, impossible.

With respect to the rationality of atheism and agnosticism, Norenzayan, Gervais and Trzeniewski offer wise counsel: 'We emphasize that our data do not suggest that disbelief solely arises through mentalizing deficits; multiple psychological and socio-cultural pathways likely lead to a complex and overdetermined phenomenon such as disbelief in God'. This is surely the conclusion to be drawn, in the study of autistic as well as non-autistic cognition.

References

American Psychiatric Association. 2013. *Diagnostic and Statistic Manual of Mental Disorders*. 5th edn. Arlington, VA: American Psychiatric Publishing.

Attwood, T. 2007. *The Complete Guide to Asperger's Syndrome*. London: Jessica Kingsley.

Baron-Cohen, S. 1995. *Mindblindness: An Essay on Autism and Theory of Mind*. Cambridge, MA: MIT Press.

Barrett, J. 1999. Theological correctness: Cognitive constraint and the study of religion. *Method and Theory in the Study of Religion* 11: 325–39.

Barrett, J. 2004. *Why Would Anyone Believe in God?* Lanham, MD: AltaMira.

Barrett, J. 2012. *Born Believers: The Science of Children's Religious Beliefs*. New York: Free Press.

Bering, J. 2002. The existential theory of mind. *Review of General Psychology* 6: 3–24.

Bird, G., and R. Cook. 2013. Mixed emotions: the contribution of alexithymia to emotional symptoms of autism. *Translational Psychiatry* 3: 1–8.

Bloom, P. 2007. Religion is natural. *Developmental Science* 10: 147–51.

Brock, J., C. B. Brown, J. Boucher and G. Rippon. 2002. The temporal binding deficit hypothesis of autism. *Development and Psychopathology* 14: 209–24.

Caldwell-Harris, C. 2012. Understanding atheism/non-belief as an expected individual-differences variable. *Religion, Brain, and Behavior* 2: 4–47.

Calver, A. 2009. The unicorn who came to stay and other stories: mothers' experiences of having a child with autism with an imaginary friend. Doctoral dissertation, University of London.

Clark, K. J. 2019. *God and the Brain*. Grand Rapids, MI: Eerdmans.

Clark, K. J., and J. Barrett. 2010. Reformed epistemology and the cognitive science of religion. *Faith and Philosophy* 27: 174–89.

Davidson, J., and M. Orsini. 2013. The shifting horizons of autism online. In *Worlds of Autism: Across the Spectrum of Neurological Difference*, ed. Davidson Joyce Orsini Michael, 285–303. Minneapolis: University of Minnesota Press.

Davis, P. E., H. Simon, E. Meins and D. L. Robin. 2018. Imaginary companions in children with autism spectrum disorder. *Journal of Autism and Developmental Disorders* 48: 1–10. http://csjarchive.cogsci.rpi.edu/proceedings/2011/papers/0782/paper0782.pdf.

Dubin, N., and J. E. Graetz. 2009. Through a different lens: spirituality in the lives of individuals with Asperger's syndrome. *Journal of Religion, Disability, and Health* 13: 29–39.

Farias, M., V. van Mulukom, G. Kahane, U. Kreplin, A. Joyce, P. Soares, L. Oviedo, M. Hernu, K. Rokita, J. Savulescu, R. Mottonen. 2017. Supernatural belief is not modulated by intuitive thinking style or cognitive inhibition. *Scientific Reports*. 7. 10.1038/s41598-017-14090-9.

Foss-Feig, J. H., L. D. Kwakye, C. J. Cascio, C. P. Burnette, H. Kadivar, W. L. Stone and M. T. Wallace. 2010. An extended multisensory temporal binding window in autism spectrum disorders. *Experimental Brain Research* 203: 381–9.

Gervais, W. M., and A. Norenzayan. 2012. Analytic thinking promotes religious disbelief. *Science* 336: 493–6.

Gervais, W. M., M. Van Elk, D. Xygalatas, R. McKay, M. Aveyard, E. Buchtel, I. Dar-Nimrod, E. Kundtová Klocová, J. Ramsay, T. Riekki, A. Svedholm-Häkkinen, J. Bulbulia. 2018. Analytic atheism: A cross-culturally weak and fickle phenomenon? *Judgment and Decision Making* 13, no. 3, May 2018: 268–74.

Guthrie, S. 1993. *Faces in the Clouds: A New Theory of Religion*. New York: Oxford University Press.

Heywood, B. T. 2010. Meant to be: how religious beliefs, cultural religiosity, and impaired theory of mind affect the implicit bias to think teleologically. Doctoral dissertation, Queens University, Belfast.

Heywood, B. T., and J. M. Bering. 2013. Meant to be: how religious beliefs and cultural religiosity affect the implicit bias to think teleologically. *Religion, Brain, and Behavior* 41: 183–201.

Jack, A. I., J. P. Friedman, R. E. Boyatzis and S. N. Taylor. 2016. Why do you believe in God? Relationships between religious belief, analytic thinking, mentalizing and moral concern. *PloS ONE* 11, no. 3: e0149989.

Kelemen, D., and E. Rosset. 2009. The human function compunction: teleological explanation in adults. *Cognition* 111: 138–43.

Kirkpatrick, L. A. 2013. Evolutionary psychology as a foundation for the psychology of religion. In *The Psychology of Religion: A Multidisciplinary Approach*, ed. R. Paloutzian and C. Park, 118–37. New York: Guilford Press.

Lindeman, M., and J. Lipsanen. 2016. Diverse cognitive profiles of religious believers and nonbelievers. *International Journal for the Psychology of Religion* 26, no. 3: 1–8.

Luhrmann, T. 2012. *When God Talks Back: Understanding the American, Evangelical Relationship with God*. New York: Vintage Books.

Maij, D. L. R., F. van Harreveld, W. Gervais, Y. Schrag, C. Mohr and M. van Elk. 2017. Mentalizing skills do not differentiate believers from non-believers but credibility enhancing displays do. *PLoS ONE* 12, no. 8: e0182764.

McCauley, R. N. 2012. *Why Religion Is Natural and Science Is Not*. Oxford: Oxford University Press.

Noranzayan, A., and W. M. Gervais. 2013. The origins of religious disbelief. *Trends in Cognitive Sciences* 17: 20–5.

Pennycook, G., R. M. Ross, D. J. Koehler and J. A. Fugelsang. 2016. Atheists and agnostics are more reflective than religious believers: four empirical studies and a meta-analysis. *PLoS ONE* 11: 1–18.

Reddish, P., P. Tok and R. Kundt. 2016. Religious cognition and behaviour in autism: the role of mentalizing. *International Journal for the Psychology of Religion* 26: 95–112.

Sanchez, S., B. Sundermeier, K. Gray and R. Calin-Jagemanl. 2017. Direct replication of Gervais & Norenzayan (2012): no evidence that analytic thinking decreases religious belief. *Plos ONE* 12, no. 2: e0172636.

Smith, A. 2009. Emotional empathy in autism spectrum conditions: Weak, intact, or heightened? *Journal of Autism and Developmental Disorders* 39: 1747–8.

Sperber, D. 1997. Intuitive and reflected beliefs. *Mind and Language* 12: 67–83.

Tremlin, T. 2005. Divergent religion: a dual-process model of religious thought, behavior, and morphology. In *Mind and Religion: Psychological and Cognitive Foundations of Religiosity*, ed. H. Whitehouse and R. N. McCauley, 69–84. Walnut Creek, CA: AltaMira Press.

Tremlin, T. 2006. *Minds and Gods: The Cognitive Foundations of Religion*. New York: Oxford University Press.

Visuri, I. 2012. Could everyone talk to God? A case study on Asperger's syndrome, religion and spirituality. *Journal of Religion, Health, and Disability* 16: 352–78.

Visuri, I. 2018. Rethinking autism, theism and atheism: bodiless agents and imaginary realities. *Archive for the Psychology of Religion* 1: 1–31.

Visuri, I. 2019. Sensory supernatural experiences in autism. *Religion, Brain, and Behavior.* Published online. doi:10.1080/2153599X.2018.1548374.

Visuri, I. 2019, in press. A room of one's own: autistic imagination as a stage for parasocial interaction and social learning. *Journal for the Cognitive Science of Religion.*

Wigger, J. B., K. Paxson and L. Ryan. 2013. What do invisible friends know? Imaginary companions, God, and theory of mind. *International Journal for the Psychology of Religion* 23: 2–14.

Winnicott, D. 1971. *Playing and Reality.* London: Tavistock.

Chapter 14

II.I *Clinical Conditions*

Personhood and Religion in People with Dementia

Julian Hughes*

It might seem natural to start with the assumption that everyone knows these days what dementia is. It is all around us as our populations age. Nevertheless, I shall start by setting out some basic facts about dementia. I do this not solely because there may be some who read this book without clear understanding of the medical facts about dementia, but also because the definition of 'dementia' is problematic. It is interesting to consider, albeit briefly, the implications of this problem, because I think they point us in two directions: towards the recognition of difference and the importance of the individual; and towards an understanding of the relevance of context. I shall then consider some of the literature that describes the neuroanatomical basis of syndromes associated with religion in the context of dementia. This neurological understanding of religion in dementia has to be set alongside the religious experience of living or working with dementia, which I shall discuss in the third section of the chapter. In the fourth, I shall suggest that some linkage between the neurological and experiential accounts of dementia might be found by considering lucid episodes, which raise profound questions about meaning and selfhood. This will lead me, in the fifth section, to discuss the importance of meaning and the broad view of personhood which can be derived from our account of meaning. In the final section, I shall discuss the implications of such a view for our understanding of religion and dementia.

Reflection on the nature of dementia for individuals leads us to consider some important facts of religious life: the role of context and meaning; the importance of coherence in terms of our general ways of living in the world; and the importance of relationships, which are essential to our being. If religion reflects, or is a manifestation of, social activity, so too dementia is a social condition, one which affects not just memory but also language and thus impedes our relationships. How do we think of religion, then, on the basis of reflections on dementia as a neurological condition? We must think of context and meaning, which imply both the given and the other. The given is the world in which we live, with all its variety and complexity; the other reflects our awareness at some level that none of this needed to exist at all.

* As well as being indebted to all those who attended and contributed to the stimulating and convivial workshop held at the Møller Centre in Churchill College, Cambridge, in September 2013, I am particularly indebted to the Reverend Dr. Alasdair Coles for initiating the event and this book. I am grateful to Dr. Kelly Clark and to the Reverend Dr. Joanna Collicutt for highlighting particular papers, which have proved useful; and especially to Dr. Clark for his very helpful criticisms of my ideas. The deficiencies in the chapter remain solely mine.

What Is Dementia Anyway?

Dementia is broadly defined as an acquired, chronic and usually progressive, global impairment of cognitive function. This defines a syndrome, that is, a collection of symptoms and signs that tend to go together, but in the case of dementia there is a huge variety of potential causes. Cognitive functions include all of the higher brain functions supporting memory, language, understanding, concentration, calculating, abstract thinking, recognition, planning and so forth. Dementia is 'acquired' in that it is not present at birth but comes on later in life. It can start surprisingly early, say in the person's 30s, but becomes more common with ageing. Dementia is 'global' because impairment in a single cognitive function (only a little bit of forgetfulness for instance) is not enough. Different centres of the brain must be damaged by the disease so that different cognitive functions are impaired. Dementia is 'chronic' in that it is not something that has only been present for a few days. Alternatively, an 'acute' confusion – a delirium – suggests a cause of confusion that, even if profound, is usually transient, such as an infection, some other illness or a problem with medication. Whereas treatment of the underlying condition will usually settle delirium, in dementia there is usually no cure for the underlying cause.

There are many diseases which cause dementia [1]. I shall briefly sketch the common four conditions that account for dementia in older people.

Alzheimer's disease is the archetypal dementia. There is loss of memory over years, which gradually worsens to include not just memory of recent events, but also memory of more distant events, as well as memory for words and meaning. As the condition progresses the person is unable to do things he or she previously undertook with ease. Practical abilities increasingly decline. In the more severe stages the person can exhibit very profound losses of memory, perhaps not recalling family members. In the end there is obvious physical deterioration, with loss of mobility, incontinence of urine and faeces, total dependence on others for personal care, with poor swallowing and increased susceptibility to infection. It is in the advanced stages of any dementia that family carers often say they feel they have lost the person they knew.

In Alzheimer's dementia, again as in other types, there can be behaviour which is found challenging, from shouting to agitation and aggression, or wandering, disinhibition and so on. However, before we regard a behaviour as indicative of brain pathology, we need to understand it; for example, 'wandering' refers to a variety of behaviours, some of which might make perfect sense given the circumstances. Other psychological and physical disturbances, such as hallucinations or seizures, can also occur. Whilst many of these symptoms and signs are common to all dementias, it is the pattern of onset that often helps to differentiate the particular types.

The pathology of Alzheimer's disease includes the deposition of amyloid, a protein, in microscopic plaques and the formation of neurofibrillary tangles within the cells, with loss of cholinergic pathways (i.e. those areas in the brain that use the neurotransmitter acetylcholine) and generalised brain shrinkage, or atrophy, caused by cell death. Initially this is more prominent in the hippocampus, the structure in the medial temporal lobe most closely associated with recall memory. In addition to plaques and tangles, there is also damage to blood vessels.

If Alzheimer's disease accounts for most cases of dementia (about 50 per cent), the next most common type is probably vascular dementia where damage to blood vessels is the prominent pathological feature. The typical history for the person with vascular dementia, therefore, is the history of the vascular disease. The person might have a sudden large stroke in which a significant area of the brain is damaged. Perhaps the individual is then left with profound language problems, but is still able to remember things reasonably, even if there are other deficits. In an alternative scenario, the blood vessel damage reflects the accumulation of multiple, small strokes, or even just poor blood flow (ischaemia), so that the onset of symptoms and signs is more gradual, but seems to be stepwise rather than a steady decline. There remains the possibility that some areas of function are better preserved. For instance, often these people have more insight into what is occurring and, perhaps for this reason, there is a higher prevalence of depression in people with vascular dementia. Many people will have a mixture of Alzheimer's and vascular dementia.

The prevalence of dementia with Lewy bodies (DLB) has been disputed, but it is not uncommon. The finding of Lewy bodies gives the diagnosis. In their classical form, these are intracellular (cytoplasmic) inclusion bodies. In DLB they are found not just in the subcortical nuclei (e.g. in the substantia nigra), as in Parkinson's disease, but diffusely in the neocortex. DLB thus affects the areas of the brain associated with (higher) cognitive function rather than only with movement and co-ordination. The hallmarks of DLB are fluctuating cognitive dysfunction (often affecting visuospatial function rather than memory), striking visual hallucinations (often involving small animals or children), parkinsonism and disturbed sleep in which people act out their dreams (a condition known as rapid eye movement (REM) sleep disorder). The condition can be associated with falls, other types of psychotic phenomena (i.e. delusions and hallucinations) and severe sensitivity to neuroleptic medication (i.e. antipsychotics).

Frontotemporal lobar degeneration is the fourth most common type of dementia, although its prevalence as a cause of dementia is low. It is somewhat more common in people who have early-onset dementia, that is dementia before the age of 65 years. It can take various forms, depending on whether it affects the frontal lobe or the temporal lobe more, so the symptoms and signs vary from language (semantic) problems to changes in personality. Stories around those with frontal lobe problems are often striking because of the changes in behaviour, which affect personality and can cause a lack of motivation, as well as sexual or other forms of disinhibition. The consequence is that these dementias are often not diagnosed quickly and are seen instead as aberrant behaviour.

Details concerning the numerous other types of dementia can be found elsewhere [2]. Much is known about dementia, and the prospect of a therapeutic breakthrough is always in the news. At present, however, drug treatments have only a modest effect and there are no specific cures (apart from in some rare types of dementia). But why did I start by suggesting that the definition of the word 'dementia' is problematic? Well, the word is problematic for at least two reasons.

First, it is stigmatising, partly because it is insulting. Secondly it does not specify anything that is useful: it does not tell us what to expect, nor how we can treat the person. Even within a type of dementia, such as Alzheimer's disease, there is significant heterogeneity. Elsewhere, I have spelt out the problems associated with the word 'dementia' [3]. I have also suggested that talk of the ageing brain is a better paradigm than talk of dementia. It is just that our brains age differently [4]. Dissatisfaction with the term 'dementia' is shown by the decision of the American drafters of the fifth edition of the *Diagnostic and Statistical Manual of Mental Disorder* (DSM-5) to replace 'dementia' by the term 'Major Neurocognitive Disorder' [5].

The Nun Study helped to show the heterogeneity of dementia [6]. Some of the nuns in the study, who had all agreed to participate and to have a post-mortem examination of their brains, showed marked pathology despite being clear of symptoms. Others had marked clinical features but little actual pathology. A different problem is to do with boundaries between mild cognitive impairment (MCI) and dementia, or between MCI and normality [3]. The problem here is about where to draw the line. What emerges is that there is no objective place to say that normal ageing has stopped and pathological ageing has begun. All of this suggests two things. First, that we need to take individual difference very seriously to see variety rather than to clump everything together as the same. Secondly, we have to look closely at context. It is the context, the full picture, surrounding symptoms and signs, which helps to establish whether or not they are pathological. In turn, context allows meaning.

Lesions, Religion and Dementia

Miller and colleagues describe five cases of frontotemporal dementia where people affected acquired new artistic skills [7]. They concluded, on the basis of neuroimaging, that loss of function in the anterior temporal lobes might 'facilitate' artistic skills. Although none of these individuals was described as religious, acquiring an increased aesthetic sense suggests that these areas of the brain might be targets to be considered in connection with religiosity. Wuerfel and colleagues scanned 33 patients with refractory epilepsy [8]. They found that having a smaller right hippocampus was correlated with increased religiosity in these patients. Recall that it is the medial temporal lobe, especially the hippocampus, that is affected by Alzheimer's disease, but also by other types of dementia (e.g. DLB). Subsequently, Chan and colleagues scanned 20 patients with predominant right temporal lobe atrophy [9]. They were found to have impairment of episodic memory, that is memory for episodes (rather than, say, semantic memory, which is memory for word meanings). They were also inclined to get lost, showing disorientation, and they demonstrated prosopagnosia, that is, failure to recognise familiar faces. There was a variety of behavioural symptoms or signs, such as depression, disinhibition and aggression. Symptoms particular to the right temporal lobe atrophy group included hyper-religiosity. Putting this together with the earlier findings it sounds as if right temporal lobe, especially hippocampal, atrophy is associated with increased religiosity.

As further evidence of the importance of the temporal lobe in connection with religiosity, a case is reported in the literature of a 65-year-old man who presented with frontotemporal dementia and Geschwind's syndrome [10]. This syndrome is usually associated with temporal lobe epilepsy, but in this case there was no evidence of epilepsy. Nevertheless, the patient did exhibit other key features of the syndrome, namely hyposexuality (loss of interest in sex), hypergraphia (copious writing) and hyper-religiosity. From the age of 55 he started attending prayer groups, reciting the prayer 'Hail Mary' 600 times a day, as well as having periodic visions, which were felt to be episodes of mystic delirium. After two years the praying decreased but his mysticism and delirium increased and he started giving significant sums of money away to charities. His brain scans demonstrated poor function in the prefrontal and middle frontal cortex (bilaterally but worse on the left) and in the left lateral and medial temporal cortices, as well as in both cordate nuclei. So the evidence, such as it is, seems to be that frontotemporal functions, but in particular the medial temporal lobes, underpin religious practice and belief. Still, as we saw, medial temporal lobe atrophy is a hallmark of Alzheimer's disease and most people with Alzheimer's do not exhibit hyper-religiosity.

A study comparing 12 healthy young adults (mean age 21) with 12 healthy elderly adults (mean age 73) and 17 people with Alzheimer's disease (mean age 84), demonstrated that the people with Alzheimer's (systematically and promiscuously) preferred teleological explanations [11]. That is, they preferred to explain things in terms of presumed purposeful functions rather than in mechanistic terms. The authors explained that children had been described as 'promiscuously teleological' in that they accept more readily the explanation that mountains exist to give animals a place to live rather than that they exist because of geological changes. In this study, questions such as 'Why are there eyes?' were posed and both a mechanistic explanation ('Because bodies have special cells that combine to produce eyes') and a teleological explanation ('So people and animals can see') were suggested. People with Alzheimer's disease preferred the teleological explanation. The study certainly raises questions (e.g. there is no comment about the significance of the difference in age between the control elderly and Alzheimer's groups). But it also raises some interesting reflections.

The hypothesis is that the promiscuous teleological tendency persists throughout life but is constrained during adult life by causal explanations. Once Alzheimer's disease erodes the person's ability to appeal to causal mechanistic explanations, the preference for teleological explanations re-emerges.

> In short, these findings provide evidence for a basic human preference to understand the world in terms of purpose. When faced with an object that supports a plausible function, humans make an immediate but defeasible inference to design, and assume a teleological explanation is warranted. [11, p. 1004]

These researchers also looked at the possibility that the appeal to function would correspond to belief in a designer. But they found that the Alzheimer's patients 'were no more likely to spontaneously invoke a designer (human or divine) than were healthy elderly participants, and healthy participants accepted teleological explanations for properties they attributed to natural selection'; they went on to suggest that 'promiscuous teleology is not a consequence of promiscuous theism'.

The implications of this research are debatable. But it does seem to show a change in terms of the person's cognitive abilities. A lot of research has confirmed that, in addition to deficits in episodic memory, there are also progressive problems in semantic memory for people with, e.g. Alzheimer's disease. Semantic memory, as suggested above, represents our cognitive store of knowledge, of words and word meanings. Lombrozo and colleagues suggest further that there are problems at the inferential level of intuitive theories [11]. It is not clear how this links to religious belief, except that it does *not* support the idea that there is an increase in religiosity as a consequence of increasing dementia. It does *not* provide good grounds for an inherent link between religiosity and cognitive deficits emanating particularly from the medial temporal lobe.

In summary, from the scanty evidence available, although we have noted an intriguing connection between the temporal (and frontal) lobes and hyper-religiosity, it is not enough to have temporal lobe dysfunction to make the person religious. Most religious people, after all, do not have cognitive dysfunction; and, it would seem, the mere presence of temporal lobe atrophy is not enough to cause hyper-religiosity, otherwise this would be a much more conspicuous sign of dementia.

Religious Experience and Dementia

Focusing on the brain provides us, potentially, with a *causal* explanation of religious belief, but it does not provide us with a *constitutive* account: it does not tell us what *constitutes* religious belief or experience in dementia. In general, we know that older people are more prone to be religious and that spirituality is regarded as contributing to various measures of life satisfaction or well-being, with some benefits in terms of both physical and mental health [12].

There has been increasing interest in religion and spirituality in connection with dementia. For example, Stuckey and colleagues noted that religion is not often discussed in the clinical setting despite the increase in literature, which they reviewed under five headings [13]. First, there is literature about how to engage people with dementia in terms of religious or spiritual expression. They mention the person's need to feel connected. Secondly, religion and spirituality are used as a resource for people with dementia and for their families. Much of the research attests to the fact that familiar religious practices can be recalled even in advanced dementia. Thirdly, there are personal accounts of dementia emphasising a religious perspective. Fourthly, literature discusses the philosophical and theological issues surrounding dementia and, finally, there is a literature looking at how clergy and communities can provide support to those living with the condition. In a series of focus groups, which involved those with dementia and their family caregivers, several themes emerged that demonstrated the relevance of religion and spirituality to dementia care.

First, the authors suggested it was better to focus on non-cognitive pathways to spirituality and religious observance. Music and other sensory modalities (including e.g. smells) may be a better way to engage the person. Secondly, religion and spirituality were seen as providing pathways to peace and acceptance in the midst of the condition. Thirdly, some carers spoke of the experience of dementia as a 'gift'. One wife expressed this as follows:

> When he had dementia, it was my greatest gift, my greatest time of being with this really wonderful man because now I got to see who he really was. He stopped using that part he had been so accustomed to using – that analyser, that intellectual. And what happened is that his heart opened up. It was just beautiful. [13, p. 204]

Fourthly, they saw relationships as spiritual connections. Finally, they felt that attention to spiritual matters should be incorporated routinely into care plans.

Lawrence suggests that, in the absence of speech, religious practices and a spiritual approach might be ways in which it is possible to continue to engage with people with dementia [14]. In which case, the person's spiritual history must have been understood fully, suggesting the need to ask questions about religious belief much sooner in the person's disease. One such approach might be to use a standardised instrument to ask questions about religion and spiritual attitudes. This has been shown to be possible and acceptable [15]. Elsewhere, Lawrence emphasises the importance of a holistic approach to the person with dementia, to include attention to spirituality and religion [16]. With this emphasis goes a focus on the nature of personhood and a need for communication.

Goodall considered the particular challenges of providing spiritual care in a care home setting [17]. She talks of the '3 Rs' – reflection, relationship and restoration – as being useful in looking at spiritual care in care homes. Familiar themes emerge:

> At its core, spirituality is in some sense not about logic or abstraction or cognition; it is ultimately the ability to connect with someone or something outside oneself, and at the same time recognize that whatever happens there is a core that remains 'oneself', a continuity of self. [17, p. 171]

In discussing the same issue – how to provide spiritual or religious care in care settings – Jolley and Moreland cite six areas that have been suggested as requiring attention: the need to value and respect the person; the importance of celebrating the person's religious heritage; the need for simplicity to engage with the person; the possibility of expression through the creative arts; the importance of spiritual care throughout the person's life, including at the end of life; and the importance of nourishing one's own spirituality to help sustain oneself [18]. Jolley and Moreland comment, 'Intuitively, these are sound propositions, but much more research is desirable to confirm the veracity and extent of such practices in care homes for people with dementia' [18, p. 389]. In connection with the point about the creative arts, bearing in mind the link between creative arts and spirituality noted elsewhere [13], it is interesting to keep in mind the association of artistic talent and the frontotemporal regions of the brain, which are also (as we have seen) associated with religiosity.

A useful systematic review looked at spirituality and dementia in long-term care and highlighted several themes [19]. Despite methodologically poor studies, there is some evidence that religious interventions might improve some aspects of cognitive function, mood and decrease agitation. Hence, guidelines suggest that formal religious interventions (e.g. prayer, spiritual reminiscence) might be useful. But we need effective strategies for assessing spiritual needs, which were summarised as preserving a sense of purpose, fostering meaningful connections with the surrounding world and maintaining a relationship with God [19].

Lucid Moments

The experience of dementia from a religious point of view has been recorded by the American Presbyterian pastor Robert Davis with help from his wife Betty [20]. More first-hand experiential accounts are emerging. But it is still difficult to understand what is occurring in the most advanced stages of dementia. One potential way to understand something of the inner life of the person with dementia is through consideration of lucid episodes. These have been defined as follows:

> episodes in the care of patients with severe dementia where the patient unexpectedly speaks or acts in a way which surprises the carer because the patient seems to be much more aware of her or his situation and to function much more adequately than usual. [21]

These authors went on to say: 'Most episodes occurred spontaneously when the patient was the subject of individual attention, or in the grip of strong emotions triggered by dislike, music and prayer' [21].

Jonathon Franzen described similar lucid episodes in his father. He wrote: 'In the two years that followed the loss of his supposed "self" I cannot stop finding it' [22]. Elsewhere, having been taken out to dinner in his family's home, Franzen was amazed to hear his father say, on their return to his nursing home, 'Better not to leave, than to have to come back' [23]. Audrey Ball, a chaplain to a NHS unit for people with severe dementia, related this story of Ellen's prayer, which was about a lady who had gradually lost most of her abilities:

> As her illness progressed, Ellen could no longer receive the sacrament and was often distracted and fidgety . . . We would sit and hold hands for a while and then I would say, 'Shall we say a prayer now?' 'That's the best', she never failed to reply. On a day I shall never forget and before I could start a prayer, Ellen, in her gentle way, said her own prayer:
>
> 'Dear God, You are all that matters,
> Help us to be happy,
> Help us to be welcoming,
> We need each other'. [24]

The worry felt by family when such lucid moments materialise out of the blue is that the real person, or the self, is still trapped in the body experiencing everything as normal people do, but unable to communicate. I doubt that this is the true situation. I think instead that lucid episodes point to two things. First they show us the complexity of the brain, which still has the potential even in severe dementia to make connections. The brain has not disappeared in dementia, even if its pathways are severely damaged. Although the person's abilities are severely compromised, we should not be so surprised if occasionally meaning can be conveyed. The ways in which people with severe dementia can still be semiotic subjects has been explored by Sabat and Harré [25]. Secondly, lucid episodes highlight how meaning is usually co-created. It requires, at least potentially, two actors to construct and to convey meaning. Meaning is not something that occurs entirely privately, it occurs in public space between people [3]. We note again that lucid episodes are more likely when the person is receiving individual attention, or is gripped by strong emotions [21]. This reminds me of an elderly woman in a care home for people with advanced dementia who was recently engaging in incoherent conversation with me, but then suddenly said: 'Whatever happens, when you are old, do not end up in a place like this'. Meaningfulness is not something that can be dissociated from context. At any event, lucid episodes bring together the neurology – what is happening in the brain – with the experiential – what is happening in the life of the person. We require both causal and constitutive (experiential) accounts to understand lucid episodes. There are both retained abilities and retained personhood, because of the possibility of meaning-making. We have also seen (again) the importance of emotions (not just cognitions) and of the creative arts (such as music).

Furthermore, there are increasing examples of meaning-making being preserved not just for moments, but for longer periods of time. This is shown in the famous video clip of Naomi Feil, the pioneer of validation therapy [26], with an elderly lady with dementia, Gladys Wilson [27]. It is noticeable that the music which stimulates Gladys Wilson is spiritual. Similarly, in another video clip involving Henry (with commentary by Oliver Sacks), although the music is not immediately spiritual, having heard it and changed from someone who is fairly inert to someone who is clearly animated, Henry says the following:

> It gives me the feeling of love, romance . . . I figure right now the world needs to come into music singing; you've got beautiful music here . . . and I feel the band of love, of dreams . . . the Lord came to me, made me holy; I am a holy man . . . so, he gave me these sounds. [28]

The striking thing for our purposes is the way music so readily facilitates communication and interaction. Similar stories are found in the work of Kate Allan and John Killick [29].

Meaning and Person

Religious practices have meaning, they are of significance for those who partake in them. Much of what we glean from reading about or observing the experience of dementia is to do with communication, which is also about meaning-making [30]. Spiritual approaches to the topic of dementia often stress both the importance of taking a holistic view that enables meaningful encounters and the importance of relationships. Sapp talks of the importance of the self's connectedness [31]. Collicutt speaks of 'targeted support of human meaning through transcendence' [32]. Allen and Coleman wished 'to show the centrality of relationship to spiritual perspectives on the person with dementia' [33, p. 218].

The underlying idea of importance here, however, is the notion of the person. As we have seen, a problem in the approach to people with dementia has often been that too narrow a view is taken of what constitutes personhood, as if personal identity is merely a cognitive matter. Emotions, conative drives, aesthetic impulses, relationships and so on are all ignored. In reaction to this narrow view, a broad view of dementia stresses situated embodied agency [3, 34]. The key notion is that we, as persons, are situated. That is, we are embedded in numerous different ways: in our culture, which includes our traditions, our norms, our history; in our particular personal histories, which involve our wishes and inclinations, our concerns and our memories; in a social context of family, friends, neighbours, geography and law; in a field of moral values and virtues; and, finally, in the context of our spiritual and our religious beliefs. Indeed, the possibilities for personhood cannot be circumscribed.

We are also embodied. So what goes on in our brains is of relevance to understanding in terms of causal explanations. Meaning, however, resides in public spaces, in our shared discourses, so that the significance of things in the world is understood not in isolation, but in terms of our connections. These connections are themselves situated, or embedded in our cultural understandings, so that the gesture or grimace of the person with advanced dementia has meaning.

We might put matters this way: neurological lesions are one thing, whether or not there is an exact correlation between the pathology and the symptoms and signs; but whether or not we think an experience has religious significance depends on the background explanations and understandings we are willing to consider. These understandings and explanations, to be plausible, must have a certain degree of coherence. The situated embodied agent view of personhood allows that causal biological accounts of brain pathology cohere with accounts of our standing as inter-connected human beings in the world and with transcendental views of the creator [35]. This lesion, in the right medial temporal lobe say, has this particular effect on my interactions in the world. But those interactions are precisely *in-the-world*. Typically, they will affect other people because of the nature of our *being-with* others. But our interactions *in-the-world* have meaning because of our shared public understandings. (I have said more about the existentialist account I am gesturing at here in the section on embodiment in [3, pp. 45–50].) Meanwhile, our situated nature can also be taken to raise questions about our existence, about the existence of anything at all, which is a way to raise the possibility of God, understood as the ineffable creator [36]. In other words, our world can be taken to raise existential questions, where the answers must inevitably be mysterious.

The same mystery surrounds dementia. It also, like any form of human suffering (but like any form of human existence actually) raises existential questions. But more than this, by its effect on personhood, dementia raises very specific questions about our being as human beings. And the account that comes from some of those who have lived with dementia is that it reveals something of the inner spiritual life of the person, which is partly constituted by interactions with others. Thus we find Barbara Pointon writing of her husband Malcolm who had Alzheimer's disease:

> Malcolm is surrounded by love. We reach out to communicate with him at a profound level – often through eye contact and gentle whispering and touch – and from him there flows a deep childlike trust, luminosity and reciprocating love – as though it were his very self, the self he was born with, that we are privileged to glimpse . . . Does it matter what we call it – spirit, soul, inner self, essence, identity – so long as we have experienced it?

> ... So the search for spirituality and the real Malcolm ends here – in the revelation of his essential self because of the loving care he receives and the trust that it engenders.
>
> ... To stand stripped of everything the world values and to see each other as we really are is a very precious and humbling experience, and one I would never have encountered were it not for the ravages of dementia. [37, p. 119]

Conclusion

Part of the difficulty in bringing together neurology and religion is that they seem to inhabit two different worlds, or what Wittgenstein would have called 'language games'. At one point Wittgenstein suggests we should not explain language games, but simply note them [38]. The thing to avoid is mixing them up. Hence, we should not expect causal explanations if we are trying to outline what constitutes religious belief and we should not expect to find meanings in the brain, even if the causal basis of meaning is in the brain. The notion of the person, however, if construed broadly, allows room both for causal and for constitutive accounts. The person as a situated embodied agent is very much a material being, but it is not the *being* of just *any thing* in the world. Human beings have a particular significance or meaning. We could go the way of social constructionism and say that we construct meaning between ourselves. But I prefer to think of meaning as immanent, as something embedded in our nature as beings of this kind. We cannot be human beings without this significance; and this is before we have co-created any thing. It is immanent; but also transcendent in the sense that it is a ground for the possibility of our being the type of beings that we are. Meaning or human significance is that without which we are not human at all.

In discourse about religion and dementia, therefore, the notion of the human person is central. If construed broadly enough – by my lights, as a situated embodied agent – there is room for physical discourse about the contribution of the body to our personhood as there is for dialogue about the social origins of our concepts. And, moreover, our embeddedness here in this world suggests the existential question about why anything should *be* at all. In addition, persons – as beings in the world of interconnectivity and interdependence – are quintessentially beings with others. Personhood, that is, suggests not just the possibility of meaning, but also the essential nature of relationships, as well as the importance of context. In one setting it makes more sense to speak of the atrophy of the hippocampus; in another, the numinous experience of a particular religious practice is more apposite as a topic of conversation.

The person is always situated in a context, is always embodied in a meaningful manner, but also (potentially at least) always acts in and on the world in a narrative which (potentially at least) must always involve others. Meanwhile, the world of persons itself raises questions about the possibility of its non-being, where the possibility of an explanation beyond the world can be contemplated in all of its mystery. But that mystery is, then, at the very heart of things: the possibility of non-existence is the upshot of meaningful existence.

Engaging with people with dementia, a condition which raises problems about the self, sets before us the need for a broad holistic view of persons and forces us to consider the ways in which we do not stand alone as persons. My personhood depends for some of its manifestations on others, just as it depends, too, on the cells in my hippocampus and other cortical areas. We see difference in dementia as we also see the need for solidarity [39]. The solidarity required to maintain the self in dementia is the same solidarity which emerges in our existential concerns about *being in the world* and the importance of *being-with;* and the same solidarity which emanates from religious concerns about community and the common good. At the same time, a religious understanding of the world, brought about by upbringing and by study or reflection, persists in dementia and can be helpful to it.

In the end, the threat to ourselves from dementia, which is a manifestation of neurotransmitter deficiencies, abnormal protein deposition and hyper-phosphorylation (among other things), forces us to see ourselves as infinitely varied, as unique beings, but as beings who interact in relationships which are meaningful and quintessential. Understanding the neurology of dementia is mundane without understanding the situated person and the multifaceted nature of personhood. And understanding persons in the human world, in which meaning is immanent, raises (especially in the context of suffering) existential questions about our being *as such*, which point us in the direction of the mystery of non-being. In this way, a religious account of dementia starts to seem as compelling as a neurological one.

References

1 Hughes, J. C. 2011. *Alzheimer's and Other Dementias: The Facts*. Oxford: Oxford University Press.

2 Ames, D., A. Burns and J. O'Brien, eds. 2010. *Dementia*. 4th edn. London: Hodder Arnold.

3 Hughes, J. C. 2011. *Thinking through Dementia*. Oxford: Oxford University Press.

4 Hughes, J. C. 2013. Dementia is dead, long live ageing: philosophy and practice in connection with 'dementia'. In *Oxford Handbook of Philosophy and Psychiatry*, eds. K. W. M. Fulford, M. Davies, R. G. T. Gipps, G. Graham, J. Z. Sadler, G. Stanghellini and T. Thornton, 835–50. Oxford: Oxford University Press.

5 Sachdev, P. S. 2013. The DSM-5 approach to dementia. In *Oxford Textbook of Old Age Psychiatry*, 2nd edn., ed. T. Dening and A. Thomas, 377–81. Oxford: Oxford University Press.

6 Snowdon, D. A. 2003. Healthy aging and dementia: findings from the Nun Study. *Annals of Internal Medicine* 139: 450–4.

7 Miller, B. L., J. Cummings, F. Mishkin, K. Boone, F. Prince, M. Ponton and C. Cotman. 1998. Emergence of artistic talent in frontotemporal dementia. *Neurology* 51: 978–82.

8 Wuerfel, J., E. S. Krishnamoorthy, R. J. Brown, L. Lemieux, M. Koepp, L. Tebartz van Elst and M. R. Trimble. 2004. Religiosity is associated with hippocampal but not amygdala volumes in patients with refractory epilepsy. *Journal of Neurology, Neurosurgery, and Psychiatry* 75: 640–2.

9 Chan, D., V. Anderson, Y. Pijnenburg, J. Whitwell, J. Barnes, R. Scahill, J. M. Stevens, F. Barkhof, P. Scheltens, M. N. Rossor and N. C. Fox. 2009. The clinical profile of right temporal lobe atrophy. *Brain* 132: 1287–9.

10 Postiglione, A., G. Milan, S. Pappatà, C. De Falco, F. Lamenza, V. Schiattarella, G. Gallotta, P. Sorrentino and S. Striano. 2008. Fronto-temporal dementia presenting as Geschwind's syndrome. *Neurocase* 14: 264–70.

11 Lombrozo, T., D. Kelemen and D. Zaitchik. 2007. Inferring design: evidence of a preference for teleological explanations in patients with Alzheimer's disease. *Psychological Science* 18: 999–1006.

12 Moberg, D. O. 2005. Research in spirituality, religion, and aging. *Journal of Gerontology and Social Work* 45: 11–40.

13 Stuckey, J. C., S. G. Post, S. Ollerton, S. J. Fallcreek and P. J. Whitehouse. 2002. Alzheimer's disease, religion, and the ethics of respect for spirituality: a community dialogue. *Alzheimer's Care Quarterly* 3: 199–207.

14 Lawrence, R. M. 2003. Aspects of spirituality in dementia care: when clinicians tune into silence. *Dementia* 2: 393–402.

15 Jolley, D., S. M. Benbow, M. Grizzell, S. Willmott, S. Bawn and P. Kingston.

2010. Spirituality and faith in dementia. *Dementia* 9: 311–25.

16 Lawrence, R. M. 2007. Dementia: a personal legacy beyond word. *Mental Health Religion and Culture* 10: 553–62.

17 Goodall, M. A. 2009. The evaluation of spiritual care in a dementia care setting. *Dementia* 8: 167–83.

18 Jolley, D., and N. Moreland. 2011. Dementia care: spiritual and faith perspectives. *Nursing and Residential Care* 13: 388–91.

19 Keast, K., C. Leskovar and R. Brohm. 2010. A systematic review of spirituality and dementia in LTC. *Annals of Long-Term Care* 18: 41–7.

20 Davis, R., and B. Davis. 1989. *My Journey into Alzheimer's Disease*. Wheaton, IL: Tyndale House.

21 Normann, H. K., K. Asplund and A. Norberg. 1998. Episodes of lucidity in people with severe dementia as narrated by formal carers. *Journal of Advanced Nursing* 28: 1295–300.

22 Franzen, J. 2001. The long slow slide into the abyss. *Guardian Weekend*, 15 December, 15–29.

23 Franzen, J. 2001. My father's brain: what Alzheimer's takes away. *New Yorker*, 10 September, 81–91.

24 Ball, A. 2006. Ellen's prayer. In *Palliative Care in Severe Dementia*, ed. J. C. Hughes, 134. London: Quay Books.

25 Sabat, S. R., and R. Harré. 1994. The Alzheimer's disease sufferer as a semiotic subject. *Philosophy, Psychiatry, and Psychology* 1: 145–60.

26 Feil, N. 1993. *The Validation Breakthrough: Simple Techniques for Communicating with People with 'Alzheimer's Type Dementia'*. Baltimore: Health Professions Press.

27 www.youtube.com/watch?v=CrZXz10FcVM&sns=em.

28 www.youtube.com/watch?v=fyZQf0p73QM.

29 Allan, K., and J. Killick. 2010. Communication with people with dementia. In *Supportive Care for the Person with Dementia*, ed. J. C. Hughes, M. Lloyd-Williams and G. A. Sachs, 217–25. Oxford: Oxford University Press.

30 Widdershoven, G. A. M., and R. L. P. Berghmans. 2006. Meaning-making in dementia: a hermeneutic perspective. In *Dementia: Mind, Meaning, and the Person*, ed. J. C. Hughes, S. J. Louw and S. R. Sabat, 179–91. Oxford: Oxford University Press.

31 Sapp, S. 2010. Spiritual care of people with dementia and their carers. In *Supportive Care for the Person with Dementia*, eds. J. C. Hughes, M. Lloyd-Williams and G. A. Sachs, 199–206. Oxford: Oxford University Press.

32 Collicutt, J. 2012. Some ethical issues in dementia care: re-membering the person. *Crucible*, October–December, 7–17.

33 Allen, F. B., and P. G. Coleman. 2006. Spiritual perspectives on the person with dementia: identity and personhood. In *Dementia: Mind, Meaning, and the Person*, ed. J. C. Hughes, S. J. Louw and S. R. Sabat, 205–21. Oxford: Oxford University Press.

34 Hughes, J. C. 2001. Views of the person with dementia. *Journal of Medical Ethics* 27: 86–91.

35 Hughes, J. C. 2011. A situated embodied view of the person with dementia: where does the spiritual come in? In *Spirituality and Personhood in Dementia*, ed. A. Jewell, 198–206. London: Jessica Kingsley.

36 McCabe, H. 1987. *God Matters*. London: Continuum.

37 Pointon, B. 2007. 'Who am I? – The search for spirituality in dementia. A family carer's perspective. In *Spirituality, Values and Mental Health: Jewels for the Journey*, ed. M. E. Coyte, P. Gilbert and V. Nicholls, 114–20. London: Jessica Kingsley.

38 Wittgenstein, L. 1968. *Philosophical Investigations*. Ed. G. E. M. Anscombe and R. Rhees. Trans. G. E. M. Anscombe. Oxford: Blackwell.

39 Nuffield Council on Bioethics. 2009. *Dementia: Ethical Issues*. London: Nuffield Council on Bioethics. www.nuffieldbioethics.org/dementia.

II.I *Clinical Conditions*

Chapter 15

Religion and Frontotemporal Dementia

Nikolas Block and Bruce Miller

If this brain model of the bicameral mind is correct, it would predict decided differences in cognitive function between the two hemispheres. Specifically, we would expect that these functions necessary for the man-side would be in the left or dominant hemisphere, and those functions necessary to the gods would be more emphasized in the right hemisphere.

Julian Jaynes, The Origin of Consciousness in the Breakdown of the Bicameral Mind

In the setting of disease, religion can play a positive role in a person's life, helping them manage their perception of an illness, bolstering the ability of the patient and their family to manage the diagnosis, day-to-day functioning and treatment [1]. Individuals who have practised religion earlier in life may show new vigour in their belief after diagnosis of a serious illness, or religion can be discovered for the first time. Increased religiosity can be a means for support and comfort through difficult periods in a person's life.

A human's relationship with the religious form may be intimate – deeply emotional, imbued through everyday experiences, motivations and decisions – and therefore is closely related to a person's sense of self.

Marked changes in religiosity can instead be due to pathological brain changes and have been described in a variety of neurological conditions. A striking upwelling or diminishment in religious practice, belief or experience can be attributed to loss of function in specific brain regions. As will be described, intensification of religious or philosophical ideas may occur in frontotemporal dementia (FTD) predominantly affecting the temporal lobes.

A Historical Perspective

Julian Jaynes, the author of the quote that introduces this chapter, attempted to understand how *Homo sapiens* began to believe in deities, entities that were responsible for, and controlled, a human's existence. He suggested auditory hallucinations, generated from the right hemisphere, were interpreted as coming from a god, or god-like presence by the language-competent left hemisphere. Albeit controversial, Jaynes' ideas captured the imagination of philosophers, psychologists and the wider public when introduced in the

1970s. Importantly, his writings represented one of the first attempts to tie religious beliefs to specific brain structures and hypothesised that the right hemisphere was the dominant hemisphere for religious experience.

Jaynes was a philosopher and psychologist, not a neuroscientist, and his work was based upon abstract concepts, not empirical data. When analysed from the perspective of modern neuroscience, his ideas about consciousness and the brain localisation of religion seem naive, even untenable. Yet, our studies of patients with FTD support the idea of distinctive contributions of the two hemispheres to religious belief and hyperreligiosity.

Around the same time that Jaynes developed his ideas about the bicameral mind and religion, Geschwind and Gastaut described intensification of religious thought in patients with temporal lobe epilepsy (TLE). Geschwind suggested that chronic seizure activity involving the temporal lobes was associated with a syndrome characterised by hyposexuality, philosophical or religious intensification, hypergraphia, viscosity and circumstantiality [2]. Bear and Fedio followed up Geschwind's studies in patients with epilepsy and described 'a distinctive profile of humourless sobriety, dependence and obsessionalism; raters discriminated temporal lobe epileptics on the basis of circumstantiality, philosophical interests, and anger' [3].

Similarly, Devinsky notes that intense religious experiences happen in 0.4–3.1 per cent of partial epilepsy patients as part of the prodrome or during a seizure, and that postictal religious experiences occur in 1.3 per cent of all epilepsy patients and 2.2 per cent of TLE patients; these experiences are more likely to occur in patients with right temporal lobe foci. Hence a relationship between heightened religious experience and temporal lobe over, or under activity is evident, but the exact neurological mechanism and lateralisation of these experiences is unknown [4, 5]. These studies are further explored in the chapter by Coles (Chapter 9).

These writings establish a rich background for the study of religious beliefs and hyperreligiosity in people with neurodegenerative conditions. Yet, nearly 40 years later, there is still a paucity of research into the religious changes found in Alzheimer's disease, FTD or other neurodegenerative disorders. While dramatic changes in religious beliefs in individuals with Alzheimer's disease, vascular dementia or dementia with Lewy body appear to be rare, we have described dramatic religious changes in patients with classical behavioural variant FTD (bvFTD) and in the semantic variant of primary progressive aphasia (svPPA), a subtype of FTD.

In 1997, in a paper on the temporal lobe variant of FTD, we described intensification of religious beliefs, sometimes in association with other features of the Geschwind-Gastaut syndrome, such as hypergraphia, in patients with focal degeneration of the right anterior temporal lobe [6]. The humourless sobriety and obsessionalism, noted by Bear and Fedio in some patients with temporal lobe epilepsy, has also been observed to be a feature of the hyperreligious behaviour associated with focal degeneration of the right anterior temporal lobe in FTD.

By contrast, in patients with bvFTD due to asymmetric degeneration of the right frontal regions, a very different religious pattern has been seen, apparently mechanistically driven by changes in a sense of self. Adapting a definition of self described by American psychologist, William James, Miller and colleagues described the sense of self as composed of three components: abstract information about one's personal attributes (semantic information), concrete, often affect-laden information (autobiographical memories) and the motivation to maintain one's prior beliefs (will) [7]. The authors noted the motivation to maintain the self had strong frontal anatomical correlates. It is reasonable that disruption of these regions would lead to dramatic shifts in the sense of self, and in turn, social, political or religious values. In patients with FTD with selective injury to the right frontal region, Miller and colleagues reported dramatic changes in religious ideas, and patients had a tendency to lose strongly established religious viewpoints, converting from one religion to another. The authors suggested that the right frontal anatomy dampened prior loyalties and diminished ties to religious and political ideologies [8]. In patients with bvFTD, for example, one woman converted to Catholicism in order to spend time with a handsome young priest. These alterations in religious beliefs contrasted greatly with the hyperreligious changes in patients with right temporal lobe disease.

Three cases are presented to illustrate the types of changes in religious behaviour associated with selective cortical degeneration in FTD. Subsequently, these cases are discussed.

Case 1: Hallucinations and Delusions

Mr A, a 67-year-old, right-handed gentleman, presented with a 15-year history of psychotic features and an accompanying diagnosis of schizophrenia. He was evaluated at the UCSF Memory and Aging Center due to progressive changes in behaviour, memory and language.

Mr A developed a gambling compulsion in the decade prior to evaluation, stealing from his clients to maintain the habit and eventually taking out a second mortgage to pay off his debts. At about the same time, Mr A had an episode of yelling at his co-workers and was under the delusion that he was an archangel. This episode was described as manic-psychotic by his psychiatrist.

Previously a frequent churchgoer, in the decade before his evaluation he increasingly spoke about religion with co-workers, family, friends and even began approaching strangers on the street to proselytise. A delusion became fixed that he was the incarnation of an archangel and he began responding to voices he described as other angels, which he reported seeing on occasion. The delusions and hallucinations were reportedly diminished after eventual hospitalisation, initiation of antipsychotic medications and electroconvulsive therapy. He received a diagnosis of late-onset schizophrenia.

Four years before his evaluation, Mr A showed increased apathy for things happening around him and began misplacing items and accusing others of their theft. He would confuse his children's names and would forget the name of objects. He also had a recent history of rising early in the morning to walk the streets until evening, becoming fixated on topics, and he was quick to anger.

Mr A's past medical history included a diagnosis of schizophrenia and appendicitis one year prior to evaluation. His family history was significant for late-onset bipolar disorder (diagnosed at age 67) and dementia in his father who died at age 94 and possible dementia in his mother who died at age 83. His physical evaluation was significant for a possible suggestion of parkinsonism, but this was attributed to his medications. The exam was otherwise normal. Neuropsychological evaluation showed predominantly executive impairment. His memory for recent events was not markedly impaired. His MRI revealed frontal-predominant atrophy (Figure 15.1). He was given a diagnosis of bvFTD.

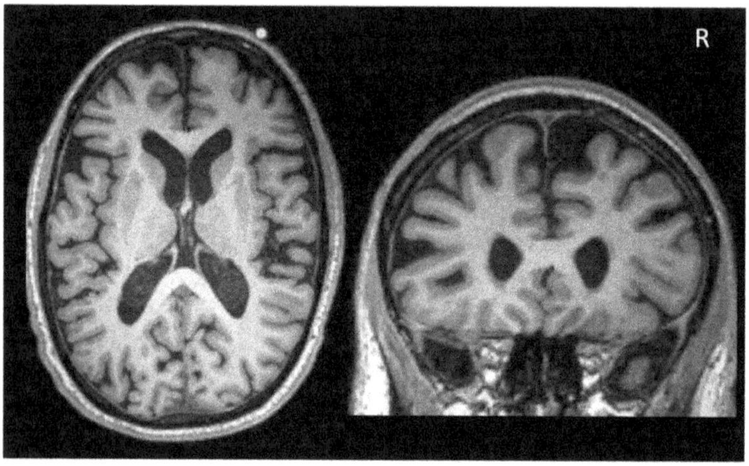

Figure 15.1 MRI of the brain from Mr A shows atrophy of the frontal lobes.

Discussion of Mr A

Mr A experienced a nearly two-decade history of hyperreligiosity that was first attributed to psychiatric illness and was either followed by a neurodegenerative process, or else the psychiatric symptoms were a prodrome of FTD. Mr A's religious behaviour was strongly driven by the delusion that he was in fact an archangel. His beliefs were bolstered by hallucinations of fellow angels who supported his religious crusade. These features, in combination with behaviours more typical of FTD – disinhibition, mental rigidity, perseveration on a topic or belief – elicited the salient religiosity in Mr A. The case of Mr A demonstrates delusions and hallucinations in the setting of FTD contributing to religious belief and practice.

Case 2: Intensification

Ms. B, a 63-year-old, right-handed woman with 13 years of education, presented with an eight-year history of progressive decline in her language as well as personality changes. Bilingual in English and German, she noticed comprehension problems at age 55 when watching English television shows. Soon after, she and her husband noticed impairment in her native language, German. She experienced word-finding difficulties, trouble with object identification and difficulty remembering the names of friends at church.

Ms. B became more withdrawn and apathetic and developed emotional blunting. At a funeral, she told a family member of the deceased, 'Well, they were old'. She exhibited decreased empathy, and when her husband cut himself and required stitches, she questioned why he was in pain and needed to go to the hospital. She made inappropriate comments about her bowel habits to strangers. She displayed obsessive-compulsive traits, like rechecking locked doors, monitoring her blood pressure repeatedly throughout the day and cleaning the house multiple times a day. She developed paranoia and covered her windows and blocked the doors with chairs when her husband left. She denied hallucinations.

Previously an avid churchgoer, after disease onset Ms. B showed increased religiosity and began composing religiously or spiritually themed songs. She showed an impulsive tendency to break out into song, which she did more than once during evaluation.

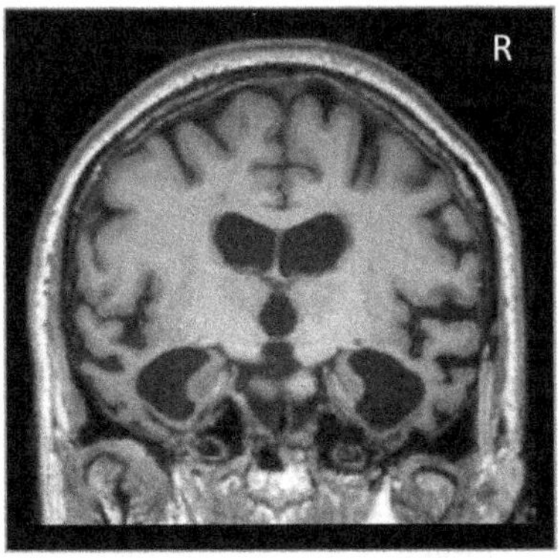

Figure 15.2 MRI of the brain of Ms B shows atrophy of both temporal lobes.

Ms. B expressed an overall greater interest in religion, finding in it great comfort and expressing that Jesus Christ would be the solution to all of her problems. At about the same time, Ms. B showed a further increase in creativity, photographing obsessively and spending considerable time organising and labelling these photographs.

Ms. B's family history showed no evidence of dementia or psychiatric illness. Her physical exam was unremarkable. She scored 11/30 on the Mini Mental State Exam (MMSE) and further cognitive testing revealed impairment in all cognitive domains, except visuospatial function. Her MRI showed bilateral temporal lobe atrophy (left > right), and insular atrophy (left > right) (Figure 15.2). She was diagnosed with svPPA.

Discussion of Ms. B

Ms. B's hyperreligious behaviour was associated with a creative surge and a compulsive tendency to compose lyrics. She also exhibited disinhibition by performing these songs in socially inappropriate settings. Her preoccupation with worship with song is interesting to note; enhanced creativity has been documented in svPPA. [9]

Case 3: Loss of Loyalty

Ms. C, a 55-year-old, right-handed woman with 18 years of education, presented with five years of progressive apathy and difficulty planning and organising, followed by three years of mild loss of empathy, compulsions, mild disinhibition, intermittently halting speech, spatial disorientation and forgetfulness. Previously a healthcare professional, she reported her first symptoms were difficulty problem solving and multi-tasking at work, as well as fatigue. She developed some rigid behaviours, including a strict laundry schedule, compulsive cleaning and the adherence to particular steps when cooking, like laying out all ingredients before food preparation. She became disinhibited, swearing for the first time and showing less concern for the appropriateness of conversation topics with her Christian friends. Interestingly, she reported decreased depression at age 52 after a long history with the illness.

Ms. C experienced progressive difficulty speaking, saying it felt like there was a disconnect between her brain and her mouth; she knew the word but had difficulty getting it out. She experienced halting speech and stuttering but no word-finding difficulty or slurred speech.

Whereas she had previously been a lifelong member of an evangelical church, she decided to leave her church to become an atheist. She also switched her political allegiance from the Republican Party to the more socially and fiscally liberal Democratic Party. When asked why she made these changes, she reported her beliefs were no longer aligned with those of the church or of the Republican Party, much to the astonishment of her husband. She developed increased apathy, reporting that she did not understand why people got so upset at the funerals she attended in the past year, and when a gruesome shooting appeared in the news, she reported not experiencing the same emotions she might have a decade prior.

Ms. C's medical history includes depression. Her family history was significant for dementia and psychiatric illness. The history included a 75-year-old mother with Alzheimer's disease (diagnosed at age 68), a 76-year-old father diagnosed with bipolar disorder, a maternal grandfather with late-life behavioural changes including depression, hypersexual behaviour, shuffling gait and dysphagia, dying at age 65 from pneumonia and carrying a pathological diagnosis of 'encephalomalacia', a maternal aunt diagnosed with bipolar disorder who also received a shunt to treat normal pressure hydrocephalus with subsequent improvement, and a 47-year-old sister diagnosed with bipolar disorder and recent personality changes, including violence and increased alcohol consumption.

On exam at age 54, Ms. C was alert but had a childlike affect and little concern for her condition. She showed mildly jerky smooth-pursuit eye movements, mildly slow, occasionally halting speech, diffuse hyperreflexia with downgoing toes, but no other significant abnormalities. On neuropsychological testing, she scored 29/30 on the MMSE and showed impairment in verbal fluency (semantic and phonemic), mildly impaired working memory, mildly impaired visual memory retrieval and mildly impaired executive control (slight slowing on Stroop inhibition). By age 55, her exam was notable for halting and stuttering speech, spastic lower extremities, hyperreflexia with jaw jerk, mild slowing of rapid alternating movements bilaterally, decreased arm swing on the right and mild retropulsion. She scored 30/30 on the MMSE by age 55. The MRI showed subtle, bilateral atrophy in the dorsomedial-frontal regions (right > left) (Figure 15.3). She was diagnosed with bvFTD.

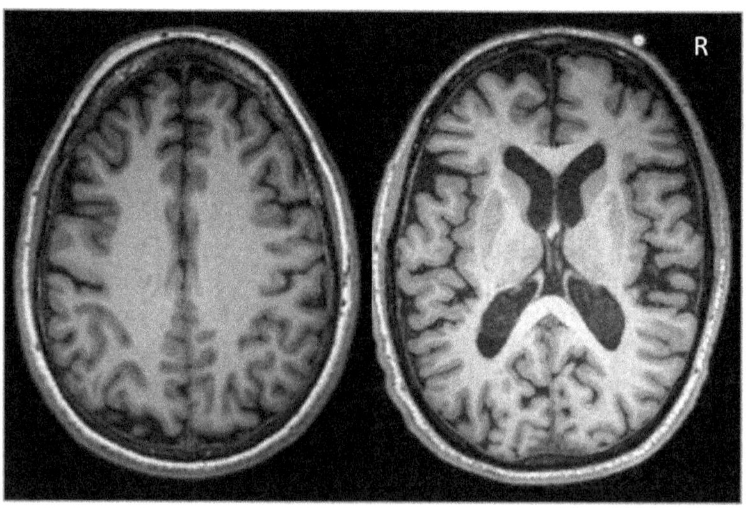

Figure 15.3 MRI of Ms C shows moderate atrophy of the dorsal part of the frontal lobe.

Discussion of Ms. C

Ms. C experienced a dramatic shift away from systems of conservative religious and political belief. She was brought up in the evangelical faith, married a man within this faith and raised her children within this religion. The retraction of a faith in God at the time of disease onset suggests a neuropathological basis for this change. What once helped to define her and her role in the world no longer provided meaning or comfort. In addition apathy – common in FTD – may have played an important role. Right medial frontal atrophy appears to be the dominant neuroanatomical correlate.

Discussion of Cases

While a single 'God region' of the brain is unlikely to exist, rather, there appears to be complex cognitive representations of the deity and of the self. From the study of FTD, it appears that the most dramatic changes in religious behaviour occur in patients with either bvFTD or the svPPA – particularly patients with more severe right temporal involvement. FTD, and other brain conditions affecting frontal brain regions, provide evidence that frontal anatomical regions are involved. Disruption of networks in these areas can cause profound changes in religious behaviour.

Cases 1 and 2 illustrate hyperreligious behaviour when particular frontotemporal brain regions are disrupted. Such cases also illustrate various co-occurring behaviours seen in FTD – impulsivity, delusions, mental rigidity – reinforce hyperreligiosity. In case 1, hyperreligiosity in FTD was associated with delusions [10]. Case 1's religiosity appears to have largely been driven by the delusions and hallucinations that he was both an archangel and that other angels presented themselves to him or spoke to him. Case 2's development of mental rigidity and impulsivity seems to have reinforced her composition of religious lyrics and her outbreaks into religious song, the impulsivity making her more prone to begin and the rigidity making her more likely to continue in the face of negative social feedback.

Unlike cases 1 and 2, case 3 illustrates different phenomenology. She divorced herself from a lifelong faith in a strict religious order, becoming anti-religious. Case 3 importantly demonstrates that disruption of FTD brain circuits can have a dramatically different effect on religious behaviour. Such opposing behavioural phenomena – release versus dampening effects – are seen in other behaviours associated with focal brain atrophy of neurodegenerative diseases (e.g. mental rigidity). Our experience suggests that intensification of religious ideas is more common with focal anterior temporal lobe degeneration. Case 3 further demonstrates that other behaviours like OCD-like behaviour, impulsivity and mental rigidity do not solely drive changes in hyperreligiosity, as case 3 demonstrated these in conjunction with *hypo*-religious behaviour. Variation in hyperreligious behaviour in patients with FTD indicates the disease may act on various levels of the self to elicit behaviour. Meanwhile, other symptoms emphasise or otherwise modulate the patient's experience of religion and the behaviours associated with hyperreligiosity.

Neuroanatomical Correlates

Work in healthy individuals has distinguished features of the God-self relationship and indicate the importance of the frontal and temporal regions. For example, increased closeness to God has been associated with increased volume in the right temporal gyrus, while increased fear of God is associated with decreased volume in the left precuneus and left orbitofrontal regions [11].

Similarly, on functional imaging tasks, religious versus non-religious individuals show varied frontal brain activity. Decreased activation is seen in the ventral medial prefrontal cortex (VMPFC) in Christian believers during tasks referencing the self [12]. The VMPFC plays an important role in evaluating whether stimuli is related to the self [13, 14]. Decreased activation in the VMPFC during self- and other judgements indicates the stimuli is less likely being referenced to the self, and is instead reappraised to determine its relevance to God's representation or opinion. Indeed, this notion is supported by greater activation in the dorsal medial prefrontal cortex (DMPFC) in those Christians, an area important for a reappraisal of stimuli as it refers to the self and for inferring others' mental states [15]. Prefrontal regions, including the VMPFC and DMPFC, are also activated during religious recitation or meditation in Buddhist, Christian and Catholic believers [16–19].

Changes in religious behaviour are associated with other brain regions as well. Late-life hippocampal atrophy is associated with those who have experienced a life-changing religious experience [20]. Hippocampal atrophy is an initial target of Alzheimer's disease and provides a possible explanation for anecdotal hyperreligiosity in some of these patients.

It follows that functional changes to the regions indicated could lead to changes to the self-deity relationship and worship behaviour. As previously described, TLE can be associated with a sudden and intense upwelling of religiosity [21, 22]. Such symptoms have been described in FTD, notably in the FTD temporal variants [9, 23]. Recent work indicates select right inferior frontal gyrus (IFG) atrophy in those individuals who have previously displayed hyperreligiosity [10]. The right IFG is implicated in aspects of self recognition and visually shifting perspectives [24, 25].

Default Mode Network and the Self

During rest, the mind automatically engages a system to explore theoretical social situations and relive past ones. The neural underpinning of this process, termed the default mode network (DMN), provides a safe environment to explore and make sense of social interactions and allows one to take on another's viewpoint [26]. Such perspective shifting, known as theory of mind (ToM), is an important social function that provides understanding of the other's intention, motivation and internal state. Theory of mind can occur even in the physical absence of the other and has more basic cognitive underpinnings; the phenomenon is seen even in chimpanzees [27], with unique frontal neural pathways with prefrontal overlap [25].

Impairment of the DMN is well documented in FTD and interferes with self-projection [26]. Disruption of the DMN not only makes it difficult to make sense of social situations, it also impairs ToM, providing opportunity for information to be misattributed to the self. The resulting disorder can lead to deception and delusional symptoms. Derangement of the DMN in FTD and the perseverative qualities inherent in the disease may play a role in the alteration in religious belief. This 'delusion of reference', attributing mundane events to be personally significant, is also described in patients with schizophrenia [28], as is the increased permeability of the line between self and other in those patients [29].

Conclusion

The focal changes to the brain caused by FTD and related brain illnesses provide a glimpse beneath higher-order behaviour and help associate features of the behaviour with brain regions. Such complexity of behaviours are only revealed as disease or trauma breaks down the fine balance needed to elicit and control them, causing astonishing departures from normal behaviour. Hyperreligiosity in FTD is a remarkable example of the intricacy of human behaviour, and one that allows for a deeper dialogue into the neuroscience of religion.

References

1 Jaynes, J. 1976. *The Origin of Consciousness in the Breakdown of the Bicameral Mind.* Boston: Houghton Mifflin.

2 Park, C. L. 2005. Religion as a meaning making framework in coping with life stress. *Journal of Social Issues* 61: 707–29.

3 Geschwind, N. 1983. Pathogenesis of behavior change in temporal lobe epilepsy. *Research Publications – Association for Research in Nervous and Mental Disorders* 61: 355–70.

4 Bear, D. M., and P. Fedio. 1977. Quantitative analysis of interictal behavior in temporal lobe epilepsy. *Archives in Neurology* 34: 454–67.

5 Devinsky, O., and G. Lai. 2008. Spirituality and religion in epilepsy. *Epilepsy and Behavior* 12: 636–43.

6 Trimble, M., and A. Freeman. 2006. An investigation of religiosity and the Gastaut-Geschwind syndrome in patients with temporal lobe epilepsy. *Epilepsy Behavior* 9: 407–14.

7 Edwards-Lee, T., B. L. Miller, D. F. Benson, J. L. Cummings, G. L. Russell, K. Boone et al. 1997. The temporal variant of frontotemporal dementia. *Brain* 120: 1027–40.

8 Miller, B. L., W. W. Seeley, P. Mychack, H. J. Rosen, I. Mena and K. Boone. 2001. Neuroanatomy of the self: evidence from patients with frontotemporal dementia. *Neurology* 57: 817–21. www.ncbi.nlm.nih.gov/pubmed/11552010.

9 Wu, T. Q., Z. A. Miller, B. Adhimoolam, D. D. Zackey, B. K. Khan, R. Ketelle et al. 2013. Verbal creativity in semantic variant primary progressive aphasia. *Neurocase*, 12 December. www.ncbi.nlm.nih.gov/pubmed/24329034.

10 Block, N. R., D. C. Perry, V. E. Sturm, Z. A. Miller and B. L. Miller. 2013. *Religious Dogmatism in Neurodegenerative Disease.* Boston: Alzheimer's Association International Conference.

11 Kapogiannis, D., A. K. Barbey, M. Su, F. Krueger and J. Grafman. 2009. Neuroanatomical variability of religiosity. *PLoS ONE* 4(9): e7180.

12 Han, S., L. Mao, X. Gu, Y. Zhu, J. Ge and Y. Ma. 2008. Neural consequences of religious belief on self-referential processing. *Social Neuroscience* 3: 1–15. doi:10.1080/17470910701469681.

13 Northoff, G., A. Heinzel, M. de Greck, F. Bermpohl, H. Dobrowolny and J. Panksepp. 2006. Self-referential processing in our brain – a meta-analysis of imaging studies on the self. *Neuroimage* 31: 440–57.

14 Northoff, G., and F. Bermpohl. 2004. Cortical midline structures and the self. *Trends in Cognitive Sciences* 8: 102–7.

15 Grèzes, J., C. D. Frith and R. E. Passingham. 2004. Inferring false beliefs from the actions of oneself and others: an fMRI study. *Neuroimage* 21: 744–50. www.sciencedirect.com/science/article/pii/S1053811903006657.

16 Azari, N., J. Nickel, G. Wunderlich, M. Niedeggen, H. Hefter, L. Tellmann et al. 2001. Neural correlates of religious experience. *European Journal* 13: 1649–52. http://onlinelibrary.wiley.com/doi/10.1046/j.0953-816x.2001.01527.x/full.

17 Newberg, A., M. Pourdehnad, A. Alavi and E. G. d'Aquili. 2003. Cerebral blood flow during meditative prayer: preliminary findings and methodological issues.

Perceptual and Motor Skills 97: 625–30. www.amsciepub.com/doi/abs/10.2466/pms.2003.97.2.625.

18 Newberg, A., A. Alavi, M. Baime, M. Pourdehnad, J. Santanna and E. d'Aquili. 2001. The measurement of regional cerebral blood flow during the complex cognitive task of meditation: a preliminary SPECT study. *Psychiatry Research: Neuroimaging* 106: 113–22. www.sciencedirect.com/science/article/pii/S0925492701000749.

19 Beauregard, M., and V. Paquette. 2006. Neural correlates of a mystical experience in Carmelite nuns. *Neuroscience Letters* 405: 186–90. www.sciencedirect.com/science/article/pii/S0304394006006392.

20 Owen, A. D., R. D. Hayward, H. G. Koenig, D. C. Steffens and M. E. Payne. 2011. Religious factors and hippocampal atrophy in late life. *PLoS One* 6, no. 3: e17006. www.pubmedcentral.nih.gov/articlerender.fcgi?artid=3068149.

21 Benson, D. F. 1991. The Geschwind syndrome. *Advances in Neurology* 55: 411–21.

22 Dewhurst, K., and A. W. Beard. 2003. Sudden religious conversions in temporal lobe epilepsy. *Epilepsy and Behavior* 4: 78–87.

23 Postiglione, A., G. Milan, S. Pappatà, C. De Falco, F. Lamenza, V. Schiattarella, G. Gallotta, P. Sorrentino and S. Striano. 2008. Fronto-temporal dementia presenting as Geschwind's syndrome. *Neurocase* 14: 264–70. doi:10.1080/13554790802269976.

24 Mazzarella, E., R. Ramsey, M. Conson and A. Hamilton. 2013. Brain systems for visual perspective taking and action perception. *Social Neuroscience* 8: 248–67. www.ncbi.nlm.nih.gov/pubmed/23350907.

25 van Veluw, S. J., and S. A. Chance. 2014. Differentiating between self and others: an ALE meta-analysis of fMRI studies of self-recognition and theory of mind. *Brain Imaging and Behavior* 8: 24–38. www.ncbi.nlm.nih.gov/pubmed/24535033.

26 Irish, M., O. Piguet and J. R. Hodges. 2011. Self-projection and the default network in frontotemporal dementia. *Nature Reviews Neurology* 8: 152–61. www.ncbi.nlm.nih.gov/pubmed/22331029.

27 Call, J., and M. Tomasello. 2008. Does the chimpanzee have a theory of mind? 30 years later. *Trends in Cognitive Science* 12: 187–92. www.ncbi.nlm.nih.gov/pubmed/18424224.

28 Frith, C. 1992. *The Cognitive Neuropsychology of Schizophrenia.* Ed. L. Erlbaum. Hove, UK: Psychology Press.

29 Dein, S., and R. Littlewood. 2011. Religion and psychosis: a common evolutionary trajectory? *Transcultural Psychiatry* 48: 318–35. www.ncbi.nlm.nih.gov/pubmed/21742955.

Chapter 16

II.II *Therapy*

Religion and Spirituality in Neuro-Rehabilitation

A Case Study

Joanna Collicutt

This chapter begins with a general consideration of the points where religion and spirituality connect with the enterprise of neuro-rehabilitation. This takes the form of a narrative that charts the chronological development of my ideas in the context of a field that is itself continually developing. It is followed by a case study of the rehabilitation of an individual with profound amnesia, whose faith was of overriding importance in his life. The case study both illustrates and elaborates several of the general themes raised in the earlier part of the chapter.

Neuro-Rehabilitation as the Re-Establishment of Meaning

In the mid 1980s I began work as a clinical neuropsychologist at Rivermead Rehabilitation Centre in Oxford.[1] At that time cognitive rehabilitation of people with acquired brain injury was in its infancy in the UK. My predecessor at Rivermead, Barbara Wilson, was about to publish her doctoral work (Wilson 1987), which drew together principles from neuropsychology, cognitive psychology and behavioural psychology to form a systematic and evidence-based approach to memory rehabilitation. It became foundational for the field.

Important as this work undoubtedly was, in the course of my daily clinical work I soon started to realise that its scope was limited. It was essentially functionalist (directed at improving task performance and independence), and largely ignored the emotional experience of affected individuals. In this it was typical of the approach of all the rehabilitation professions in the multi-disciplinary team (medicine, psychology, therapies, nursing and social work), which each worked mainly on discrete functionalist programmes in its largely independent silo, keeping other disciplines informed of its work, but only occasionally collaborating with them.

This approach felt fragmented and uncoordinated, and the overall aims of the rehabilitation process (beyond maximising independence or possibly increasing employability) were not clear to me. After much reflection on this issue, my assistant psychologist Alison Davis and I published a paper entitled 'Rehabilitation: Where Are We Going and How Do We Get There?' (McGrath and Davis 1992), which put forward some suggestions as to how it might be addressed within the framework of the WHO model of impairments, disabilities

[1] At that time, this was a 30-bed unit specialising in the multidisciplinary rehabilitation of people with complex disabilities following severe acquired brain injury (due mainly to trauma, cerebrovascular accident or cerebral hypoxia). The unit also had a significant number of outpatients and day patients.

and handicaps (Wood 1980).[2] From this beginning, a complex and sophisticated system of patient-centred, interdisciplinary goal planning was developed at Rivermead (McGrath et al. 1995), that subsequently had a wide influence on rehabilitation practice (see e.g. Dean et al. 2012). This was based around an assessment tool that we named the Rivermead Life Goals Questionnaire (RLGQ) (Wade 1999; Collicutt McGrath 2008).[3]

The RLGQ was distinctive because, instead of simply asking a patient what she wanted to get out of the rehabilitation process, it asked her to rate different areas of her life in terms of how important they were to her. The questionnaire items emphasised meaningful roles and relationships rather than functional abilities and, unusually for the time, they included 'my religion or life philosophy'. We were trying genuinely to see things from the patient's point of view; we reckoned that if we could see what motivated her, we could target our rehabilitation more effectively and also achieve greater cooperation. As a result of pilot studies we found that the questionnaire on its own did not always give us this information in a useful form, so we augmented it with a short structured interview (McGrath et al. 1995, 323).

One of the questions in this interview proved to be key: 'What makes (or used to make) your life enjoyable/meaningful/worthwhile?' The inclusion of this question and the heavy use we subsequently made of it in the rehabilitation process indicates that we were gradually and unconsciously moving towards an existential model of neuro-rehabilitation, one that was aiming to re-establish some sort of *meaning* in the life of our patients.

Neuro-Rehabilitation as the Reconstruction of Identity

In parallel with these developments I was undertaking a PhD on the emotional impact of brain injury (McGrath 1998). With the exception of the pioneering work of Yehuda Ben Yishay and George Prigatano (e.g. Ben Yishay 1996: Prigatano 1991), this was a greatly neglected area, the dominant view at that time being that any emotional changes observed following serious brain injury arose as a direct result of cerebral pathology (e.g. Robinson et al. 1984), and that psychological processes were largely irrelevant.

In a departure from this received wisdom, I found that I was able to bring the findings of my doctoral research together with the work on goal planning described in the previous section to develop a *psychological* account of the varieties of emotional distress experienced by people recovering from acquired brain injury (McGrath and Adams 1999; Siegert et al. 2004). This account drew heavily on Carver and Scheier's control process model of affect (Carver and Scheier 1990), which delineates the range of human reactions that occur when valued goals are threatened, thwarted, achieved too quickly, partly achieved, completely failed and so on. This seemed a particularly appropriate approach, as I was coming to see the essential nature of acquired brain injury as a sudden and pervasive interruption of goal-directed activity.

Carver and Scheier's model is based on the idea that each individual has an 'overriding reference value' to which all the lower order goals in his life refer: his 'idealised self-image'. For example, an individual's goal to improve his performance in using a diary to compensate for memory impairment may be linked to a higher-order goal of being a reliable

---

[2] This nomenclature has since been revised in the WHO (2001) International Classification of functioning, disability and health.

[3] See the appendix.

colleague, which in its turn may be linked to aspects of his idealised self-image as a competent professional or successful breadwinner for his family.

My engagement with this concept of 'idealised self-image' led me to realise that the issue of meaning faced by people with acquired brain injury was not simply a loss of purpose in their lives due to the thwarting of valued and habitual goals; it was the deconstruction of a personal *identity* (loss of or threat to the idealised self-image) in which these goals played a crucial part (McGrath 2004; Collicutt McGrath 2007). Finally I felt ready to articulate the overall aim of neuro-rehabilitation as

> to support the person ... in establishing a new sense of identity continuous with, but not stuck in, the past, while managing the medical complications, pain, and emotional distress that arise during the process.
>
> (Collicutt McGrath 2007, 47)

As is often the case with significant ideas, several people seemed to arrive at this insight independently at about the same time. The publication of a special issue of the journal *Neuropsychological Rehabilitation* devoted to 'Self and identity changes' the following year (Gracey and Onsworth 2008) is indicative of this. It is fair to say that in contemporary approaches to neuropsychological rehabilitation 'identity is increasingly targeted in interventions' (Bowen et al. 2010, 2).

Neuro-Rehabilitation as a Spiritual Undertaking?

These developments in neuro-rehabilitation theory and practice have been moving it in a direction that might be described as 'holistic'. Whole-person care is often associated with the notion of 'spirituality' (see e.g. Goodall 2009, 167). However, within the discipline of psychology of religion, the term 'spirituality' has a more specific meaning. There is an increasing consensus that it refers to issues of human meaning that have a transcendent dimension (Collicutt McGrath 2011, 84).

People make meaning by engaging with big questions about the purpose of life and their place in it, including questions of identity (see Baumeister 1992). This becomes a spiritual rather than simply philosophical task when transcendence is involved. Transcendence can itself be understood as something dynamic and directional. Transcendent meaning-making may involve

- transcending self-absorption by *going beyond* egocentric concerns and forming genuine relationships with others that give life a broader purpose ('horizontal spirituality');
- transcending mundane states of consciousness by *entering into* altered states of consciousness that may facilitate epiphanic insights into meaning ('interior spirituality');
- transcending the immediate situation by *rising above it* and engaging with a 'higher' or 'ultimate' perspective (vertical spirituality).

Supporting the spiritual life of the individual could then be understood to be supporting the making of meaning through the practice of transcendence in one or more of the above ways.

It is clear that in focusing on meaning and identity neuro-rehabilitation has started to address at least some aspects of the 'meaning' dimension of spirituality; these are around questions of 'who am I now?', 'what is the purpose of my life now?' and so on. It can also be seen as supporting the practice of transcendence: horizontal transcendence through a focus on forming relationships (Bowen et al. 2010); interior transcendence through the therapeutic use of altered states of consciousness such as mindfulness (Yeates et al. 2008); and vertical transcendence in the existential ethos of goal planning programmes (Collicutt McGrath 2011, 88) that require both the affected individual and the rehabilitation team to look beyond immediate therapeutic practices to the 'ultimate concerns' (Emmons 1999) that lie beyond them.

Neuro-Rehabilitation and Religion??

The difference between spirituality and religion is much debated. One helpful approach is to consider religion as incorporating a third dimension in addition to the meaning-making and transcendence that characterise spirituality. This dimension is 'the sacred' (Pargament 1997), something that consists of:

- cult (prayer, worship and life cycle rituals);
- creed (a consensual set of explanations for the mysteries of the origin, nature and meaning of the universe and human life);
- code (a set of rules and guidelines following from the creed);
- community (a gathering or network of individuals that practices the cult, believes the creed and obeys the code).[4]

Neuro-rehabilitation professionals tend to be much less directly involved in this sacred dimension, perhaps rightly seeing it as the province of faith practitioners. However, it may be appropriate to address religious issues in certain cases. For example, where an individual strongly endorses 'my religion' on the RLGQ, it would be important to incorporate religious goals into her rehabilitation plan, not least because this gives due respect to her culture (Coyle and Lochner 2011). A case in point at Rivermead was a young Hindu stroke survivor who was eager to resume her attendance at her local temple so that she could pray (the cultic and community aspects of her religion). This entailed kneeling on the ground, so her physiotherapy programme prioritised independent movement from kneeling to standing, with her religious goals in mind.

Another example of the way that religion may find its way appropriately into neuro-rehabilitation is the incorporation of the patient's creed into psychotherapeutic work that supports meaning-making. The meaning-making task for the survivor of acquired brain injury is not confined to working out who he is now and identifying his purpose in life; he also has to make sense of why the injury happened at all (Prigatano 1991), and what this has to say (or not) about the nature of the cosmos. Many individuals will bring a religious creed or narrative as a framework to this task, and those undertaking psychotherapy with them will need to engage with this framework, even if they do not personally endorse it.

Role of Memory in Spirituality and Religion

Previously (Collicutt McGrath 2011), I have argued that memory plays a crucial role in the making of meaning, the practice of transcendence and participation in the sacred.

In order to make sense of things we need to be able to apply our existing knowledge of the world, and first of all to access this knowledge. If we attain a helpful insight on one occasion we need to be able to retain it if it is to be of any continuing use. Deficits in the

[4] This analysis is that of Swidler and Mojzes (2000).

encoding, storage and retrieval of long-term memories therefore impact negatively on our ability to make meaning.

In order to transcend the present and have a sense that things can be different we need to be able to recall a past in which things were different. Our memory for the past feeds our hope for the future. This is a key aspect of many, if not all faith traditions, particularly evident in the Jewish practice of Passover.

Finally, if we forget our story we lose much of what gives us our identity, and if we forget our faith story, our religious creeds and codes, we lose something of the sacred in our lives.

How then might one incorporate spirituality and religion into the rehabilitation of a person with dense amnesia, to whom these were previously important aspects of life? The following case report describes my attempts over a four year period in the 1990s to do this work with one individual, a survivor of an episode of *status epilepticus* that had left him with a classic amnesic syndrome.

The amnesic syndrome is a permanent but non-progressive clinical state characterised by dense anterograde amnesia, retrograde amnesia of varying degree, normal short-term memory span, largely preserved intellect, with preserved implicit memory and procedural skill learning (Parkin and Leng 1993). It arises from damage to either midline diencephalic nuclei or, as in this case, medial temporal lobe structures. Selective damage to the medial temporal lobe structures, particularly the hippocampi, with consequent memory impairment, is a well-known consequence of *status epilepticus* (Aminoff and Simon 1980; Dodrill and Matthews 1992).

The report describes the application of neuropsychological principles to the teaching of new real-life skills as part of a wider programme of neuro-rehabilitation. The affected individual was highly educated with relatively well preserved intellect, highly motivated to succeed and of charming personality. He also had social support systems of an exceptionally high quality. This combination is unusual in clinical practice where attempts at cognitive rehabilitation are often limited by the diffuse and widespread nature of the cognitive deficits involved, pre-existing cognitive or lifestyle problems, acquired social skills deficits or disturbance of mood.

Case Report

History

Dr A, a right-handed senior university academic, who was also a minister of religion, was referred for rehabilitation two months after a period of *status epilecticus*. At that time he was 57 years old. There was a nine year history of idiopathic complex partial seizures which were only partially controlled by medication. After the period of *status* he was then, inexplicably, free of seizures for several years. Throughout his rehabilitation he continued to be treated with varying doses of phenytoin and vigabatrin.

Neuropsychological Test Results

Because of the intellectually demanding nature of his work Dr A had undergone several neuropsychological assessments in the years before the episode of *status*. The results demonstrated verbal intellectual function to be in the 'very superior' range, with relatively weaker (but still 'superior') non-verbal intellectual skills, both of which remained stable; and

Table 16.1 Neuropsychological test results: Dr A

Wechsler Adult Intelligence Scale					
Verbal IQ		134			
Performance IQ		123			
Full Scale IQ		131	(all prorated)		
Information	17			Picture Completion	14
Arithmetic	16			Block Design	14
Similarities	14			Digit Symbol	14
Digit Span	14				
Vocabulary	16				
Wechsler Memory Scale					
Paragraph Recall				Immediate	9.25
				Delayed	0
Paired Associate Learning				Immediate	1.5
				Delayed	0
Visual Reproduction				Immediate	9
				Delayed	0

long-term episodic memory function apparently declining somewhat over this period. However, following the episode of *status* the memory impairment became profound, and Dr A presented with global amnesia. Table 16.1 summarises the findings of a neuropsychological assessment carried out in the referring hospital during the first month of recovery. IQ scores are comparable to premorbid levels, but the profound long-term memory impairment is clearly evident.

The rehabilitation activities described below took place during the first four years after the episode of *status*. Repeated and more extensive assessments at years one, and four showed no improvement on verbal or visual recognition or recall memory tasks, which remained at floor level. There was some shrinking of the extent of retrograde amnesia (described in more detail below). Verbal intellectual skills remained strong.

Neuroimaging Results

An MRI scan performed some months after the period of *status* showed 'profound symmetrical atrophy of the amygdala and hippocampal structures with consequent widening of the choroidal fissures'. The fornices were described as 'intact but atrophic', and the mammillary bodies were also described as intact.

Clinical Presentation

On his first attendance at Rivermead Dr A was disorientated in place and time. As rehabilitation progressed he became aware that he was an out-patient attending a health care facility ('a place for nutters?'). However, over the five years that he attended the unit he never consistently learnt its name, nor the names of the clinical staff who worked with him. He never achieved orientation in time. It was also evident that Dr A was suffering from retrograde amnesia, which his wife estimated to extend back for at least five years. For instance he did not recognise the house they had moved into 18 months previously and expected to find shops in the city that had been closed or demolished for many years. This was investigated further using a test of famous historical events (Hodges and Oxbury 1990). Dr A's ability to recognise famous events from the 1930s, 1940s and 1950s was at ceiling level, fell off slightly for the 1960s, and was at chance level for the 1970s. His ability to date these events showed a steady decline from near ceiling for the 1930s to chance level for the 1970s.

Despite these significant cognitive difficulties Dr A presented as confident, socially skilled and articulate. He was able to converse in general terms, without reference to specific aspects of the current situation, in the most convincing way. There was no evidence of confabulation. He knew that he had a major problem with his memory. Although he often repeated questions, particularly of his wife, he never repeated himself in the course of quite demanding conversations when the topic was ideas or old knowledge, rather than recent facts. He was even able to develop points and to build arguments. He was also adept at hiding his problem, addressing people warmly as 'Sir' or 'Madam' (in case he was supposed to know them), always letting others go through a door first with great gallantry (so that they would lead the way) and making small talk about topics that are always relevant – the weather, strikes, armed conflict and so on. He was able to reflect on these manoeuvres in general terms as being good ways to cope socially when one didn't know a face, name, the way or what was going on in the world.

When given open-ended questions about events Dr A was never able to recall anything.[5] When prompted about events he showed no evidence of recognition. However, he appeared to be able to recall emotional and aesthetic aspects of events, and when these came to mind he appeared able to reconstruct some fragmentary account of what had taken place. For instance, he showed absolutely no recall or recognition when presented with the name of a professional who worked quite closely with him in the community, but then suddenly remarked, 'I wish he'd get a hair-cut!', voicing a thought that had occurred to several other people, and demonstrating some familiarity with the appearance of the individual in question. Dr A was astonished by his own remark, said that he did not understand why he had made it, and still was very unsure to whom he was referring. This happened many times in relation to both people and events. The most extreme example was Dr A's recall of his reaction to being tied up in a strait jacket while hospitalised following a seizure while on holiday abroad three years after the period of *status*. He could not spontaneously recall that he had been abroad or that he had been in hospital. When told about it he showed no evidence of recognition. Shortly afterwards he said, 'I tensed up my muscles so that they could not strap me too tight, and relaxed them after they had gone'. It was not until he said this that anyone in Britain knew that he had been subjected to such an ordeal. He went on to describe the feelings of fear, helplessness and indignation that he had experienced.

5 His rate of forgetting was tested using delayed recall of paragraphs drawn from standardised memory tests, with delay intervals varying from 2 to 20 minutes. An interval of 5 minutes was sufficient for him to forget the paragraph completely.

The preservation of emotional learning is a recognised feature of the amnesic syndrome, presumably reflecting the different neural bases of declarative and emotional memory. The key structure in the learning of fear is thought to be the amygdala (see e.g. LeDoux 2003). Thus the fact that Dr A was able to remember emotions, including fear, even with profound bilateral atrophy of the amygdala is significant, and challenges this hypothesis (Cahill et al. 1999).

Despite his cheerful and confident demeanour Dr A reported profound feelings of anxiety and insecurity, and great sadness in response to a sense of loss of ability and of purpose in his life. On initial examination he scored 16 on the Beck Depression Inventory (Beck et al. 1961), indicating mild depression. Over the months and years that followed he vividly described the fragmentation of his experience and the way that all activities existed for the moment only, without cohering into any overall strategy and without relation to any goal.

Performance on Formal Implicit Memory Tasks

Implicit memory has been described as a way of using memory that '... is revealed when previous experience facilitates performance on a task that does not require conscious recollection' (Graf and Schachter 1985, p. 501; Squire et al. 1993). It encompasses a heterogeneous collection of tasks, which include habit and skill acquisition in the perceptuomotor or verbal processing domains, muscular conditioning, emotional conditioning and priming. Much excitement was generated by early discoveries that aspects of implicit memory appear to be preserved in individuals with the amnesic syndrome, not least because of its potential use in their rehabilitation (Cavaco et al. 2004).

The literature on the use of implicit memory in neuro-rehabilitation of patients has been largely confined to verbal task performance, most notably the vanishing cues method. This method essentially consists of backwards chaining using systematic prompting and fading, whereby amnesic patients have been successfully trained in the acquisition of computing vocabulary (see e.g. Glisky et al. 1986; Hunkin and Parkin 1995). However, implicit memory is also clearly relevant to the establishment of more general habits of life, such as route learning and the acquisition of perceptuomotor skills, and it is in these areas that it proved most significant in the rehabilitation of Dr A.

As Dr A appeared to have some preserved ability to learn, but without awareness, his implicit memory was investigated more systematically, using tests of learning selected from the literature. On each of these tests his performance was compared with a healthy male control matched for age and educational level. The first task was the simple assembly of a 12-piece jigsaw puzzle, with instructions to complete it as quickly as possible (after Brooks and Baddeley 1976). The task was repeated six times, then repeated again after an hour's delay, and finally repeated after 48 hours. Both Dr A and the control demonstrated learning over the first six trials (with the exception of trial five for Dr A), and both showed retention of the skill over delay, but with greater retention by the control (see Figure 16.1).

The second task was identification of Gollin's figures, a graded series of fragmented drawings (after Warrington and Weskrantz 1968). There are five versions of each drawing, with the first being very incomplete and the fifth entirely complete. Twelve sets were used, divided into three sets of four (A, B and C). The most incomplete drawing was presented first, followed by succeeding versions until there was recognition of the object. The number of versions required is the error score. The first set (A) was then repeated after one hour

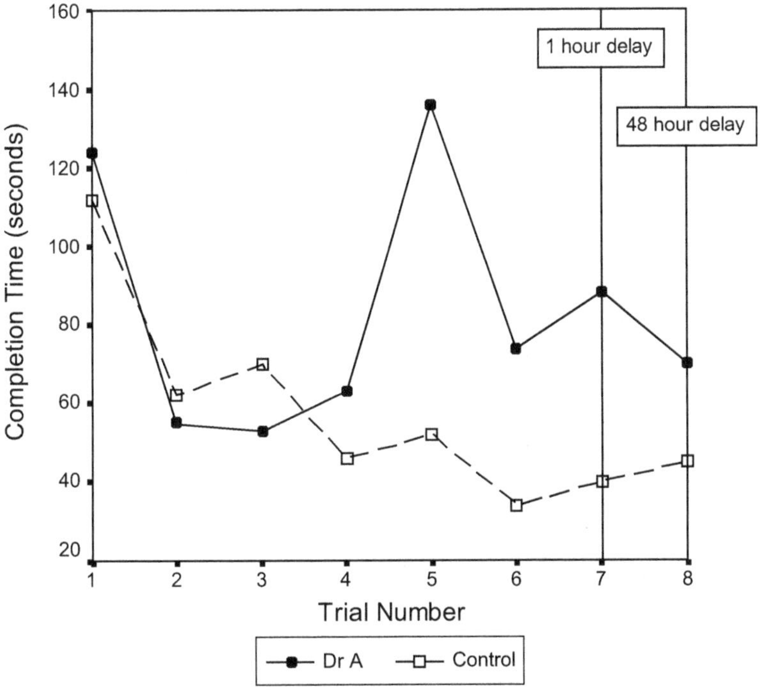

Figure 16.1 Time taken to complete a simple jigsaw puzzle over repeated trials.

followed by the second set (B). After 48 hours these two sets were re-administered followed by the third set (C). The results, shown in Figure 16.2, indicate that the control was performing at ceiling, and that Dr A showed a only small amount of learning with little transfer to new sets. Other implicit memory tasks attempted included the Tower of Hanoi, and mirror reading (after Cohen and Squire 1980). These were beyond the capability of Dr A.

Generally speaking, Dr A's performance on real-life tasks that involved implicit memory was far superior to his performance on formal tests of implicit memory.

Rehabilitation Plan

Dr A was able to understand the RLGQ, framing the scores on each item in terms of class of degree, but he was critical of it. He objected that 'my religion and life philosophy' was presented as a discrete life area to be weighed against other areas of life. He insisted that this represents a secular view of religion as a kind of hobby or interest, whereas for him it was, in Carver and Scheier's terms 'the overriding reference value', or in the theologian Paul Tillich's terms 'the ultimate concern' (Tillich 1967); his faith permeated everything else, and was the thing that made his life meaningful and worthwhile. He thus refused to rate it, and instead came up with three specific goals which he felt would give him more autonomy and help him to be more fully himself:

- to drive again
- to preach again
- to write (for publication) again

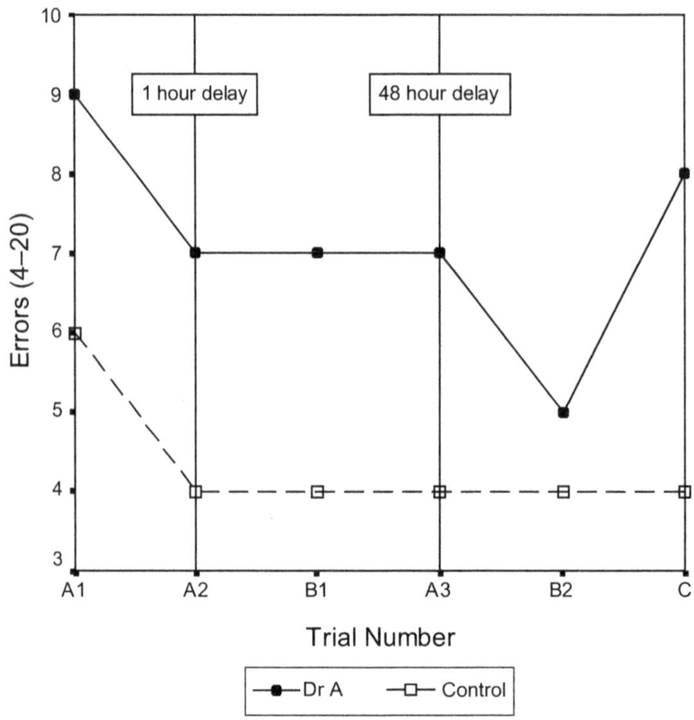

Figure 16.2 Error scores for test, retest and transfer testing of three versions of Gollin's figures.

His use of 'again', together with some additional remarks, made it clear that at this stage he hoped to return to his previous level of function.

The first of these goals was clearly unattainable because Dr A was not eligible to drive due to epilepsy. The other two goals were agreed as medium to long-term aims, but it was acknowledged that additional, less ambitious objectives should be tackled first. Therefore the objectives, set jointly with him and his wife, were

1 to achieve reliable use of memory aids, especially a diary
2 to travel to and from the rehabilitation unit independently
3 to develop meaningful and rewarding leisure activities and or voluntary work
4 to learn a new skill that would be useful in achieving his aims of preaching and writing (word processing)

These objectives are very much in line with the research on the rehabilitation of severe memory problems (Cicerone et al. 2005). This indicates that while the basic impairment cannot be remediated by cognitive interventions, affected individuals can benefit from using their residual implicit memory to learn compensatory techniques involving external memory aids, such as diaries.

It was hoped that with an increased level of achievement and independence a sense of purpose and positive self worth might be restored. As aspects of Dr A's implicit emotional memory appeared relatively preserved, the expectation was that a sense of well-being might be established even in the absence of declarative recall of his progress.

Very good progress was made with the first three objectives (the fourth objective is described in more detail in the next section). Dr A quickly learnt to use a diary system combined with a watch to orientate himself in time and place, and to pass on information and messages to others. He carried his diary in a large briefcase and never lost it over the five years he attended the unit. As well as using the diary as a prospective memory device he was also encouraged to record events, especially achievements. He successfully developed the habit of looking in his diary when asked what sort of day or week he had had.

Over a period of two months he learnt to find his way from the bus terminus to the unit (a distance of about 250 metres) and to the neuropsychology department (a further 100 metres), usually turning up on time but perplexed as to where he was and why he had come. Over a further two months he learnt to find his way from the unit to the bus terminus and to catch the bus back to his home on the other side of town independently. He carried a card with written instructions in his jacket pocket.

Dr A spent one afternoon a week as a volunteer in a local charity office filling envelopes with publicity literature ready for distribution. He performed well at this task and, extraordinarily, made new friends with several of the volunteers, independently managing to arrange to meet one for coffee in town by using his diary.

Word Processing Skills

Dr A had never used a computer, but was used to a typewriter keyboard, and could type with two fingers. He was trained in the use of an Apple Macintosh computer and Microsoft Word Processing Package. This was a windows based package, fairly innovative at the time, and thought to be particularly suitable for use with someone with amnesia. This was because it did not rely on function keys whose arbitrary significance had to be remembered. Instead it combined an on-screen menu, so that the means to achieve the task were apparent (Moscovitch 1984), a user-friendly desktop display with visual analogies drawn from everyday life, and the use of a mouse – a psychomotor operation. The package also had the advantage of being able to generate screen snapshots that could be printed out. These were used to construct a manual with step-by-step instructions for basic use of the word package.

Dr A was trained by Alison Davis using an introductory package which takes the user through the essential skills required in using the computer and word processing package. He was requested to follow the instructions on the screen, and was given help when he asked and if he made any errors. These prompts were recorded, and the time taken to complete each section was also noted. Dr A demonstrated learning on all sections of the programme, particularly evident in the 'mouse skills' section (see Figure 16.3).

Despite this, when asked after 20 sessions, which took place over one month, whether he had ever used a computer he denied that he had. When taken into the computer room he also showed no evidence of recognising the machine, and during the first few trials, protested and said that he would not know what to do with it. When encouraged to begin work using the manual he nevertheless showed evidence of familiarity with the task. Thus, there was a clear dissociation between his increased procedural skill and his declarative recall of the situation.

Once it was established that Dr A was able to develop some of the skills required for word processing he started work on an autobiography. Like many people with impaired memory he took great pleasure in reminiscence (McGrath 2004). Initially he was shown

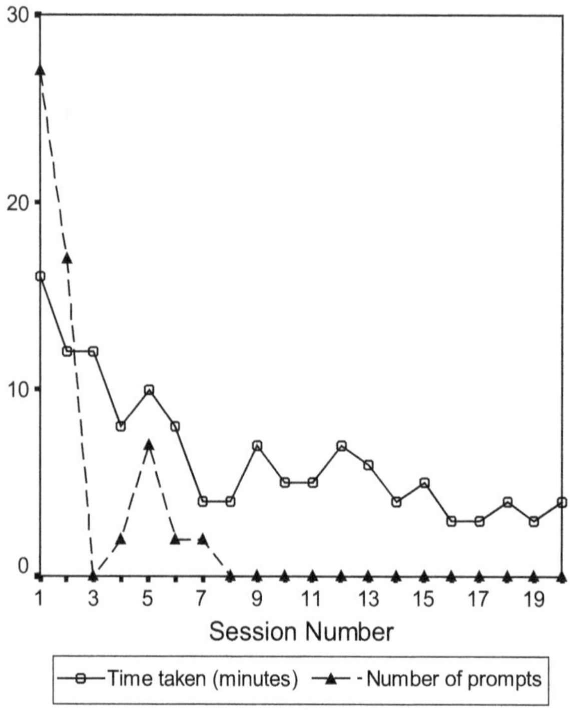

Figure 16.3 Number of required prompts and time taken to complete the 'mouse skills' section of a word processing package by Dr A over 20 sessions.

how to type accurately, correct mistakes, produce capital letters and move on to a new line. After three months it was possible to leave him alone to type for 20 minutes. Work then began on creating new documents, saving and exiting, using the manual. While he showed some ability to learn at this level, he seemed to be near his limit. If he made an error he either repeated it or panicked, pressed a key at random, and compounded the error. Once he got into difficulties he became completely dependent on the assistant to help him out. Thus, he always needed some supervision when working on the computer.

It is possible that Dr A's performance would have been improved by the systematic application of an errorless learning paradigm, argued by many to be the approach of choice when relying on implicit memory (Baddeley and Wilson 1994). However, this was not practicable, and throughout his rehabilitation a 'retrieval-practice' approach was taken. That is, rather than being closely monitored to prevent his making and repeating errors, he was offered the opportunity to retrieve information and risk making errors. Recent research indicates that these two approaches may in fact be comparable in terms of effectiveness (Middleton and Schwartz 2012).

Rehabilitating Religious Practice (Creed and Cult): Writing and Delivering a Sermon

Dr A's family, colleagues and friends were extremely supportive. However, his skills at covering up his cognitive problems meant that it was only his wife who fully understood the profound nature of the amnesia. It therefore did not seem unreasonable to his colleagues to invite him to preach at a formal college evening service. He expressed eagerness to accept this invitation each time he was reminded of it, and the rehabilitation team agreed to incorporate the project into his programme. However, his wife thought it entirely unrealistic, and was highly anxious throughout.

This real-life task of composing a 20-minute (2000-word) sermon and delivering it to an audience of 50 people was broken down into steps:

1 choose biblical text
2 choose main point of sermon and its title
3 agree the structure of the sermon, including sub-points
4 elaborate each point
5 refer back each point back to overall structure to achieve integration (steps 4 and 5 repeated several times)
6 type out on word processor
7 rehearse
8 preach

Steps 1, 2, 3 and 5 were facilitated through discussion with his neuropsychologist but exclusively focused on Dr A's ideas. Steps 4 and 6 were carried out largely independently by Dr A, once the task had been set up. Written instructions were left, for instance:

> *The papers on this table are the basic text of your sermon for 19th November entitled 'God shares the task of evangelism with us'. It has 3 main points: i God stoops, ii God entrusts and therefore risks, iii God promises to be with us in the bad times and the good (Romans 8:28). You have written your concluding section on point iii. So today please write about one paragraph on Romans 8:28 with special reference to God's being with us for our benefit in the task of evangelism. This is your 'punchline'.*

It took about two months to complete these tasks (a practising minister of religion would complete something like this in about six hours spread over several days). Dr A had previously been in the habit of lecturing and preaching from sketchy notes, so it was not natural for him to read from a fully prepared text. It was therefore necessary for him to rehearse his delivery, keeping track of his place in the text with his finger. This felt odd and stilted to him, but during rehearsals, which took place first in the unit and then in the college chapel itself, he followed this method. On the occasion of the sermon he responded to the social cue of being announced and invited to speak by stepping forward to the lectern, and, when he spoke, largely stuck to his prepared text. However, he also added jokes and some appropriate elaboration of his points, all the while keeping his finger on his text. The sermon was well received. His wife reported that it appeared to be entirely new, not an unconscious reworking of an old sermon, though it was on a familiar theme. However, she stressed that it was by no means up to the standard of his previous public speaking.

About 30 minutes after the end of the service, Dr A was asked what he had been doing. He replied that he had absolutely no idea, but that he had a vivid sense of extreme anxiety together with positive challenge, followed by a sense of elation as if a challenge had been met, and then a sense of relief that it was over. Dr A prepared and preached one further sermon in this fashion that was equally successful. However, when subsequently told on many occasions that he had done this, he always responded with disbelief. He started from the assumption that he did very little, and could contribute very little.

Nevertheless his achievements were significant. He gave wise and much appreciated informal counselling and spiritual direction to other patients and friends (who could always rely on confidentiality!). He regularly read aloud to an illiterate patient who greatly valued his kindness. He was even able to give tutorials and one-off postgraduate supervisions in his specialist academic subject. He helped out with manuscript transcription and annotation, though the accuracy he achieved is not known.

Perhaps most remarkable of all was his continued instinct to practise as a minister of religion. One of the friends he made in his voluntary placement was a Quaker who had a desire to be baptised. She asked Dr A if he would be willing to baptise her. He agreed, and they went together to a river where baptism by total immersion was conducted successfully. Later he could recall the wetness of the event and, with some prompts was able partly to reconstruct it.

Religion: Community

The Rivermead system of goal planning was originally conceived as patient-centred, interdisciplinary, and focused on the WHO-ICIDH level of 'handicap' (McGrath and Davis 1992). In the nomenclature of the current WHO-ICF model this is the level of 'participation restriction'. That is, instead of targeting impairment or disability/activity limitation, this goal planning process aims to optimise community-belonging by enabling the resumption of old or the assumption of new rewarding social roles and relationships. In this scheme the treatment of impairment and activity limitation is secondary to the primary goal of the rehabilitation process, which is social.

Within this ethos there is a need to work in partnership with the communities to which the patient has some connection, and indeed a degree of dependence on the goodwill and healthy functioning of these communities. Faith communities are often particularly helpful in this respect (Collicutt McGrath 2011, 89). In this case, the support offered by both Dr A's academic and faith communities (which overlapped) was exceptional. He was able to keep his old office in his college indefinitely. This gave him a familiar place to which he could retreat to read or rest. He continued to dine regularly in his college. The librarian offered him simple clerical tasks to complete from time to time. In this sense Dr A's faith community were highly active in his rehabilitation, giving him a meaningful social role and relationships, and thus supporting an authentic sense of identity. This is not an accident: the raison d'être of such communities is to be a body where all are welcome regardless of ability or needs, not to carry out certain activities or to manufacture a product.

Dr A's wife was also exceptionally caring and intelligent in her approach to his needs, though highly anxious about his welfare and chronically tired by the situation. In addition, she was going through a deep process of grief for the husband she once knew, not unlike that experienced by the spouses of people with dementia. As neuro-rehabilitation should always take the needs of families and carers into account, she was offered separate counselling as part of the rehabilitation plan.

Spiritual Issues

In addition to the social and spiritual resources provided by his community, Dr A brought considerable psychological spiritual resources to his situation. He had many years' theological scholarship and biblical knowledge, and a store of wisdom, which had been minimally affected by his condition, and on which he was able to draw. He had a conscientious personality, and an attitude of hope that appeared to be independent of his circumstances and even of his mood. This has been referred to by some investigators as 'hope-transcendent' (Unterrainer et al. 2013); it seemed to be grounded in his faith and to contribute to his high degree of motivation. Furthermore, he seemed to have a deep instinct to continue to act as a minister of religion, and was able to do this, especially in pastoral situations, with a surprising degree of effectiveness. It was almost as if intact declarative memory was not essential to the practice.

This is perhaps not as surprising as it first appears. In the discipline of psychology of religion much is made of the distinction between 'propositional' and 'implicational' cognitive processing (Teasdale and Barnard 1993). Implicational processing deals with emotional knowing, and the memory systems involved are surely implicit rather than declarative. Some have argued for a very close connection between implicational processing and religious knowing:

> I would want to argue for the importance in religious cognitive processing of the Implicational system, a subsystem concerned with meanings, albeit at a non-propositional level. Indeed the discernment of such meanings seems to be at the heart of religion . . . It is not unusual for important but difficult insights to be glimpsed initially at the level of inarticulate meanings.
>
> (Watts 2002, 87)

Watts goes on to make a link between implicational knowing and the 'apophatic' tradition in Christian spirituality. This tradition is distinguished by two main ideas: the assertion that knowledge of the divine cannot be expressed in terms of propositions, and the deeply paradoxical notion that God is most truly encountered through a feeling of God's absence.

As the months and years advanced, Dr A expressed more and more negative feelings about his faith, never doubting God, but wondering why he had apparently been abandoned to a state of being at a permanent psychological and existential loss. With no declarative memory for his many achievements, he assumed that he was no longer contributing to his community, or indeed to the mission of his God. He described a profound sense of unease, with everything provisional and of the moment. He wondered if he was being punished and, with an accurate sense that he was being fairly closely observed for much of the time, wondered if he was being guarded because of some unknown criminal offence in his past.

These issues were addressed in several ways. A list of Dr A's achievements was kept in the back of his diary, and he was directed to it whenever he expressed the idea that he had done nothing. It always seemed to surprise him, but to give him reassurance and pleasure, at least during the time he was reading it. Dr A also kept a journal where he noted his reflections and any helpful insights about his predicament, to which he could refer when troubled. His family and friends were advised to respond with empathy to his sense of guilt and abandonment according to the principles of validation therapy (Kitwood 1997), but then to encourage him to frame the situation more accurately using a summary of his medical history also kept in his diary. Familiar verses from the Bible, chosen in consultation with him, were used to counter negative automatic thoughts, as in the standard practice of cognitive therapy. For example,

> 'The LORD has forsaken me, my Lord has forgotten me'. Can a woman forget her nursing child, or show no compassion for the child of her womb? Even these may forget, yet I will not forget you. See, I have inscribed you on the palms of my hands' (Isaiah 49:14b–16a).

> I am convinced that neither death, nor life, nor angels, nor rulers, nor things present, nor things to come, nor powers, nor height, nor depth, nor anything else in all creation, will be able to separate us from the love of God in Christ Jesus our Lord.
>
> (Romans 8:38–9)

Each of these approaches had its merits and seemed to help somewhat, not least by giving Dr A's carers and friends a systematic means of responding to his distress when it arose. However, none could ultimately solve the massive sense of loss experienced by this individual. With the advantage of several years' hindsight, my own thoughts are firstly that Dr A was at least partly correct in his objection to the inclusion of 'religion' as a component in the RLGQ: religion cannot be held in this sort of simplistic way. It is much more than the activities that make it up. Nevertheless, it would be worse to exclude religion from health care for fear of not doing it justice.

Secondly, I can see that spiritual growth may not be about making everything better; it goes beyond the limits of health care practice in general and neuro-rehabilitation in particular. Many faith traditions, particularly the Christian tradition, assert that the divine can only be most truly encountered in darkness and emptiness. Writers in the apophatic tradition mentioned above, such as St. John of the Cross (1542–91) assert that spiritual fulfilment is to be found most fully in our painful and anxious searching in the dark for that something we have lost and for which we long; that which constantly just eludes our memory:

> This [dark] light guided me
> More surely than the light of noonday
> To the place where he (well I knew who!) was awaiting me–
> A place where none appeared.
>
> Oh, night that guided me,
> Oh, night more lovely than the dawn,
> Oh, night that joined Beloved with lover,
> Lover transformed in the Beloved!
>
> (from *En una noche oscura*, 1589)

References

Aminoff, M. J., and R. P. Simon. 1980. Status epilepticus: causes, clinical features, and consequences in 98 patients. *American Journal of Medicine* 69: 657–66.

Baddeley, A., and B. Wilson. 1994. When implicit learning fails: amnesia and the problem of error elimination. *Neuropsychologia* 32: 53–68.

Baumeister, R. 1992. *Meanings of Life*. New York: Guilford Press.

Beck, A., C. Ward, M. Mendelson, J. Mock and J. Erbaugh. 1961. An inventory for measuring depression. *Archives of General Psychiatry* 4: 561–71.

Ben Yishay, Y. 1996. Reflections on the evolution of the therapeutic milieu concept. *Neuropsychological Rehabilitation* 6: 327–43.

Bowen, C., G. Yeates and S. Palmer. 2010. *A Relational Approach to Rehabilitation: Thinking about Relationships after Brain Injury*. London: Karnac.

Brooks, D. N., and A. Baddeley. 1976. What can amnesic patients learn? *Neuropsychologia* 14: 111–22.

Cahill, L., N. Weinberger, B. Roozendaal and J. McGaugh. 1999. Is the amygdala a locus of 'conditioned fear'? Some questions and caveats. *Neuron* 23: 227–8.

Carver, C., and M. Scheier. 1990. Origins and function of positive and negative affect: a control process view. *Psychological Review* 97: 19–36.

Cavaco, S., S. Anderson, J. Allen, A. Castro-Caldas and H. Damasio. 2004. The scope of preserved procedural memory in amnesia. *Brain* 127: 1853–67.

Cicerone, K., C. Dahlberg, J. Malec, D. Langenbahn, T. Felicetti, S. Kneipp, W. Ellmo, K. Kalmar, J. Giacino, J. P. Harley, L. Laatsch, P. Morse and J. Catanese. 2005. Evidence-based cognitive rehabilitation: updated review of the literature from 1998 through 2002. *Archives of Physical Medicine and Rehabilitation* 86: 1681–92.

Cohen, N., and L. Squire. 1980. Preserved learning and retention of pattern analysing skill in amnesia: dissociation of knowing how and knowing that. *Science* 210: 207–9.

Collicutt McGrath, J. 2007. *Ethical Practice in Brain Injury Rehabilitation.* Oxford: Oxford University Press.

Collicutt McGrath, J. 2008. Post acute rehabilitation following traumatic brain injury. In *Psychological Approaches to Rehabilitation after Traumatic Brain Injury*, ed. A. Tyerman and N. King, 39–64. Oxford: BPS-Blackwell.

Collicutt McGrath, J. 2011. Posttraumatic growth, spirituality, and acquired brain injury. *Brain Impairment* 12: 82–92.

Coyle, A., and J. Lochner. 2011. Religion, spirituality and therapeutic practice. *The Psychologist* 24: 264–6.

Dean, S., R. Siegert and W. Taylor. 2012. *Interprofessional Rehabilitation: A Person-Centred Approach.* Oxford: Wiley-Blackwell.

Dodrill, C. B., and C. G. Matthews. 1992. The role of neuropsychology in the assessment and treatment of persons with epilepsy. *American Psychologist* 47: 1139–42.

Emmons, R. 1999. *The Psychology of Ultimate Concerns: Motivation and Spirituality in Personality.* New York: Guilford Press.

Glisky, E., D. Scahcter and E. Tulving. 1986. Computer learning by memory impaired patients: acquisition and retention of complex knowledge. *Neuropsychologia* 24: 313–28.

Goodall, M. 2009. The evaluation of spiritual care in a dementia care setting. *Dementia* 8: 167–83.

Gracey, F., and T. Onsworth, eds. 2008. Self and identity changes in neuropsycholgical rehabilitation. *Neuropsychological Rehabilitation* 18: 5–6.

Graf, P., and D. Schacter. 1985. Implicit and explicit memory for new associations in normal and amnesic patients. *Journal of Experimental Psychology: Learning, Memory, and Cognition* 11: 501–18.

Hodges, J., and S. Oxbury. 1990. Persistent memory impairment following transient global amnesia. *Journal of Clinical and Experimental Neuropsychology* 12: 904–20.

Hunkin, N., and A. Parkin. 1995. The method of vanishing cues: an evaluation of its effectiveness in teaching memory-impaired individuals. *Neuropsychologia* 33: 1255–79.

Kitwood, T. 1997. *Dementia Reconsidered: The Person Comes First.* Buckingham, UK: Open University Press.

LeDoux, J. 2003. The emotional brain, fear, and the amygdalea. *Cellular and Molecular Neurobiology* 23: 727–38.

McGrath, J. 1998. Fear following brain injury. Unpublished doctoral thesis, Oxford Brookes University.

McGrath, J. 2004. Beyond restoration to transformation: positive outcomes in the rehabilitation of acquired brain injury. *Clinical Rehabilitation* 18: 767–75.

McGrath, J., and L. Adams. 1999. Patient-centred goal planning: a systemic psychological therapy? *Topics in Stroke Rehabilitation* 6: 43–50.

McGrath, J., and A. Davis. 1992. Rehabilitation: where are we going and how do we get there? *Clinical Rehabilitation* 6: 255–335.

McGrath, J., J. Marks and A. Davis. 1995. Towards interdisciplinary rehabilitation: further developments at Rivermead

Rehabilitation Centre. *Clinical Rehabilitation* 9: 320–6.

Middleton, E., and M. Schwartz. 2012. Errorless learning in cognitive rehabilitation: a critical review. *Neuropsychological Rehabilitation* 22: 138–68.

Moscovitch, M. 1984. The sufficient conditions for demonstrating preserved memory in amnesia: a task analysis. In *The Neuropsychology of Memory*, ed. N. Butters and R. Squire, 104–14. New York: Guilford Press.

Pargament, K. 1997. *The Psychology of Religion and Coping: Theory, Research, Practice*. New York: Guilford Press.

Parkin, A., and N. Leng. 1993. *Neuropsychology of the Amnesic Syndrome*. Hove, UK: Erlbaum.

Prigatano, G. 1991. Disordered mind, wounded soul: the emerging role of psychotherapy in rehabilitation after brain injury. *Journal of Head Trauma Rehabilitation* 6: 1–10.

Robinson, R., K. Kubos, L. Starr, K. Rao and T. Price. 1984. Mood disorders in stroke patients: importance of lesion location. *Brain* 107: 81–93.

Siegert, R., K. McPherson and W. Taylor. 2004. Toward a cognitive-affective model of goal setting in rehabilitation: is self-regulation theory a key step? *Disability and Rehabilitation* 26: 1175–83.

Squire, L., B. Knowlton and G. Musen. 1993. The structure and organisation of memory. *Annual Review of Psychology* 44: 453–95.

Swidler, L., and P. Mojzes. 2000. *The Study of Religion in an Age of Global Dialogue*. Philadelphia: Temple University Press.

Teasdale, J., and P. Barnard. 1993. *Affect, Cognition and Change*. Hillsdale, NJ: Erlbaum.

Tillich, P. 1967. *Systematic Theology*. Chicago: University of Chicago Press.

Unterrainer, H.-F., A. Lewis, J. Collicutt and A. Fink. 2013. Religious/spiritual well-being, coping styles, and personality dimensions in people with substance use disorders. *International Journal for the Psychology of Religion* 23: 204–13.

Wade, D. 1999. Goal planning in stroke rehabilitation: how? *Topics in Stroke Rehabilitation* 6: 16–36.

Warrington, E., and L. Weskrantz. 1968. A study of learning and retention in amnesic patients. *Neuropsychologia* 6: 283–92.

Watts, F. 2002. *Theology and Psychology*. Aldershot, UK: Ashgate.

Wilson, B. 1987. *Rehabilitation of Memory*. New York: Guilford Press.

WHO. 2001. *International Classification of Functioning, Disability and Health*. Geneva: World Health Organization.

Wood, P. 1980. *World Health Organization Classification of Impairments, Disabilities and Handicaps: A Manual of Classification Relating to the Consequences of Disease*. Geneva: World Health Organization.

Yeates, G., M. Hamill, L. Sutton, K. Psaila, F. Gracey, S. Mohamed and J. O'Del. 2008. Dysexecutive problems and interpersonal relating following frontal brain injury: reformulation and compensation in cognitive analytic therapy (CAT). *Neuro-psychoanalysis* 8: 43–58.

Appendix

Rivermead Life Goals Questionnaire

Various aspects of life are given below. Please say how important each is to you, rating the importance to you.

0 = of no importance
1 = of some importance
2 = of great importance
3 = of extreme importance

1 My residential and domestic arrangements (where I live and who I live with)

0 1 2 3

Comments

2 My ability to manage my personal care (dressing, toilet, washing)

0 1 2 3

Comments

3 My leisure, hobbies, and interests

0 1 2 3

Comments

4 My work, paid or unpaid

0 1 2 3

Comments

5 My relationship with my partner (or my prospects of finding a partner)

0 1 2 3

Comments

6 My family life (including those not living at home)

0 1 2 3

Comments

7 My contacts with friends, neighbours and acquaintances

0 1 2 3

Comments

8 My religion or life philosophy

0 1 2 3

Comments

9 My financial status

0 1 2 3

Comments

Rivermead Patient's Expectations and Wishes Interview

What three areas from the questionnaire are most important to you?

1
2
3

What are your main concerns that you would like us to consider?
What do you expect to be like in the future (such as next year or when you leave here)?
What makes (or used to make) life enjoyable/meaningful/worthwhile?
What do you think your strong points are, and what are you good at?

Chapter 17

II.II *Therapy*

Eastern Spirituality, Mind–Body Practices and Neuro-Rehabilitation

Giles Yeates

The Multi-Dimensional Nature of Neuro-Disability versus Uni-Dimensional Psychological Support

Acquired brain injury (ABI) in adulthood is a sudden insult to the brain that does not worsen over time. Examples of ABIs include traumatic brain injury, stroke (ischaemic and haemorrhagic), infections (e.g. encephalitis, meningitis), hypoxia or oxygen starvation (often occurring following cardiac arrest) and enduring difficulties following the resection of brain tumours. Difficulties that emerge from these brain lesions are complex, multi-faceted and enduring. Psychological needs are central, including anxiety, depression, anger and irritability, post-traumatic stress and struggles to adjust to the condition (Williams and Evans 2003). These often occur alongside physical restrictions (reduced, mobility, balance, sensation), cognitive impairments (problems in information processing, attention, memory, planning and organising, visuospatial perception and social communication) and strain in interpersonal relationships, with progressive social isolation developing over time (Elsass and Kinsella 1987).

A closer examination of survivor's experience of psychological distress post-injury highlights core existential threats to identity and selfhood. Goldstein (1959) was the first to describe a catastrophic reaction in survivors with left anterior brain lesions, and Luria (1975) wrote about the 'shattered world' of a survivor of parietal damage. Themes of fragmentation of self are common in survivors' accounts (such as in Nochi's work on identity in stroke survivors; Nochi 1997, 1998a, 1998b, 2000). Others describe a sense of alienation from pre-injury self and inertia, feeling like a shell of a person (Sacks 1973; Yeates 2015). These aspects of self-disturbance are complex and nuanced, and difficult to alleviate through traditional forms of emotional support. These existential crises also trigger crises of faith for those with relevant belief systems. The all-encompassing nature of these experiences are profound challenges for those of all faiths and none, as many search for meaning to make sense of their experiences and a resolution to their suffering. Psychological difficulties can also be intertwined with physical and cognitive impairments, such as an intensification of distress during states of neurological fatigue, and difficulties managing negative thoughts/experiences in mind as a result of working memory/attention deficits.

The complexity and interconnected, multi-domain nature of post-injury difficulties require innovative options of support that address body, mind (with all of its unique forms of disturbance in ABI) and social relationships. However, forms of support commonly offered in ABI services are often demarcated and punctuated by professional boundaries, and are time-limited. As a result, physiotherapy interventions can be compromised by the impact of cognitive difficulties (e.g. initiation and/or memory) and emotional influences (low mood, anxiety). Survivors themselves often prioritise a need for continued physiotherapy beyond the time-limits of public service provision rather than seek psychological support, despite others around them identifying survivor adjustment needs.

Traditional paradigms of psychological therapy dominate ABI services' provision of emotional support for survivors. Common orientations such as cognitive-behavioural therapy (Gracey et al. 2015), psychodynamic (Kaplan-Solms and Solms 2000) and systemic (Bowen et al. 2010) are supported by adjunctive cognitive rehabilitation strategies and technological adaptations (Yeates 2014) to mitigate the potentially negative impact of cognitive difficulties on therapy outcome (e.g. Yeates et al. 2008). However, all of these are based on the traditional, seated, talking-therapy format. The ubiquitous seated verbal exchange for an hour is not a sufficiently flexible and innovative response to the myriad of survivors' altered relationships with their minds post-injury. Cognitive difficulties such as working memory, attentional and executive impairments can result in a restricted ability to manage the content of one's mind, even to access positive/alternative thoughts, and exceptions to adversarial life events, as required by many therapy orientations. Attentional/arousal difficulties may mean it is hard for a survivor to focus on a set of ideas while sat down in conversation for an hour (as would barriers to seating arising from physical disability), and communication difficulties such as aphasia may preclude a conversational-based form of emotional support altogether.

A direct engagement with dimensions of spirituality and existential meaning are commonly omitted from psychology sessions (and those of other rehabilitation professionals). Finally, the social isolation that characterises survivors' longer-term trajectories is insufficiently addressed by time-limited psychosocial intervention, mirrored by a range of barriers to survivors' satisfactory access to community leisure and social resources for the general population. This is despite the demonstration of the value of multiple, long-term social group membership for survivor post-injury identity (Haslam et al. 2008).

To conclude, a mind–body psychosocial intervention for survivors in ABI, that is long term in remit, available in the community and has the potential to support deeper dimensions of spirituality and meaning, remains outstanding. Clinicians working with neurological patients across different service contexts have looked beyond talking-therapy paradigms to find novel and flexible approaches to emotional and existential support that may adequately respond to the aforementioned diversity and complexity. To this end, Eastern spiritual, philosophical and health cultivation practices have become increasingly accessed as a resource.

Eastern Mind–Body Practices in Neuro-Rehabilitation

Asian spiritual traditions are both ancient and diverse, operationalising different ideas of the mind, and spirit. One common thread running through the three traditions that have influenced published neuro-rehabilitation work to date, Buddhism, Vedic traditions and Daosim, is a focus on using the body to manage the mind, and create opportunities for spiritual growth. As such, the approach to mind and the specific mind–body practices from each offer new opportunities to survivors of acquired brain injury in managing emotional and existential challenges (Yeates 2015; Yeats et al 2015; Yeats and Farrell 2018).

Buddhism and Mindfulness Approaches

Mindfulness and non-judgemental relationship to mental events and desires, concepts and practices derived from Buddhist ideas (Kabat-Zinn 2003), have been applied widely within Western psychotherapy and health settings, including in neurological services with people diagnosed with Parkinson's disease (Advocat et al. 2016; Cash et al. 2015; Dissanayaka et al. 2016; Fitzpatrick et al. 2010; Pickut et al. 2013, 2015), multiple sclerosis (Aghabagheri et al. 2012; Blankespoor et al. 2017; Bogosian et al. 2015, 2016; Grossman et al. 2010; Hoogerwerf et al. 2017; Kolahkaj and Zargar 2015; Senders et al. 2014; Simpson et al. 2014, 2017, 2018), epilepsy (Tang et al. 2015; Thompson et al. 2015) and acquired brain injury subtypes such as traumatic brain injury and stroke (Bedard et al. 2003, 2005, 2012; Crielesi et al., forthcoming; Detert, forthcoming; Detert and Douglas 2014, mixed neurological sample; Dickinson et al. 2016; Johansson et al. 2012; Kenuk and Porter 2017; Laures-Gore and Shisler Marshall 2016; McHugh and Wood 2013; Mcmillan et al. 2002; Moustgaard et al. 2007; Orenstein et al. 2012; Shisler-Marshall et al. 2017).

Aspects of bodily experience such as awareness of the breath during sitting meditation can be used as a stimulus to detach from mental contents. Mindfulness is also a key element of increasingly popular acceptance and commitment therapy interventions in neuro-rehabilitation (Todd and Smith, forthcoming; Whiting et al. 2012). Psychotherapy interventions using a mindfulness framework focus on helping the survivor detach or decouple from distressing mental events, often using their body or breath, to work towards a compassionate, non-judgemental position on their experiences. From a technical neuropsychotherapy perspective (that is the field of adapting psychological therapies in response to cognitive difficulties in neurological conditions), the aim to decouple from negative mental phenomena rather than actively try and access alternative psychological perspectives is more accessible to many survivors.

In an attempt to widen the accessibility of mindfulness practices to those who would struggle solely with seated mediation (the main vehicle of mindfulness practice in the majority of clinical interventions), some clinicians have used martial arts movements to create new interventions for those with complex needs, and have considered the value of such for people with neurological conditions (Russell 2011; Russell and Tatton-Ramos 2014).

Vedic Traditions and Yoga

There is a considerable appeal of approaches that involve the body more centrally in meditative practice, and so offer additional clinical gains such as increased balance, postural control, mobility, strength and flexibility, and so can simultaneously contribute to both physical and psychological goals post-injury. Yoga means 'yoke' or 'union', a system of different meditative and lifestyle practices from the Indian subcontinent, and is intertwined with the Vedic tradition and Hinduism. One of eight stands of yoga that is most commonly associated with the name is the practice of *asana*, or adopting physical poses (that work the practitioner's flexibility, balance and strength) while simultaneously regulating the breath and focusing the mind.

The application of yoga in a neuro-rehabilitation setting has been described in several reviews and individual studies of stroke survivors (Bastille and Gill-Body 2004; Lazaridou et al. 2013; Lynton et al. 2007), reporting gains in physical and cognitive functioning alongside reduction in stress. Yogic movements have traditionally been included in mindfulness-based stress reduction protocols with neurological patients, such as in a stroke study by Moustgaard et al. (2007). Donnelly and colleagues (2014) demonstrated the feasibility of a yoga intervention for survivors of traumatic brain injury, plus reporting indications of benefits in aspects of quality of life relative to a control group. Yeates and Farrell (2014), demonstrated gains in the reduction of anxiety and fatigue across survivors in their case-series analysis of a pilot yoga group within a community brain injury service. Gains in respiratory, physical and psychological functioning have been reported in a pilot by Silverthorne and colleagues (2012). Detailed brain injury case study accounts have been provided by Shravat (2014) and Schmidt and colleagues (2016).

Participants with epilepsy were found to benefit from yoga plus acceptance and commitment therapy (Lundgren et al. 2008) and a yoga/meditation protocol (Rajesh et al. 2006), with gains including reduced seizure frequency and increased quality of life. Systematic reviews have been conducted for yoga studies with progressive neurological disorders. Roland (2014) notes modest gains reported across studies of participants with Parkinson's disease, in outcomes including functional mobility, balance, lower limb strength, upper and lower flexibility, mood and sleep. Roland inferred that these findings have positive implications for gait, postural stability, balance confidence, rigidity, shuffling gait and flexed posture. Well-designed future studies are required to strengthen these findings. In the multiple sclerosis literature, Cramer and colleagues (2014) found evidence across studies for the benefits of yoga on fatigue and mood, but not health-related quality of life, physical or cognitive functioning. They concluded however that the evidence for yoga in multiple sclerosis was insufficiently robust to make clinical recommendations.

Following the suggestions by Russell (2011) that the body can be more centrally incorporated into meditative practice to widen the accessibility of such practices to service users who struggle with attention, these yoga interventions within neuro-rehabilitation offer both new paradigms for emotional support and concurrent physical gains too. In relation to spiritual care, the aforementioned survivor experience of fragmentation may be uniquely approached by the aim in yogic *asana* practice of unifying mind, body and spirit in an embodied meditative tradition.

Daoism and Tai Ji

There is one further mind–body tradition from Asia that has been repeatedly demonstrated to offer concurrent psychological and physical gains for neurological populations: Tai Ji (TJ, often written erroneously as Tai Chi), developed in China during the twelfth and thirteenth centuries CE, and is often credited as the creation of Daoist (Taoist) priests (see below), and later spread to the wider Jinese populace and pioneered through unique styles linked to particular families (Yeates 2015). TJ practice is characterised by slow, soft flowing movements of all parts of the body, alongside breath regulation and deep psychological immersion in the movements. It is practised as both a martial art (and is indeed the world's most popular martial art) and health cultivation practice. TJ will form the main focus of this chapter going forward, but here I will introduce the main findings from the rapidly growing clinical evidence-base of the use of TJ with different neurological populations. In the subsequent sections of this chapter, I will explore the theological and psychological dimension of TJ practice, and how this may inform future use of TJ within neuro-rehabilitation.

The scientific study of TJ in the general population has demonstrated gains in physical, cognitive and emotional functioning plus biophysical structural differences for regular practitioners (Jahnke et al. 2012). A review of TJ group trials with long-term complex conditions concluded there was evidence of both physical and psychological gains of TJ practice within these groups (Zhang et al. 2011). The strongest and most established evidence-base for the use of TJ with specific neurological conditions is with Parkinson's disease and stroke, and primarily evidence of gains in physical functioning from participation in TJ groups.

In the Parkinson's disease literature, large-sample group studies (Gao et al. 2014; Li et al. 2012) have demonstrated gains in balance, postural stability and differing aspects of mobility for TJ practitioners relative to control groups, validating similar findings in smaller sample studies (Hackney and Earhart 2008). These findings are consistent with conclusions drawn from broader reviews of both English and Chinese literature studies (Mazzarin et al. 2017; Ni et al. 2014; Toh 2013; Radder et al. 2017; Yang et al. 2014; Zhou et al. 2015).

A lower incidence of falls was reported in a post-TJ intervention follow-up period by Gao and colleagues (2014), compared to controls. A systematic review and meta-analysis by Winser and colleagues (2018b) concluded that there is strong evidence for improvement in balance and reduction in falls in people with either Parkinson's or stroke, with weaker evidence for this outcome in other conditions.

With regards to reviews of the stroke rehabilitation literature, Lyu and colleagues (2018) found TJ to have an overall beneficial effect on activities of daily living, balance, limb motor function, walking quality, mood and sleep from low quality evidence-based studies. Zheng et al. (2016) found that when compared with standard physically orientated rehabilitation, TJ conferred significant gains in the areas of balance function, gait speed, anxiety and quality of life, In their meta-analysis of 15 eligible studies from both the English and Chinese language scientific literature. In contrast no advantages were evident for survivor levels of depression or functional walking quality. Ding (2012) concluded from a review of five studies that TJ confers advantageous gains to stroke survivors in the domains of balance, mobility, quality of life, anxiety and depression. Gains in balance is the most replicated outcome across studies, concluded in reviews by Wu and colleagues (2018), Yan Li and workers (2018) and Zou and colleagues (2018a, 2018b). Similar practices, such as Baduanjin Qi Gong, have also been shown across studies to improve balance and other aspects of physical functioning, while reducing levels of depression, among other indices (Zou et al. 2018a, 2018b).

In terms of specific studies, a large-sample ($n = 244$) study by Xie and colleagues (2018) identified gains in motor functioning, fear of falling and depression when compared with a balance training control intervention. Taylor-Piliae et al. (2014) found an older stroke survivors (>50) Yang style TJ group had fewer falls than aerobic and treatment as usual control groups. Both TJ and aerobic control groups had better aerobic endurance than treatment as usual. No group effect was found for perceived mental health. Wang and colleagues (2010) found a positive effect for a TJ stroke group on measures of sleep quality/daytime dysfunction (including fatigue) and depressive symptoms. TJ interventions have been shown to improve standing balance in an older adults sample (Au-Yeung et al. 2009), and a sample of community-based stroke survivors reported gains in both general functioning and mood, alongside no adverse effects for participants (Hart et al. 2004). Hwang and colleagues (2017) found that an adapted TJ group for stroke survivors with hemiplegia that lasted for one year (10 participants completed all sessions) was characterised by improvements in balance, self-efficacy and flexibility on quantitative measures, alongside qualitative interviews highlighting positive improvements for participants in physical and psychological functioning, social support and activities of daily living. In a case study of a stroke survivor with expressive aphasia, Yeates and colleagues (forthcoming) reported clinically significant and reliable gains on measures of depression and fatigue-related psychosocial functioning, plus detailed qualitative data following the survivor's attendance at a 6-month TJ group. A qualitative analysis of stroke survivor experiences in a TJ group by Desrochers and colleagues (2016) highlighted simultaneous perceived physical and psychological benefits by participants. Interestingly, TJ has been applied to intentionally reduce risk factors to prevent the incidence of stroke in those who are at risk (Chan et al. 2017).

Another key subgroup of acquired brain injury, traumatic brain injury (TBI) has been investigated in TJ studies, but using much smaller samples. Gemmell and Leathem (2006) have studied the psychosocial benefits for nine TBI survivors from a brief (six weeks) TJ group intervention, and reported participants' improved levels of sadness, confusion, anger, tension, fear and increased energy on visual analogue scales. Blake and Batson (2006) used a randomised design to demonstrate improvements in mood and self-esteem but not physical functioning in a TJ versus control group (20 participants in each condition). The authors concluded that their results were inconclusive as a recommendation for the use of TJ with TBI survivors. Finally Shapira and colleagues (2001) report three case studies where TBI survivors who had participated in TJ reported gains in mobility and feelings of security while walking.

Other neurological conditions have also been studied in the TJ literature. A systematic review of studies investigating TJ for people with multiple sclerosis concluded that it is safe, and confers both physical and psychological benefits (Taylor and Taylor-Piliae 2017). In a twice weekly TJ group for people with multiple sclerosis, Burschka and colleagues (2014) found a small effect size (sample of 32 participants) for therapeutic gains in balance, co-ordination and levels of depression relative to a treatment as usual group. Tavee and colleagues (2011) found improvements in ratings of pain, physical and mental health functioning in a two-month TJ group for people with multiple sclerosis (n=22) relative to a control intervention. These findings are consistent with those reported by smaller sample studies conducted by Mills and Allen (2000; Mills et al. 2000).

Gains from TJ have also been reported for people with mild cognitive impairment (reduction of falls; Sungkarat et al. 2017) and cerebellar ataxia (balance and functional independence; Winser et al. 2017, 2018a). Finally, Quinn and Jones (2012) reported a range of psychosocial gains following completion of a TJ group for people with a variety of neurological conditions. Yeates and colleagues (forthcoming) also report positive single-case outcomes for a small group of survivors of ABI following a six-month TJ group, but also draw attention to significant diversity in this group and the influence of such on the range of outcomes within the group

In summary, the existing literature points reliably to a range of physical functioning gains across neurological conditions, although the evidence is strongest and most reliable in Parkinson's disease and stroke. Conclusions for other conditions are limited by small sample sizes and differing outcome measures. There are two key problems with this literature as a whole however. A general critique is that the most rigorously designed studies have optimised participant homogeneity by excluding those participants with significant cognitive difficulties alongside their physical impairments (e.g. Taylor-Piliae et al. 2014). This then creates a barrier to applying the findings of these studies to the users of services described earlier in this chapter, who are struggling with multiple domains of disability (Yeates 2015, 2018, forthcoming). More recently, Hwang and colleagues (2017) have been the first to describe physical adaptations to a TJ group for stroke survivors with hemiplegia.

Furthermore, most studies have operationalised physical functioning measures as the primary outcome only. Where psychological functioning has been additionally studied, it is clear from the findings above that frequent gains in anxiety and depression are found by investigators. However these have not been the main focus of each study, nor have investigators offered explanatory frameworks to explain the link between performing TJ movements and emotional well-being. Burschka and colleagues (2014) did offer mindfulness as a possible explanatory framework for these empirical associations, but as we will explore below, this is not the key mind–body framework that TJ experts use themselves to guide their practice.

Daoist Frameworks for Tai Ji, Qi Gong and Flow-Based Practices

The omissions in the scientific literature described above are all the more significant when one considers that those expert TJ practitioners who practise the most, for the longest and prioritise this discipline above other aspects of life all hold the internal, subjective (psychological) dimension to be central to their practice. *Taijiquan* means the representation of the universe (in the Daoist view) through bodily movement. It is still practised by the Daoist monastic community to this day, as well of millions of other practitioners worldwide, of all ages, backgrounds and abilities. For the Daoist monk TJ masters, despite their mastery and prowess of physical movements, balance and co-ordination, their focus is on their internal experience in harmony with both their bodily movements and wider universal natural processes, all connected within their view of natural laws and organisation. This is a unique biopsychosocial–spiritual–ecological framework, which will be explored here.

Daoism is a key indigenous religion of China. Practised by at least 20 million people in China and worldwide, Daoism was formalised in the second century CE, but is thought to have developed from preceding shamanic beliefs and co-developed in reciprocal dialogue with Chan Buddhism and Confucianism, the other two main spiritual-philosophical traditions in pre-communist China. The Daoist view of the divine is an emanating universal force that proceeds and evolves, underlying all the manifestations of change and transition in the natural world and wider universe. This process is called *Dao*, which translates as the 'way' or 'path'. Nature is a key source of inspiration to connect with the divine in Daoism, through the witnessing and harmonising one's lifestyle with changing seasons, differing states and qualities of essential elements such as water (ice, fog, mist, rivers and lakes). This harmonisation of lifestyle is done via horticultural practices, herbology, musical and architectural styles and mind–body practices. The body is viewed as a manifestation of nature and subject to its laws (*yin* – receiving, embracing, yielding forces – and *yang* – emanating, protruding, opening forces). As such one's body, and the interrelationship between the body and the embodied mind (see below) is seen as a domain in which a Daoist can intentionally promote harmony with nature.

This harmonisation and health cultivation process in the level of body, mind and spirit is referred to as *Neidan*, or 'Inner Alchemy'. The practitioner aims to self-harmonise with natural processes and facilitate a key process of conversion – from their bodily essence/physical properties (*Jing*) their physical attributes are used in service of breath regulation to stimulate and circulate a flow of vitality and life energy (*Qi*) around the body. This circulation alters the mind and subjective experience of the practitioner, leading to expanded states of consciousness. These final processes are conceived as the domain of spirit (*Shen*), but different qualities of mind-spirit are anchored to specific mind–body physiological networks, with links to specific organs (including the heart, lungs, kidneys and liver). This echoes more contemporary developments in neuroscience that highlight interoceptive processes mediated by subcortical-viscera networks that are generative of consciousness (Damasio 1999). This conversion of body-breath/life energy-spirit is completed by the highest converted essence being put back into the universe. As such the body, breath, mind and spirit are all vehicles and containers for a never-ending flow of universal change processes that permeate all things. The aim then, is to minimise blocks and desynchronies that would obstruct this process.

The *Neidan* process is a core focus of seated Daoist meditational practices, but is also the organiser for a range of mind–body practices such as TJ, *qi gong* (still or moving yogic practices that typically involve greater repetition of fewer movements than TJ), and *gong fu* (kung fu – faster and more dynamic practices with a clear martial focus). Furthermore, music, chanting of hymns and scriptures, horticulture, cooking and eating, architecture, divination and sleeping are also used as lifestyle vehicles for Neidan to aim towards a constant trend towards harmonisation with nature and the divine.

Poetry and literature are also key *mediums* for the Daoist philosophical exploration of divine change, famously including the *Dao De Ching*, attributed in Chinese folklore to a semi-historical/mythological figure, Lao Tzu (Kaltenmark 1969). In ancient Daoist writings, philosophical ideas were communicated powerfully through imagery and allegory, famously including Zhuangzi's (fourth century BCE) Butterfly Dream:

> Once upon a time, I, Chuang Chou, dreamt I was a butterfly, fluttering hither and thither, to all intents and purposes a butterfly. I was conscious only of my happiness as a butterfly, unaware that I was Chou. Soon I awoke, and there I was, veritably myself again. Now I do not know whether I was then a man dreaming I was a butterfly, or whether I am now a butterfly, dreaming I am a man. Between a man and a butterfly there is necessarily a distinction. The transition is called the transformation of material things.
>
> (cited in Merton 1969)

In Daoist practice, these ideas of mind–body work and harmonisation with change are then located within a broader environmental context, the surrounding natural world and universe. Five Element Theory (*Wuxing*) is a framework that is constantly used to link parts of the body, emotions, the changing seasonal environment and diet to promote synchronisation. For example, I am writing this chapter in Autumn, where the leaves falling from the bare trees remind the Chinese of the structure of a lung, so body movements are chosen to stimulate respiration, along with the increased consumption of spices. The key element is metal, consistent with the sensory properties of lung tissue and the smell of decaying leaf matter in the ground. The prominent emotion and subjective state is sorrow and sadness, with nature providing lessons of loss and exposed vulnerability.

Nature provides inspiration for a model of mind, behaviour and interaction with others. For example, the bending of the willow under the weight of snowfall is contrasted with a rigid tree such as a fir that seems stronger on the surface, but in its rigidity does not yield and so breaks under the weight of the snow. Thus, the concept of *Wu Wei* is a guiding principal – a Daoist tried to respond to external stimulation and challenge through initially yielding and accommodating – not jumping forwards with judgements, preconceptions and bulldozing into situations. The sage or hermit in harmony with nature and not overly organised by societal expectations is a key archetypal template for Daoist psychological and social life. TJ is practised within this biopsychosocial–spiritual–ecological framework. Given this brief overview of the Daoist view of the embodied mind and spirit within the cosmos, the physiological reductionism of TJ research becomes stark.

Flow Psychology

Therefore in contrast to TJ as a physical practice only, we have a rich range of Daoist concepts that both guide internal experience during bodily practice, and situate such within a wider ecological and lifestyle context. One limitation is that these concepts are esoteric and not easily accessible. These core concepts do, however, overlap significantly with some key ideas within Western positive psychology, a broad contemporary influence on neuro-rehabilitation (Cullen et al. 2018; Evans 2011; Evans and Cullen, forthcoming). Mihály Csíkszentmihályi (1990, 1997) has developed the concept of Flow, a concept which can potentially offer an explanatory bridge between Daoist terminology and scientific-clinical discourse (Yeates 2015, 2018). Indeed, Csíkszentmihályi (1990) has explicitly identified another eastern mind–body tradition, yoga, as a purposefully designed flow activity:

> The similarities between Yoga and flow are extremely strong; in fact it makes sense to think that (Patanjali's system of) Yoga is a very thoroughly planned Flow activity.
>
> (105)

> Therefore it is not unreasonable to perform Yoga as one of the oldest and most systematic methods of producing the Flow experience.
>
> (105)

Csíkszentmihályi has primarily studied intense states of absorption in the domains of sport, music, creativity and work. Flow states are routinely described by practitioners as involving the dissolving of a self-state and loss of normal self-boundaries (loss of reflective self-consciousness), distortion of temporal experience, a merging of action and awareness where intention is not effortful and the activity concerned seems to flow forth of its own accord. Practitioners feel intense well-being, ecstatic experiences at the time and part of something bigger than themselves. Importantly, those experiencing flow states in a particular activity have attained some level of mastery over that activity through practice and experience, such that there is a dimension of automaticity and diminution of effort. Practitioners across diverse fields consistently use a metaphorical language of creativity and action flowing forth, hence Csíkszentmihályi's term Flow states. Many of us know what it is to be 'in the flow', and the value of such, when we think about optimal times for our own performance and productivity. Flow has been associated with optimal psychological well-being (Csíkszentmihályi 1990, 1997), and a specific focus on flow has been included in a positive psychotherapy intervention that was shown to be acceptable for survivors of acquired brain injury, with a recommendation for a future trial of this approach in ABI (Cullen et al. 2018).

Csíkszentmihályi acknowledged historical precursors to his psychological study of flow, notably religious thought from near and far eastern traditions. Many faiths have historically articulated and practised a desired goal to be at oneness with something greater, via dissolution of the boundaries of present sensory experience. In addition to Daoism these include in Islam, Sufi Dervishes' practice of spinning and whirling; in Vedic/Hindu thought, a form of flow-like psychological absorption in an object of meditation, Samyama, aimed for in Raja Yoga, and in fast forms of physical yoga, flow states are explicitly the desired vehicle for self-transcendence (Pattni 2016); in Christianity flow has been linked with the Ignatian spiritual exercises (Dawson and Austin 2014). The concept of flow is explicitly mentioned by exponents of the Daoist world view, famously Bruce Lee:

> Be like water . . . empty your mind, be formless, shapeless like water. If you put water in the cup, it becomes the cup. You put water in the bottle, it becomes the bottle. You put it in the teapot, it becomes the teapot. Now, water can flow or it can crash. Be water my friend.
>
> (Little and Lee 2000)

> We are always in a process of becoming and nothing is fixed. Have no rigid system in you, and you'll be flexible to change with the ever changing. Open yourself and flow, my friend. Flow in the total openness of the living moment. If nothing within you stays rigid, outward things will disclose themselves. Moving, be like water. Still, be like a mirror. Respond like an echo.
>
> (Lee 2000, 13)

While there is clearly overlap between Daoist and positive psychological conceptualisation of Flow states, the latter differs in emphasising explicit appraisal as a critical dimension. This includes assertions of flow components and conditions for flow such as an individual's sense of personal control or agency, involvement in a task with a clear set of goals and progress, and which provides immediate feedback, simultaneous perception of high task challenges alongside high personal skill (Csíkszentmihályi et al. 2005; Schaffer 2013). While Daoist masters clearly have mastery of highly skilled practices such as martial arts, accounts of their subjective experiences during practice indicate a diminution of explicit appraisal processes generally and subjective absence of perceived challenge or personal skill (see 'The Taijiquan Classics'; Davis 2004). Furthermore, the psychological study of people in flow states has focused on those who have specific goals around performance (be this athletic or work productivity), with flow states being a dimension towards these outcomes. The Daoist TJ masters aspire specifically to enter into flow states and the opportunities for transcendence and wider harmony, irrespective of their performance (although it is clear that their physical and psychological abilities exceed most in the general population).

Liminality and Psychological Growth

With transformation processes afforded such psychological and spiritual significance, the dimension of change is seen as the domain in which personal development occurs. This is commensurate with the focus across cultures and human experience on *liminality*, which has become an area of transdisciplinary academic and applied clinical interest. Liminal experiences occur within a phase of transition (between what someone once was and what they are becoming) and being of psychological value. Anthropologists have noted the centrality of liminal experience in rites of passage across cultures, where this phase (such as adolescent transition between childhood and adulthood) is marked by ceremony and symbolism. Narratives of passing through gates and portals permeate all of the major religions, be these processes of change in behaviour and learning or the unlocking of centres within the body. Psychotherapy too has been conceived as an arena where

> a new set of circumstances involve the dissolution of a former identity and the formation of a new identity. Between these two states, the condition of liminality suspends a person or system in what may appear to be an amorphous or ill-defined state.
>
> (Elliot 2011)

Growth and adaptation are viewed as emergent from such conditions. To link back to the experiences of ABI survivors, adjustment, awareness and post-injury growth can be limited by a rigid investment in pre-injury identity in a way that devalues post-injury change and closes down growth opportunities (Tyerman and Humphrey 1984). An Daoist-focused exploration of the course of change itself rather than the privileging of one particular state in that journey may create new rehabilitation opportunities. An example would be comparing the relative attributes and limitations of different values and abilities at different points in time, in response to varying life conditions and demands post-injury

Using Flow States to Guide Tai Ji Groups in Neuro-Rehabilitation

The extrapolation of concepts from Daoist psychology, by way of a translation with the Western concept of Flow, has provided us with a new psychological tool to be used in clinical application. As there was once a time before people were using the mindfulness concept across a range of sectors, the concept of Flow awaits a future explosion of clinical application. It is argued here (and in Yeates 2015, 2018), that Flow provides the core operationalisation of a psychological (and for some a spiritual) dimension in the formulation and implementation of TJ groups for people with neuro-disability. Flow is significant for TJ clinical interventions in two main ways.

First, it links the bodily movements with the evidenced psychological gains from TJ practice, consistent with positive psychology's identification of an association between well-being and flow states. This may offer a unique response to the existential disturbances to self-experience described above. To use the Daoist inspirations from the natural world, think of leaves floating in a stream. They are individual elements, but when moved simultaneously in the flow of currents and eddies in the stream, they are held in unison by a higher level of process or organisation. Similarly, the survivor of ABI, initially experiencing themselves as fragmented, 'in pieces', can be temporarily held together by the TJ movement sequence, also perhaps held together by moving in unison with fellow TJ practitioners (akin to a murmuration of starlings or a shoal of fish), and for some there may be an experience of synchrony and union with a higher principle – a transcendent experience.

Secondly, TJ can provide the specificity to optimise flow experience (with associated conditions of improved psychological well-being and the possibility of transcendence) for each practitioner in a bespoke fashion. If flow emerges from the optimal ratio of perceived challenge and perceived ability to meet that challenge, then specific movements are chosen that fit this ratio for each survivor (with their unique constellation of physical, cognitive, emotional and social needs). Furthermore, specific compensatory rehabilitation strategies are included as adjuncts to optimise the learning and practice of TJ (see Table 17.1 for examples), again to promote and optimise flow.

The systematic use of Flow in this way to optimise psychological well-being within TJ practice for survivors of ABI and people with other forms of disability would result in two different practitioners performing very different movement sequences (each with varying physical and psychological demands) and using very different compensatory strategies, but both entering into a similar state of flow within their practice (having arrived at it, entered

Table 17.1 Examples of adaptations to Tai Ji learning and practice for different post-stroke difficulties

Area of difficulty	Suggested adaptation
Mobility	Chair-based sequences and/or restricted standing TJ forms
Balance	Chair-based sequences and/or TJ forms that have minimal weight and direction changes
Hemiplegia	Use therapy bands, sticks and bilateral hand connection to mobilise mirroring upper-body movements, visual imagery of paralysed limb movement and focus on trunk movement to amplify functional movement of ipsilateral limbs
Fatigue	Do short sequences of instruction and movement, slowly increasing over time, with regular breaks
Dyspraxia	Use tactile feedback and physical adjustments rather than relying on visual demonstration alone
Communication	Emphasise visual and kinaesthetic teaching as opposed to verbally based
Attention	Do short sequences of instruction and movement, slowly increasing over time, with regular breaks; use key phrases and words for optimal alerting qualities
Episodic memory/new learning	Focus on errorless learning in class to minimise the introduction of mistakes into the learning process; for those who want to learn sequences at home, use DVDs/internet videos to provide a guide between session times and promote a greater number of repetition learning experiences, also supporting the autonomous learning of a sequence through backwards chaining rather than traditional instruction
Topographical disorientation/visuospatial difficulties in using allocentric or egocentric cues	Use grids marked on the floor to assist with changing directions of movement and posture shapes
Anxiety	Use relaxing music and short teaching sequences; teach body-tension reduction and breath regulation strategies at the beginning of the class; reduce the learning/practice demands of the movements initially to increase confidence, then gently introduce progressively more challenging sequences
Low mood	Use shorter learning/practice phases; pace the progressive challenge of sequences as above, supporting achievements with praise and encouragement and emphasising the group fellowship and identity aspects of attendance; draw comparisons to embodied experience at the end of the session versus the beginning

into it, through different routes). Within a TJ group intervention (a Flow Group; Yeates 2015), the session would be structured to offer both time devoted to individual learning of bespoke movements and also an additional segment of group movement sequences (accessible to all attendees) to facilitate the experience of group cohesion with others, plus a dedicated time for socialising and peer connection during a tea break.

This model of a TJ intervention for individuals or groups of ABI survivors is very different in scope and character from those protocols described in published studies. This is the author's current approach to TJ use as a clinical neuropsychologist, and awaits future controlled studies to confirm the core hypothesis – that optimising Flow via the bespoke selection of TJ movements and use of compensatory strategies will result in more significant psychological gains for more practitioners than unadapted TJ groups. To provide more details on the value of TJ and the experience of Flow for a survivor of ABI, a case study will be described below.

Case Example: Raymond

Raymond is a 48 –old survivor of a right-sided haemorrhagic stroke (a bleed on the brain involving the right middle cerebral artery territory), which occurred four years ago. He sustained enduring physical difficulties (he used a wheelchair, with hemiparesis on his left side affecting both lower and upper limbs, plus longstanding difficulties with fatigue), plus changes in cognition (he struggled with challenges to initiation, planning and organising, and attentions to/representations of visual stimuli on the left side). His marriage ended within the year of his stroke and he became socially isolated. He was initially supported by acute stroke services, early-supported discharge team (six weeks of physiotherapy and occupational therapy support) and then periodic physiotherapy and psychology reviews within his local community neuro-rehab service. He struggled with fluctuating levels of anxiety and depressed mood as he struggled to come to terms with the impact of the stroke on his life, his new limitations and the increased social isolation (apart from his wife, his other main relationships were with work colleagues, who slowly discontinued social contact after he was medically retired from his job as an IT programmer). Fluctuating levels of fatigue exacerbated his levels of psychological distress, and in these moments in particular he would question the absence of meaning in his life (experiencing suicidal ideation on occasion). His one source of support was his ageing mother, with whom he moved in to live following the separation from his wife. However his mother lived in a village, and Raymond was dependent on transport schemes to travel into the nearest town and access community and leisure facilities (Raymond had to relinquish his driving licence as a result of his difficulties).

New social and leisure opportunities started to emerge three years post-stroke, when Raymond started to be supported by a charity that enabled people with disabilities to increase their social participation. This same organisation co-ran a pilot of an unadapted six-month weekly TJ group (Yeates et al., forthcoming) with the author's NHS clinical service and Raymond agreed to participate in the study, which involved single-case repeated-measures data collection of mood, fatigue and quality of life questionnaires plus qualitative focus group interviews with all participants at the half-way and end points during the six months of weekly TJ group attendance. Raymond's questionnaire scores prior to the group and immediately after the last session of the six-month programme are provided in Table 17.2, followed by graphs (Figures 17.1, 17.2 and 17.3) depicting detailed scores on each measure and its subscales across the schedule of repeated questionnaire administration every fourth group session.

The reader will see that he was very committed to the group, attending 92 per cent of the sessions. In terms of clinical change during these six months, Raymond's anxiety and depression scores (Hospital Anxiety and Depression Scale; Zigmond and Snaith 1983) fluctuated but remained roughly the same – hovering around the cut-off point between the normal range and mild levels of both forms of distress. His engagement with the charity and increase in a range of social activities in the year prior to the TJ group had already been a big influence in reducing levels of distress. Overall Quality of Life also remained constant over the six months (evident in scores on the Quality of Life Brain Injury Inventory, Von Steinbüchel et al. 2010), but with significant increases in the psychological and physical

Table 17.2 Raymond's mood, fatigue and quality of life data

Measure	Pre-TJ	Post-TJ	Significance?
HADS Anxiety	8	6	Mild to normal, not reliable
HADS Depression	6	8	Mild to normal, not reliable
MFIS Total	51	39	Clinically significant and reliable
MFIS Physical Subscale	20	14	n/a
MFIS Cognitive Subscale	27	22	n/a
MFIS Psychosocial	4	3	n/a
QoLiBRI Total	60	59	No change

Note: HADS = Hospital Anxiety and Depression Scale; MFIS = Modified-Fatigue Impact Scale; QoLIBRI = Quality of Life in Brain Injury Scale.

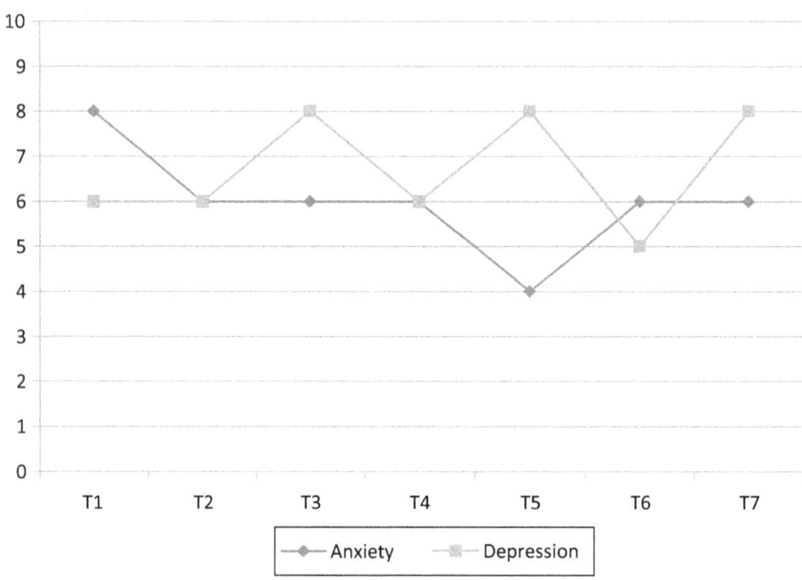

Figure 17.1 Raymond's Anxiety and Depression (HADS) scores across sessions during the six-month Taiji Group.

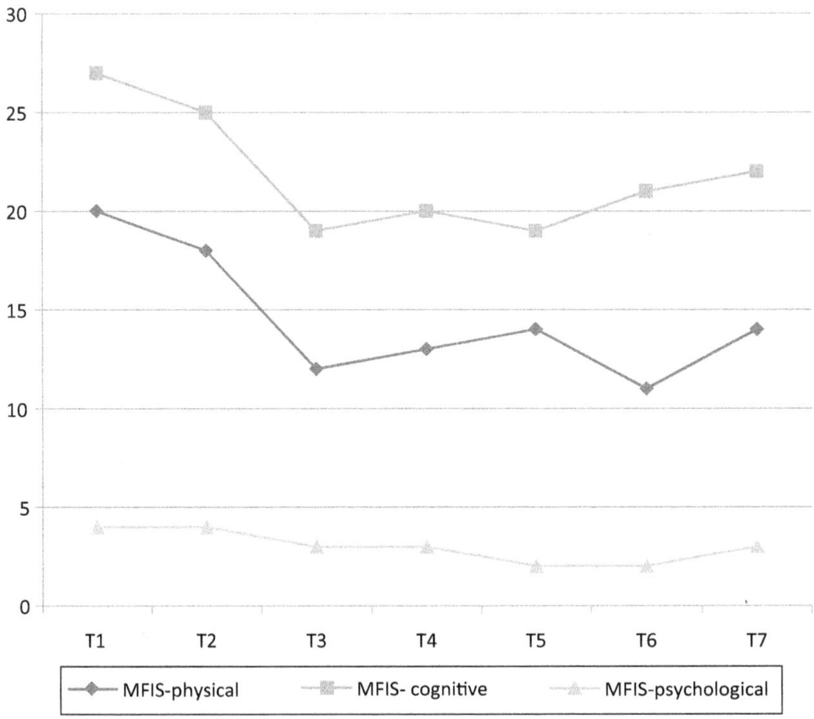

Figure 17.2 Raymond's Fatigue (MFIS) scores across sessions during the six-month Taiji Group.

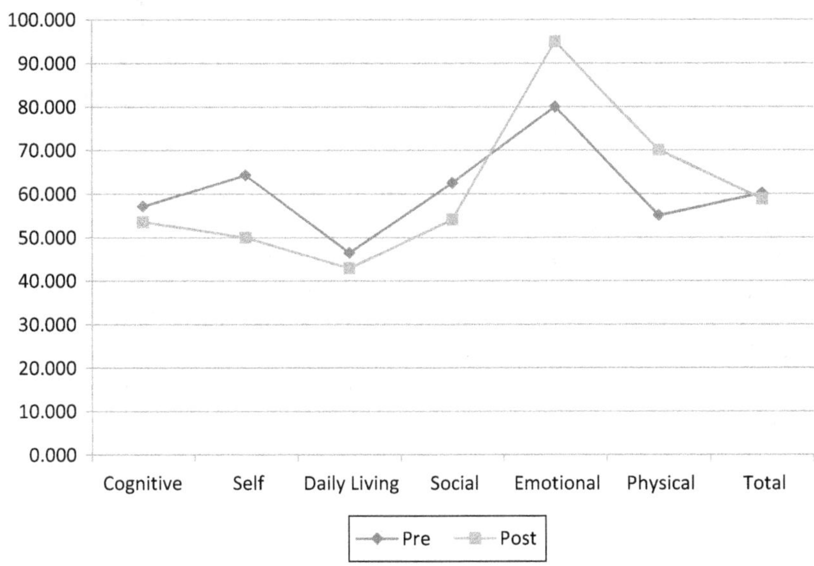

Figure 17.3 Raymond's Quality of Life (QoLIBRI Subscales) scores before and after the six-month Taiji Group.

aspects of Quality of Life. His levels of fatigue were a key change however (on the Modified-Fatigue Impact Scale; Fisk et al. 1994). Both a clinically significant and statistically reliable change was evident for total levels of fatigue (using the Reliable Change Index method of Jacobson and Truax (1991)), and a trend of reduced fatigue was evident across physical, cognitive and psychosocial subscales.

Raymond was able to learn a chair-based TJ sequence over the six months, where the upper-body movements synched with other members of the group who were performing whole-body forms. He loved the way in which his right arm moved in ways that he learned could be generated from his whole trunk, and so involve parts of his left affected side too (shoulder, hip). In addition to the TJ, having tea with his training group in the mid-session break was a key point of social contact for him. He felt equal to the others, who were all struggling with the task of learning new and increasingly difficult movements. Raymond felt that in contrast to his life at home, where he experienced himself as limited, isolated and imprisoned, he experienced himself during his 90-minute TJ session each week as free, connected and stimulated. Towards the end of the six months, Raymond reported improvements in levels of fatigue across the week between each sessions, with a positive and stabilising impact on his mood as a result.

Conclusion

This chapter has argued for the use of Eastern mind–body approaches as a new paradigm for simultaneous physical, psychological and spiritual support for survivors of ABI and for those with other neurological conditions. Following a brief overview of published application of Vedic yoga and Buddhist mindfulness approaches with this clinical group, the chapter proceeded to explore Daoist Tai Ji specifically as a suitable mind–body intervention. In response to omissions within the literature, the Daoist concept of *Neidan* and its close counterpart in positive psychology, Flow states, have been introduced to operationalise a psychological dimension to both explain existing findings in the literature and guide the design and implementation of future TJ protocols in research to come. It is hypothesised that these suggested adaptations will increase the level of psychological and spiritual gains from TJ practice for more people with neuro-disability. The case study above offers a detailed example of the clinical value from these ideas.

Future research is required to evaluate the proposed TJ model in a systematic and controlled way, attending to both standardised outcome measures and subjective experience of participants. Further ideas to adapt TJ in order to optimise Flow are welcome. Inherent to an evaluation of Flow and its role in TJ is the need for an object measurement methodology, both questionnaire measures and the identification of reliable physiological markers of Flow state experience (such as the proposals put forward by Yeates (2015, 2018)). In anticipation of such developments however, it conceivable that mind–body practices used to optimise Flow states may uniquely offer physical and psychological benefits for ABI survivors, along with the possibility of transcendence for survivors of all faiths and none.

References

Advocat, J., J. Enticott, B. Vandenberg, C. Hassed, J. Hester and G. Russell. 2016. The effects of a mindfulness-based lifestyle program for adults with Parkinson's disease: a mixed methods, wait list controlled randomised control study. *BMC Neurology* 16: 166.

Aghabagheri, H., P. Mohammadkhani, S. Omrani and V. Farahmand. 2012. Mindfulness based group therapy on increase in subjective well-being and hope to MS patients. *Clinical Psychology* 4: 23–33.

Au-Yeung, S. S. Y., C. W. Y. Hui-Chan and J. C. S. Tang. 2009. Short-form Tai Chi improves standing balance of people with chronic stroke. *Neurorehabilitation and Neural Repair* 23: 515–22.

Bastille, J. V., and K. M. Gill-Body. 2004. A yoga-based exercise program for people with post-stroke chronic hemiparesis. *Physical Therapy* 84: 33–48.

Bedard, M., M. Felteau, D. Mazmanian, K. Fedyk, R. Klein, J. Richardson, W. Parkinson and M. B. Minthorn-Biggs. 2003. Pilot evaluation of a mindfulness-based intervention to improve quality of life among individuals who sustained traumatic brain injuries. *Disability and Rehabilitation* 25: 722–31.

Bedard, M., M. Felteau, C. Gibbons, R. Klein, D. Mazmanian, K. Fedyk and G. Mack. 2005. A mindfulness-based intervention to improve quality of life among individuals who sustained traumatic brain injuries: one-year follow-up. *Journal of Cognitive Rehabilitation*, Spring, 2–7.

Bedard, M., M. Felteau, S. Marshall, S. Dubois, C. Gibbons, R. Klein and B. Weaver. 2012. Mindfulness-based cognitive therapy: benefits in reducing depression following a traumatic brain injury. *Advances in Mind–Body Medicine* 26: 14–20.

Blake, H., and M. Batson. 2006. Exercise intervention in brain injury: a pilot randomized study of Tai Chi Qigong. *Clinical Rehabilitation* 23: 589–98.

Blankespoor, R. J., M. P. J. Schellekens, S. H. Vos, A. E. M. Speckens and B. A. de Jong. 2017. The effectiveness of mindfulness-based stress reduction on psychological distress and cognitive functioning in patients with multiple sclerosis: a pilot study. *Mindfulness*. Published online. doi:10.1007/s12671-017-0701-6.

Bogosian A., P. Chadwick, S. Windgassen, S. Norton, P. McCrone, I. Mosweu, E. Silber and R. Moss-Morris. 2015. Distress improves after mindfulness training for progressive MS: a pilot randomised trial. *Multiple Sclerosis Journal* 21: 1184–94.

Bogosian, A., A. Hughes, S. Norton, E. Silber and R. Moss-Morris. 2016. Potential treatment mechanisms in a mindfulness based intervention for people with progressive multiple sclerosis. *British Journal of Health Psychology* 21: 859–80.

Bowen, C., G. Yeates and S. Palmer. 2010. *A Relational Approach to Rehabilitation: Thinking about Relationships after Brain Injury*. London: Karnac.

Burschka, J. M., P. M. Keune, U. Oy, P. Oschman and P. Kuhn. 2014. Mindfulness-based interventions in multiple sclerosis: beneficial effects of Tai Chi on balance, coordination, fatigue and depression. *BioMedCentral Neurology* 14: 165–174.

Cash, T., V. Ekouevi, C. Kilbourn and S. Lageman. 2015. Pilot study of a mindfulness-based group intervention for individuals with Parkinson's disease and their caregivers. *Mindfulness* 7: 361–71.

Chan, A. W., J. W. Sit and S. Y. Chair. 2017. Tai Chi exercise reduces stroke risk factors: a randomized controlled trial. *Stroke* 48: AWP416.

Cramer, H., R. Lauche, H. Azizi, G. Dobos and J. Langhorst. 2014. Yoga for multiple sclerosis: a systematic review and meta-analysis. *PLoS One* 9: e112414.

Crielesi, M., G. Monopoli, G. N. Yeates and S. Monte. Forthcoming. A mindfulness group intervention for people with aphasia: a pilot study. In *Neuro-disability and Psychotherapy, Specialist Topics: Vol. 2. Psychotherapy and Aphasia: Supporting Emotions and Relationships*, ed. G. N. Yeates and K. Meredith. Oxford: Routledge.

Csikszentmihalyi, M. 1990. *Flow: The Psychology of Optimal Experience*. New York: Harper and Row.

Csikszentmihalyi, M. 1997. *Finding Flow: The Psychology of Engagement with Everyday Life*. New York: Basic Books.

Csikszentmihalyi, M., S. Abuhamdeh and J. Nakamura. 2005. Flow. In *Handbook of Competence and Motivation*, ed. A. Elliot, 598–698. New York: Guilford Press.

Cullen, B., J. Pownall, J. Cummings, S. Baylan, N. Broomfield, C. Haig, D. Kersel, H. Murray and J. Evans. 2018. Positive PsychoTherapy in ABI rehab (PoPsTAR): a pilot randomised controlled trial. *Neuropsychological Rehabilitation* 28: 17–33.

Damasio, A. 1999. *The Feeling of What Happens*. San Diego, CA: Harcourt.

Davis, B. 2004. *The Taijiquan Classics: An Annotated Translation*. Berkeley: North Atlantic.

Dawson, R., and Austin, N. 2014. The consolation of character strength in Ignatian spirituality and positive psychology. *The Way* 53(3): 7–21.

Desrochers, P., D. Kairy, S. Pan, H. Corriveau and M. Tousignant. 2016. Tai Chi for upper limb rehabilitation in stroke patients: the patient's perspective. *Disability and Rehabilitation* 39: 1313–19.

Detert, V. Forthcoming. Mindfulness in neurological conditions. In *Psychological Therapies in Neuropsychological Rehabilitation*, ed. G. N. Yeates and F. Ashworth. Hove, UK: Psychology Press.

Detert, N., and L. Douglas. 2014. Mindfulness MBSR/MBCT improves general psychiatric symptom severity, depression, anxiety and perceived stress in neurological disorders in an NHS clinical setting. *Neuro-disability and Psychotherapy* 2: 137–156.

Dickinson, J., P. Friary and C. M. McCann. 2016. The influence of mindfulness meditation on communication and anxiety: a case study of a person with aphasia. *Aphasiology* 31: 1044–58.

Ding, M. 2012. Tai Chi for stroke rehabilitation: a focused review. *American Journal of Physical Medicine and Rehabilitation* 91: 1091–6.

Dissanayaka, N. N., F. Idu Jion, N. A. Pachana, J. D. O'Sullivan, R. Marsh, G. J. Byrne et al. 2016. Mindfulness for motor and nonmotor dysfunctions in Parkinson's disease. *Parkinson's Disease*. Published online. doi:10.1155/2016/7109052.

Donnelly, K. Z., K. Linnea, D. A. Grant and J. Lichtenstein. 2014. The feasibility and impact of a yoga pilot programme on the quality-of-life of adults with acquired brain injury. *Brain Injury* 31: 208–14.

Elliot, B. 2011. Arts-based and narrative inquiry in liminal experience reveal platforming as basic social psychological process. *The Arts in Psychotherapy* 38: 96–103.

Elsass, L., and G. Kinsella. 1987. Social interaction following severe closed head injury. *Psychological Medicine* 17(1): 67–78.

Evans, J. J. 2011. Positive psychology and brain injury rehabilitation. *Brain Impairment* 12: 117–27.

Evans, J. J., and B. Cullen. Forthcoming. Positive psychotherapy for neurological conditions. In *Psychological Therapies in Neuropsychological Rehabilitation*, ed. G. N. Yeates and F. Ashworth. Hove, UK: Psychology Press.

Fisk, J. D., P. G. Ritvo, L. Ross, D. A. Haasem, T. J. Marrie and W. F. Schlech. 1994. Measuring the functional impact of fatigue: initial validation of the fatigure impact scale. *Clinical Infectious Disease* 18(Suppl. 1): s79–83.

Fitzpatrick, L., J. Simpson and A. Smith. 2010. A qualitative analysis of mindfulness-based cognitive therapy (MBCT) in Parkinson's disease. *Psychology and Psychotherapy* 83: 179–92.

Gao, Q., A. Leung, Y. Yang et al. 2014. Effects of tai chi on balance and fall prevention in Parkinson's disease: a randomized controlled trial. *Clinical Rehabilitation* 28: 748–53.

Gemmell, C., and J. M. Leathem. 2006. A study investigating the effects of Tai Chi Chuan: individuals with traumatic brain injury compared to controls. *Brain Injury* 20: 151–6.

Goldstein, K. 1959. Notes on the development of my concepts. *Journal of Individual Psychology* 15: 5–14.

Gracey, F., C. Ford and K. Psaila. 2015. A provisional transdiagnostic cognitive behavioural model of post brain injury emotional adjustment. *NeuroDisability and Psychotherapy* 3: 154–85.

Grossman, P., L. Kappos, H. Gensicke, M. D'Souza, D. Mohr, I. Penner and C. Steiner. 2010. MS quality of life, depression and fatigue improve after mindfulness training. *Neurology* 75: 1141–9.

Hackney, M. E., and G. M. Earhart. 2008. Tai Chi improves balance and mobility in people with Parkinson disease. *Gait and Posture* 28: 456–60.

Hart, J., H. Kanner, R. Gilboa-Mayo, O. Haroeh-Peer, N. Rozenthul-Sorokin and R. Eldar. 2004. Tai Chi Chuan practice in community-dwelling persons after stroke. *International Journal of Rehabilitation Research* 27: 303–4.

Haslam, C., A. Holme, S. A. Haslam, A. Lyer, J. Jetten and W. H. Williams. 2008. Maintaining group memberships: social identity continuity predicts well-being after stroke. *Neuropsychological Rehabilitation* 18: 671–91.

Hoogerwerf, A. E. W., Y. Bol, J. Lobbestael, R. Hupperts and C. M. van Heugten. 2017. Mindfulness-based cognitive therapy for severely fatigued multiple sclerosis patients: a waiting list controlled study. *Journal of Rehabilitation Medicine* 49: 497–504.

Hwang, I., R. Song, S. Ahn, M. Lee, P. Wayne and M. K. Sohn. 2017. Exploring the adaptability of Tai Chi to stroke rehabilitation. *Rehabilitation Nursing*. Published online. doi:10.1097/rnj.0000000000000110.

Jacobson, N. S., and P. Truax. 1991. Clinical significance: A statistical approach to defining meaningful change in psychotherapy research. *Journal of Consulting and Clinical Psychology* 59: 12–19.

Jahnke, R., L. Larkey, C. Rogers, J. Etnier and F. Lin. 2012. A comprehensive review of health benefits of Qi Gong and Tai Chi. *American Journal of Health Promotion* 24: e1–e25.

Johansson, B., H. Bjhur and L. Rönnbäck. 2012. Mindfulness-based stress reduction (MBSR) improves long-term mental fatigue after stroke and traumatic brain injury. *Brain Injury* 26: 1621–8.

Kabat-Zinn, J. 2003. Mindfulness-based interventions in context: past, present and future. *Clinical Psychology: Science and Practice* 10: 144–56.

Kaltenmark, M. 1969. *Lao Tzu and Taoism*. Trans. Roger Greaves. Stanford, CA: Stanford University Press.

Kaplan-Solms, K., and M. Solms. 2000. *Clinical Studies in Neuro-Psychoanalysis: An Introduction to a Depth Neuropsychology*. London: Karnac.

Kenuk, S., and H. Porter. 2017. The outcomes for mindfulness-based interventions for adults who have experienced a traumatic brain injury: a systematic review of the literature. *American Journal of Recreation Therapy* 16.

Kolahkaj, B., and F. Zargar. 2015. Effect of mindfulness-based stress reduction on anxiety, depression and stress in women with multiple sclerosis. *Nursing and Midwifery Studies* 4: e29655.

Laures-Gore, J., and R. Shisler Marshall. 2016. Mindfulness meditation in aphasia: a case report. *NeuroRehabilitation* 38: 321–9.

Lazaridou, A., P. Philbrook and A. A. Tzika. 2013. Yoga and mindfulness as therapeutic interventions for stroke rehabilitation: a systematic review. *Evidence-Based Complementary and Alternative Medicine* 2013: 357108.

Lee, B. 2000. *Striking Thoughts: Bruce Lee's Wisdom for Daily Living*. New York: Tuttle.

Li, F., P. Harmer, K. J. Fitzgerald, E. Eckstrom, R. Stock, J. Galver, G. Maddalozzo and S. S. Batya. 2012. Tai Chi and postural stability in patients with Parkinson's disease. *New England Journal of Medicine* 366: 511–19.

Little, J., and B. Lee. 2000. *Bruce Lee: A Warrior's Journey*. TV documentary. CA, USA: Warner Home Video.

Lundgren, T., J. Dahl, N. Yardi and L. Melin. 2008. Acceptance and commitment therapy and yoga for drug-refractory epilepsy: a randomized controlled trial. *Epilepsy and Behaviour* 13: 102–8.

Luria, A. R. 1975. *The Man with a Shattered World*. Harmondsworth, UK: Penguin Books.

Lynton, H., B. Kligler and S. Shiflett. 2007. Yoga in stroke rehabilitation: a systematic review and results of a pilot study. *Topics in Stroke Rehabilitation* 14, no. 4: 1–8.

Lyu, D., X. Lyu, Y. Zhang, Y. Ren, F. Yang, L. Zhou, Y. Zou and Z. Li. 2018. Tai Chi for stroke rehabilitation: a systematic review and meta-analysis of randomized controlled trials. *Frontiers in Physiology* 9: 983. doi:10.3389/fphys.2018.00983.

Mazzarin, C. M., S. R. Valderramas, F. M. de Paula, E. Tiepolo, L. Guérios, D. Parisotto and V. L. Israel. 2017. Effects of dance and of Tai Chi on functional mobility, balance, and agility in Parkinson disease. *Topics in Geriatric Rehabilitation* 33: 262–72.

McHugh, L., and R. Wood. 2013. Stimulus over-selectivity in temporal brain injury: mindfulness as a potential intervention. *Brain Injury* 27: 1595–9.

Mcmillan, T., I. H. Robertson, D. Brock and L. Chorlton. 2002. Brief mindfulness training for attentional problems after traumatic brain injury: a randomised control treatment trial. *Neuropsychological Rehabilitation* 12: 117–25.

Merton, T. 1969. *The Way of Chuang Tzu*. New York: New Directions.

Mills, N., and J. Allen. 2000. Mindfulness of movement as a coping strategy in multiple sclerosis: a pilot study. *General Hospital Psychiatry* 22: 425–31.

Mills, N., J. Allen and S. Carey-Morgan. 2000. Does Tai Chi/Qi Gong help patients with multiple sclerosis? *Journal of Bodywork and Movement Therapies* 4: 39–48.

Moustgaard, A., M. Bedard and M. Felteau. 2007. Mindfulness-based cognitive therapy (MBCT) for individuals who had a stroke: results from a pilot 90 study. *Journal of Cognitive Rehabilitation* 25: 4–10.

Ni, X., S. Liu, F. Lu, X. Shi and X. Guo. 2014. Efficacy and safety of Tai Chi for Parkinson's disease: a systematic review and meta-analysis of randomized controlled trials. *PloS One*, June 13. https://doi.org/10.1371/journal.pone.0099377.

Nochi, M. 1997. Dealing with the 'void': traumatic brain injury as a story. *Disability and Society* 12: 533–55.

Nochi, M. 1998a. Struggling with the labelled self: people with traumatic brain injuries in social settings. *Qualitative Health Research* 8: 665–81.

Nochi, M. 1998b. 'Loss of self' in the narratives of people with traumatic brain injuries: a qualitative analysis. *Social Science and Medicine* 7: 869–78.

Nochi, M. 2000. Reconstructing self-narratives in coping with traumatic brain injury. *Social Science and Medicine* 51: 1795–1804.

Orenstein, E., A. Basilakos and R. Shisler Marshall. 2012. Effects of mindfulness meditation on three individuals with aphasia. *International Journal of Language and Communication Disorders* 47: 673–84.

Pattni, R. 2016. A psychological understanding of the *Yogasūtra of Patanjali* (1–6) with a comparative phenomenology of *Sāmādhi* and flow. Unpublished doctoral thesis, University of Oxford.

Pickut, B. A., W. Van Hecke, E. Kerckhofs, P. Mariën, S. Vanneste, P. Cras and P. M. Parizel. 2013. Mindfulness based intervention in Parkinson's disease leads to structural brain changes on MRI: a randomized controlled longitudinal trial. *Clinical Neurology and Neurosurgery* 115: 2419–25.

Pickut, B., S. Vanneste, M. A. Hirsch, W. Van Hecke, E. Kerckhofs, P. Marien et al. 2015. Mindfulness training among individuals with Parkinson's disease: neurobehavioral effects. *Parkinson's Disease*. Published online. doi:10.1155/2015/816404.

Quinn, D., and K. Jones. 2012. Tai chi movement (TMW) and embodied mindfulness in mental and physical health. Inservice presentation for Herefordshire Primary Care Trust, UK.

Radder, D. L., I. H. Sturkenboom, M. van Nimwegen, S. H. Keus, B. R. Bloem and N. M. de Vries. 2017. Physical therapy and occupational therapy in Parkinson's disease. *International Journal of Neuroscience* 1e14.

Rajesh, B., D. Jayachandran, G. Mohandas and K. Radhakrishnan. 2006. A pilot study of a yoga meditation protocol for patients with medically refractory epilepsy. *Journal of Alternative and Complementary Medicine* 12: 367–71.

Roland, K. P. 2014. Applications of yoga in Parkinson's disease: a systematic literature review. *Journal of Parkinsonism and Restless Legs Syndrome* 4: 1–8.

Russell, T. A. 2011. Body in mind training: mindful movement for severe and enduring mental illness. *British Journal of Wellbeing* 2, no. 4: 13–16.

Russell, T. A., and T. Tatton-Ramos. 2014. Body in mind training: mindful movement for the clinical setting. *Neuro-disability and Psychotherapy* 2: 108–36.

Sacks, O. 1973. *Awakenings*. New York: Random House.

Schaffer, O. 2013. *Crafting Fun User Experiences: A Method to Facilitate Flow*. Fairfield, IA: Human Factors International.

Schmidt, A. A., K. K. Miller, M. Van Puymbroeck and N. Schalk. 2016. Feasibility and results of a case study of yoga to improve physical functioning in people with chronic traumatic brain injury. *Disability and Rehabilitation* 38: 914–20.

Senders, A., D. Bourdette, D. Hanes, Y. Vijaysgree and L. Shinto. 2014. Perceived stress in multiple sclerosis: the potential role of mindfulness in health and well-being. *Journal of Evidence-Based Complementary and Alternative Medicine* 19: 104–11.

Shapira, M. Y., M. Chelouche, R. Yanai, C. Kaner and A. Szold. 2001. Tai Chi Chuan practice as a tool for rehabilitation of severe head trauma: 3 case reports. *Archives of Physical Medicine and Rehabilitation* 82: 1283–5.

Shisler-Marshall, R., J. Lores-Gore and K. Love. 2017. Brief mindfulness meditation group training in aphasia: exploring attention, language and psychophysiological outcomes. *International Journal of Language and Communication Disorders* 53: 40–54.

Shravat, A. 2014. The role of a Yoga group within a holistic rehabilitation setting for ABI using compassion focused therapy approach: a qualitative case illustration. *Neuro-disability and Psychotherapy* 2: 100–7.

Silverthorne, C., S. B. Khalsa, R. Gueth, N. DeAvilla and J. Pansini. 2012. Respiratory, physical, and psychological benefits of breath-focused yoga for adults with severe traumatic brain injury (TBI): a brief pilot study report. *International Journal of Yoga Therapy* 22: 47–51.

Simpson, R., J. Booth, M. Lawrence, S. Byrne, F. Mair and S. Mercer. 2014. Mindfulness 21 based interventions in multiple sclerosis: a systematic review. *BMC Neurology* 14: 15.

Simpson, R., F. S. Mair and S. W. Mercer. 2017. Mindfulness-based stress reduction for people with multiple sclerosis – a feasibility randomised controlled trial. *BMC Neurology* 17: 141.

Simpson, R., S. Byrne, K. Wood, F. S. Mair and S. W. Mercer. 2018. *Optimising Mindfulness-Based Stress Reduction for People with Multiple Sclerosis*. London: Sage.

Sungkarat, S., S. Boripuntakul, N. Chattipakorn, K. Watcharasaksilp and S. R. Lord. 2017. Effects of tai chi on cognition and fall risk in older adults with mild cognitive impairment: a randomized controlled trial. *Journal of the American Geriatrics Society* 65: 721–7.

Tang, V., W. S. Poon and P. Kwan. 2015. Mindfulness-based therapy for drug-resistant epilepsy: an assessor-blinded randomized trial. *Neurology* 85: 1100–7.

Tavee, J., M. Rensel, S. M. Planchon, R. S. Butler and L. Stone. 2011. Effects of meditation on pain and quality of life in multiple sclerosis and peripheral neuropathy. *International Journal of MS Care* 13: 163–8.

Taylor, E., and R. E. Taylor-Piliae. 2017. The effects of Tai Chi on physical and psychosocial function among persons with multiple sclerosis: a systematic review. *Complementary Therapies in Medicine* 31: 100–8.

Taylor-Piliae, R. E., T. M. Hoke, J. T. Hepworth, L. D. Latt, B. Najafi et al. 2014. Effect of Tai Chi on physical function, fall rates and quality of life among older stroke survivors. *Archives of Physical Medicine and Rehabilitation* 95: 816–24.

Thompson, N. J., A. H. Patel, L. M. Selwa, S. C. Stoll, C. E. Begley, E. K. Johnson et al. 2015. Expanding the efficacy of Project UPLIFT: distance delivery of mindfulness-based depression prevention to people with epilepsy. *Journal of Consulting and Clinical Psychology* 83: 304–13.

Todd, D., and M. Smith. Forthcoming. Acceptance and commitment therapy. In *Psychological Therapies in Neuropsychological*

Rehabilitation, ed. G. N. Yeates and F. Ashworth. Hove, UK: Psychology Press.

Toh, S. F. M. 2013. A systematic review on the effectiveness of Tai Chi exercise in individuals with Parkinson's disease from 2003 to 2013. *Hong Kong Journal of Occupational Therapy* 23: 69–81.

Tyerman, A., and M. Humphrey. 1984. Changes in self concept following severe head injury. *International Journal of Rehabilitation Research* 7: 11–23.

Von Steinbüchel, N., L. Wilson, H. Gibbons, G. Hawthorne, S. Höfer, S. Schmidt, J. Truelle et al. 2010. Quality of Life after Brain Injury (QOLIBRI): scale development and metric properties. *Journal of Neurotrauma* 27: 1167–85.

Wang, C., R. Bannuru, J. Ramel, B. Kupelnick, T. Scott and C. H. Schmid. 2010. Tai Chi on psychological well-being: systematic review and meta-analysis. *BMC Complementary Alternative Medicine* 10: 23.

Whiting, D., G. Simpson, J. Ciarrochi and H. McLeod. 2012. Assessing the feasibility of acceptance and commitment therapy in promoting psychological adjustment after severe traumatic brain injury. *Brain Injury* 26: 588–9.

Williams, W. H., and J. J. Evans. 2003. Brain injury and emotion: an overview to a special issue on biopsychosocial approaches in neurorehabilitation. *Neuropsychological Rehabilitation* 13(1/12): 1–11.

Winser, S. J., P. Kannan, M. Pang and W. W. Tsang. 2017. Tai Chi for improving balance in cerebellar ataxia: a feasibility. *Archives of Physical Medicine and Rehabilitation* 98, no. 10: e113–14.

Winser, S. J., P. Kannan, M. Pang, C. Smith and W. W. Tsang. 2018a. Potential benefits and safety of T'ai Chi for balance and functional independence in people with cerebellar ataxia. *Journal of Alternative and Complimentary Medicine* 24: 1221–3.

Winser, S. J., W. W. Tsang, K. Krishnamurthy and P. Kannan. 2018b. Does Tai Chi improve balance and reduce falls incidence in neurological disorders? A systematic review and meta-analysis. *Clinical Rehabilitation* 32: 1157–68.

Wu, S., J. Chen, S. Wang, M. Jiang, X. Wang and Y. Wen. 2018. Effect of Tai Chi exercise on balance function of stroke patients: a meta-analysis. *Medical Science Monitor Basic Research* 24: 210–15.

Xie, G. L., T. Rao, L. Lin, Z. Lin, T. Xiao, M. Yang, Y. Xu, J. Fan, S. Lin, J. Wu, X. Feng, L. Li, J. Tao and L. Chen. 2018. Effects of Tai Chi Yunshou exercise on community-based stroke patients: a cluster randomized controlled trial. *European Review of Aging and Physical Activity* 15: 17.

Yan Li, G., G. L. Liu and Y. Zhang. 2018. Effects of Tai Chi on balance and gait in stroke survivors: a systematic meta-analysis of randomized controlled trials. *Journal of Rehabilitation Medicine* 50: 582–8.

Yang, Y., X.-Y. Li, L. Gong, Y.-L. Zhu and Y.-L. Hao. 2014. Tai Chi for improvement of motor function, balance and gait in Parkinson's disease: a systematic review and meta-analysis. *PLoS ONE* 9(7): e102942.

Yeates, G. N. 2014. Using pagers and alerts as adjuncts to psychological therapies following acquired brain injury. In *Telerehabilitation and Adaptations: Assistive Technology for People with Neuropsychological Impairments*, ed. Anna Cantagallo. Milan: francoAngeli.

Yeates, G. N. 2015. Flow state experiences as a biopsychosocial guide for Tai Ji intervention and research in neuro-rehabilitation. *Neuro-disability and Psychotherapy* 3: 22–41.

Yeates, G. N. 2018. Flow state experiences as a biopsychosocial guide for Tai Ji intervention and research in neuro-rehabilitation. In *Neuro-disability and Psychotherapy, Specialist Topics: Vol. 1. Eastern Influences on Neuropsychotherapy: Accepting, Soothing and Stilling Cluttered and Critical Minds in Neurological Conditions*, ed. G. N. Yeates and G. Farrell, 210–19. Oxford: Routledge.

Yeates, G. N. Forthcoming. Mind–body interventions for neurological conditions. In *Psychological Therapies in Neuropsychological Rehabilitation*, ed. G. N. Yeates and F. Ashworth. Hove, UK: Psychology Press.

Yeates, G. N., and G. Farrell. 2014. Editorial for special issue: 'Accepting,soothing and stilling cluttered and critical minds in neurological conditions: The influence of Eastern practices'. *Neuro-disability and Psychotherapy* 2: 1–2.

Yeates, G. N., and G. Farrell. 2018. Editors' foreword. In *Neuro-disability and Psychotherapy, Specialist Topics: Vol. 1. Eastern Influences on Neuropsychotherapy: Accepting, Soothing and Stilling Cluttered and Critical Minds in Neurological Conditions*, ed. G. N. Yeates and G. Farrell, Oxford: Routledge.

Yeates, G. N., M. Hamill, L. Sutton, K. Psaila, S. Mohamed and J. O'Dell. 2008. Dysexecutive problems and interpersonal relating following frontal brain injury: reformulation in cognitive-analytic therapy. *Neuro-Psychoanalysis* 10: 43–58.

Yeates, G. N., M. Murphy, J. Baldwin, J. Wilkes and M. Mahadevan. 2015. A pilot evaluation of a yoga group for survivors of acquired brain injury in a community setting. *Clinical Psychology Forum* 267: 46–51.

Yeates, G. N., S. Nagrani, A. Smith, J. Dorney-Savage, J. Whitman and E. Khan. 2008. Diversity of needs Tai Chi (Taiji) group interventions following acquired brain injury: a mixed methods study. Unpublished manuscript.

Yeates, G. N., S. Nagrani, A. Smith, J. Dorney-Savage, J. Whitman and E. Khan. Forthcoming. Mind–body interventions following expressive aphasia and stroke a single case study. In *Neuro-disability and Psychotherapy, Specialist Topics: Vol. 2. Psychotherapy and Aphasia: Supporting Emotions and Relationships,* ed. G. N. Yeates & K. Meredith. Oxford: Routledge.

Zhang, L., C. Layne, T. Lowder and J. Liu. 2011. A review focused on the psychological effectiveness of Tai Chi on different populations. *Evidence-Based Complementary and Alternative Medicine*. Published online. doi:10.1155/2012/678107.

Zheng, G., W. Zhou, R. Xia, J. Tao and L. Chen. 2016. Aerobic exercises for cognition rehabilitation following stroke: a systematic review. *Journal of Stroke and Cerebrovascular Disease* 25: 2780–9.

Zhou, J., T. Yin, Q. Gao and X. C. Yang. 2015. A meta-analysis on the efficacy of Tai Chi in patients with Parkinson's disease between 2008 and 2014. *Evidence Based Complementary and Alternative Medicine* 2015: 593263.

Zigmond, A. S., and R. P. Snaith. 1983. The Hospital Anxiety and Depression Scale. *Acta Psychiatrica Scandinavica* 67: 361–70.

Zou, L., C. Wang, X. Chen and H. Wang. 2018a. Baduanjin exercise for stroke rehabilitation: a systematic review with meta-analysis of randomized controlled trials. *International Journal of Environmental Research and Public Health* 15: 600.

Zou, L., A. Yeung, N. Zeng, C. Wang, L. Sun, G. Thomas and H. Wang. 2018b. Effects of mind–body exercises for mood and functional capabilities in post-stroke patients: an analytical review of randomized controlled trials. *International Journal of Environmental Research and Public Health,* 15: 721.

Chapter 18

II.III *Death and the Brain*

Examining the Continuum of Life to Determine Death

A Jewish Perspective

Aron Buchman*

Medical and technological advances have enhanced our ability to sustain life, while simultaneously calling into question criteria for determining when life has irrevocably ceased. Controversy surrounding the determination of death, and to what extent irreversible brain damage needs to be established, has continued unabated for more than 50 years, raising concerns as to whether and how it can ever be resolved. These controversies will be discussed in the light of ongoing discussions in the medical literature and Halakha, Jewish legal teachings, on the diagnosis and criteria for death.

The stakes are ready to get even higher. Rapid advances in neuroscience have facilitated our understanding of brain function and together with increases in computational power and miniaturisation of technology, have led to the development of new diagnostic and therapeutic tools. Just as the development of artificial respiration enhanced our ability to sustain life, advances in brain-machine interface technology have the potential to profoundly transform many other aspects of our daily lives. And just as the availability of artificial ventilation led to a debate that persists to today about how we determine death, the spread of technology-enhanced central nervous system (CNS) function will confront society with a new host of complex ethical issues [1–2].

Availability of these technologies will force society to examine a wide range of questions about the nature of human life including personal identity, agency, personhood, privacy and the limits of medical treatments. These questions rival the complexity of issues that underlie determination of death. In fact, they are likely to be even more difficult to resolve due to their novelty, extensive supplantation or enhancement of human functions and the lack of precedents. The rapid pace of medical discovery and technology development and adoption will not allow society the latitude to leave these issues unresolved for another 50 years.

Isolating issues which have contributed to the prolonged controversy about determining death have important implications for clarifying future efforts to integrate complex medical and technologic advances into our daily lives in an ethical way.

* This work has been supported in part by the National Institute of Health grants R01AG17917, P30AG10161, RF1AG22018, R01NS078009, R01AG040039. I would like to thank the following individuals for helpful comments and discussions in the preparation of this paper including: Tova R. Osofsky, MBA, David A. Bennett, MD, Rabbi Gedaliah A. Rabinowitz, Rabbi A. Walfish, PhD, David J. Landes, PhD, Berachyahu Lifshitz, PhD and Shmuel Weinberger, PhD.

Medical Disease: Continuum versus Discrete Category

According to traditional principles of medicine, diseases are diagnosed according to strictly delimited and differentiated categories. Clear, rigorous definitions are essential for managing cases and have contributed greatly to the success of modern epidemiology and therapeutic interventions. In contrast, evidence from epidemiologic research indicates that many diseases are best characterised as continua without clear natural boundaries [3]. As far back as the 1950s it was suggested that hypertension did not exist as a hard-edged category, but was best thought of as a continuum in which low blood pressure merged imperceptibly with 'normal' pressure and 'normal' pressure merged into elevated pressure.

This model also applies to common chronic conditions such as osteoporosis, chronic obstructive pulmonary disease and cardiovascular disease which develop slowly and insidiously over years to decades. Concepts of chronic age-related neurologic diseases have evolved similarly: Pathologies of Alzheimer's disease (AD), Parkinson's disease (PD) and cerebrovascular disease (CVD) are common in persons without clinically diagnosed dementia, PD or stroke and are associated with different levels of deficits affecting both motor and cognitive function, pointing to a continuum of progressive accumulation of these pathologies [4–6].

Increasingly, cases meeting established clinical criteria are being recognised as the 'tip of the iceberg' in that they are so severe that the diagnosis cannot be missed. However, a much larger number of older adults are likely to be suffering from milder, not yet fully developed diseases that have not yet reached the point at which a traditional diagnosis is possible.

Establishing and Applying Clinical Cut-Off Points

Despite the gradual, often imperceptibly progressive nature of the biological continuum from health to illness, for practical reasons clinicians must create and apply cut-offs for diagnostic and therapeutic decisions. But these cut-offs should not be misconstrued as indicating biological distinct states. They simply reflect the fact that many medical decisions are binary. Is a medical test positive or not? Should a therapeutic intervention be initiated or not?

For example, neuroscientists and researchers of ageing recognise a wide range of cognitive and non-cognitive symptoms along the continuum of cognitive decline. They have not identified a precise, quantifiable biologic boundary that distinguishes between mild cognitive impairment and dementia and are unlikely to ever do so. Nonetheless, available information enables development of a consensus about the clinical criteria that will serve as cut-off points for diagnoses of dementia, PD and stroke.

Public policy and medical treatment decisions require unambiguous labels. The fact that cut-off points are superimposed on the biological continuum does not minimise their practical or operational necessity. However, these cut-off points must not be misconstrued as objective boundaries between the absence of a disease or biologic entity on the one hand, and its presence on the other.

While scientific knowledge is essential for establishing cut-off points, the manifestations and consequences of disease in patients' daily lives are more important determinants of where the points should be placed. Furthermore, as technologies and therapies advance, manifestations and consequences evolve and diagnostic thresholds change. For example, a diagnosis of pulmonary tuberculosis used to require the clinical signs of consumption. Today, a positive PPD test will lead to the diagnosis of tuberculosis and a therapeutic intervention. Thus, both medical and non-medical communities face the challenge of creating valid procedures for constructing cut-off points along the underlying biologic continuum to replace previous definitions of disease.

When developing cut-off points, a wide range of expertise is required to represent diverse social, economic, psychological, religious, philosophic and legal concerns, and to integrate them with the best available medical information. Medical expertise is also essential to determine optimal means for the practical application of cut-off points.

The determination of a cut-off point, along with the development of a procedure for its implementation may often give rise to the faulty notion that the cut-off point represents a hard and fast boundary between two different biologic entities. Finally, given the diverse scientific and non-scientific information essential for developing clinical cut-off points, these cut-off points change as our knowledge and social sensibilities change.

Reframing the Brain Death Controversy

Death: Discrete Event versus a Continuum

Until very recently, death, like disease, was conceptualised as a discrete event. From time immemorial, bodily functions and life ceased when a patient's oxygen supply was interrupted for more than a very limited time.

Circulation of adequately oxygenated blood throughout the body depends on blood first being pumped by the heart to the lungs to be oxygenated. Prior to the advent of artificial respiration, a predictable sequence of events would occur if an individual's heart or lungs stopped working. Within minutes of the failure of either organ system, the other would irrevocably cease to function as well due to the lack of oxygen (anoxia). Since the brain is very sensitive to anoxia, the patient would lose consciousness and be rendered immobile within less than a minute from when the heart stopped pumping [7]. Persistence of anoxia would lead to inevitable loss of function in other tissues and organs.

Prior to the advent of mechanical ventilation, this sequence of events was inevitable and could not be altered. Therefore, cessation of a heartbeat and spontaneous breathing were recognised and universally applied as reliable and reproducible signs of the cessation of human life.

Like disease, death was viewed as a discrete event or well-defined category [8–9]. The question of which human characteristics ceased when the heart and lung stopped working was not articulated, since the cessation of all human activity and bodily function was inevitable and appeared to onlookers to end simultaneously, for all intents and purposes.

Tissues and organs vary in their sensitivity to loss of oxygen (anoxia). When the heart and lung have stopped working, other tissues and organs may continue to function for periods of time that vary with their sensitivities to anoxia. This belies the traditional conceptualisation of the cessation of heart and lung function as a biologically 'discrete event' of death and is consistent with the idea that the biologic continuum underlying dying does not include a natural boundary before the complete cessation of ALL organ functions.

The dissociation of cardiac and lung function through the use of mechanical ventilation began in the 1950s. Since that time, it has become increasingly clear that artificial ventilation has rendered the age-old procedure for identifying the cessation of life inadequate. While human physiology has, of course, not been altered by advances in medical technology, the advances undermined the perceived inherence of the physiological link between heart, lung and brain function.

With widespread adoption of ventilators, an uninterrupted supply of oxygen can be provided mechanically for patients whose respiration has failed as long as their hearts continue to beat, disrupting the inexorable progression from respiratory failure to anoxia, heart failure and death. Previously, heart, lung and brain function failed in such rapid succession that they seemed simultaneous, lending support to idea of death as a discrete event. The availability of mechanical ventilation, however, led to a new reality. Since blood continues to be oxygenated and to circulate despite respiratory failure, the brain and other organs need not fail. Halting the domino effect of anoxia enabled organs to fail at different points in time as would be expected in a biologic continuum.

Categorising Individuals When Mechanical Ventilation Is Available

The use of mechanical ventilation allowed a host of individuals who would have previously died to survive for extended periods of time. As experience with ventilators increased, more clinical data became available about the consequences of dissociation of cardiac respiratory and brain functions. Physicians began to categorise the location, severity and likely impact of an individual's injuries based on their respiratory and brain function.

Loss of respiration can occur in individuals who have normal heart function and are fully conscious. Respiration is controlled by centres located in the lower brainstem (medulla) which, if damaged can cause the permanent loss of independent breathing. A host of other nerve, muscle or primary lung disorders can cause loss of breathing without affecting heart function or consciousness [10]. For example, individuals with high cervical spinal cord injury cannot breathe and are quadriplegic, but are conscious and can be kept alive with ventilatory support. The very rare individual with locked-in-syndrome due to a focal brainstem injury which spares the arousal centres, who retains consciousness and cognitive function but can only control eye movements, can be kept alive with mechanical ventilation [11].

By contrast, individuals may become unconscious yet still retain normal respiration and heart function. The respiratory centres in the lower brainstem (medulla) are anatomically distinct from arousal centres located in the upper brainstem. Injuries to the upper brainstem or both hemispheres spare the respiratory centres in the lower brainstem, but cause persistent unconsciousness (coma). Nonetheless, since the breathing centres remain intact, the individual would retain the capacity to breathe without a ventilator and has normal heart function despite being unconscious and in coma. The recovery of comatose individuals varies widely, so it is difficult to predict the extent of recovery in any individual case with any degree of certainty. However, in many cases, the clinical status of patients in coma is not irrevocable.

Recent studies using PET and fMRI suggest that bedside testing alone is insufficient to determine the depth of coma, i.e. whether an individual is experiencing unresponsive wakefulness (vegetative state) versus minimally conscious state [12]. Further work is needed to develop accurate procedures that can assess whether an individual with severe brain injury has sufficient residual brain function to return to a conscious state [13].

In a minority of cases, loss of consciousness occurs in conjunction with loss of capacity to breathe. These individuals have more extensive brain damage, including damage to both the arousal centres in the upper brainstem (pons) and breathing centres in the lower brainstem (medulla). These injuries cause the loss of brainstem reflexes, consciousness and the capacity to breathe. The patients who fall into this category require ventilatory support to prevent anoxia and cessation of heart function, although the maintenance of adequate oxygenation cannot revive the damaged brain.

The widespread and severe damage to the brain in these cases can increase pressure in the cranial cavity to the degree that it exceeds systemic blood pressure and prevents oxygenated blood from entering the skull. Advances in imaging modalities such as transcranial Doppler and CT angiography confirm that many cases of brain death are characterised by the absence of blood flow to the brainstem and brain [10]. Documentation of the lack of cerebral blood flow to the brain is important since it can provide evidence that the brain damage is irrevocable. Thus, in such cases, even continued cardiac function and circulation of adequately oxygenated blood outside of the brain will not enable the brain itself to recover.

Do Traditional Indicators of Death Need Updating?

Prior to the advent of mechanical ventilation, the absence of brainstem respiratory drive lead quickly to the loss of systemic oxygenation necessary to maintain a beating heart. Physicians only began to encounter individual's whose heart continued beating, despite persistent irrevocable loss of cerebral and brainstem function, with the widespread clinical use of mechanical ventilation. As physicians, medical ethicists and even family members accumulated experience with individuals who required mechanical ventilation and manifested this novel clinical combination, many came to believe that a new standard for determining death was needed [14].

Since clinical examination documented irrevocable cessation of function in the brain and brainstem, this clinical state scenario was termed brain death. A variety of other terms have been used to describe the same state including, whole brain death, total brain failure or brainstem death [15]. In contrast to cases of persistent coma (chronic vegetative state) that sometimes improve, there has never been a documented case of recovery when clinical findings consistent with loss of brainstem function (a key feature of all definitions of brain death) have been documented by experienced clinicians [16–17].

Advocates of the brain death concept consider irrevocable cessation of brain function sufficient for indicating the cessation of human life. Opponents of brain death dispute the necessity of a new standard for determining death. They believe that an individual with a beating heart cannot be a corpse. In their view, as long as the heart and other bodily functions have not stopped, human life has not ceased. Advocates of this view would argue that the brain can fail like any other organ system, and its failure alone without the cessation of the heart is not synonymous with death. In this view, brain death cannot be equated with the death of the person and until his heart stops beating an individual is not dead.

Is Clinical Brain Death an Adequate Indicator of the Irrevocable Cessation of Life?

Since the concept of brain death was initially proposed, the efficacy of cardiac transplantation and cardiopulmonary bypass has improved dramatically. These medical advances lend further support to the notion that the absence of cardiopulmonary function does not now and never did constitute a natural boundary for defining death. However, prior to the availability of efficacious interventions, the absence of cardiopulmonary function served as a reliable indicator of the cessation of human life.

But if cardiopulmonary function indicates the cessation of human life, what are the essential characteristics of that life? For millennia, the inextricable linkage of heart, lung and brain function and their near-simultaneous cessation rendered the question moot. Today, however, medical advances which enable us to uncouple these clinical functions set the stage for a new reality in which the absence of cardiopulmonary function, for instance, can no longer serve as a reliable indicator for the irrevocable cessation of brain function. In an age when we can artificially replace heart and lung function, the absence or continued functioning of the brain and its manifold networks no longer depends on natural heart and lung function.

The brain is essential for myriad automatic and volitional behaviours which underlie human life – so many, in fact, that it is hard to pinpoint the human characteristics that are essential to our concept of life and whose absence could definitively separate the living from the dead.

Loss of consciousness, language and other predominantly cortical mediated behaviours, or even persistent coma with intact brainstem function have all failed to garner proponents as cut-off points, perhaps because these observed behaviours cannot be characterised as irrevocable since in a small number of cases variable recovery occurs [18].

Furthermore, it is unclear how definitions of death which focus on cortical brain functions would be applied at the beginning of life. Take, for example, the case of a baby born with anencephaly (absent telencephalon) who is blind, deaf, unable to perceive pain and will never interact cognitively with his environment. Nonetheless, this baby can breathe and control other vegetative functions. Few would advocate that this baby with anencephaly is 'dead'.

The clinical criteria for brain death were initially justified as representing 'whole brain death' and later reconceptualised as the loss of 'integrative brain function'. However, today, there is increasing recognition that individuals who fulfil the clinical criteria for brain death do not necessarily show irrevocable loss of all integrative central nervous system (CNS) functions. Temperature regulation, energy balance, the maintenance of systemic blood pressure, metabolic functions and even the ability to support gestation of a fetes may all be present in patients who fit the clinical definition of brain death, suggesting residual central nervous system integrative functions [15, 17].

The presence of residual brain function in individuals who meet current clinical criteria for brain death does not change the fact that no brain dead individual has ever recovered [16]. The heterogeneity of residual brain function in cases meeting clinical criteria for brain death suggests that there is not a natural boundary for current brain death criteria. Furthermore, the fact that these other integrative function as well as other bodily functions will eventually fail in individuals meeting the criteria of clinical brain death is consistent with a biologic continuum.

Nonetheless, the presence of residual brain functions in cases meeting current clinical brain death criteria underscores the necessity to justify the choice of the clinical functions chosen for determining brain death. Why should loss of respiration be chosen as the clinical indicator of a brain death cut-off point rather than employing loss of temperature regulation or loss of maintenance of systemic blood pressure? This question is difficult to answer for advocates of current brain death criteria, but in fact critics of the brain death criteria would have the same difficulty in justifying the standard cardiopulmonary criteria for determining death [19–20].

Developing a Cut-Off Point for Death as a Precondition for Identifying a Clinical Indicator

Medical advances have rendered traditional cardiopulmonary indicators inadequate as the exclusive standard for determining death. These advances have expanded our knowledge about the biologic continuum at the end of life. Nonetheless, the rapidly growing body of scientific knowledge will not provide answers regarding where to place a cut-off point for the cessation of life. Determining a cut-off point must start with development of a consensus about which human characteristics must be present for an individual to be considered alive.

The ongoing conversation about brain death focuses largely on the practical issue of determining biologic markers or clinical functions to employ for determining death. This persistent focus skirts the daunting task of developing a conceptual consensus for a cut-off point for death. Development of a conceptual consensus should precede discussion about the most efficacious indicator for demarcating the cut-off point for cessation of human life. The lack of a conceptual grounding for indicators of when life ends makes it difficult to reassess the efficacy of traditional indicators as medical knowledge and technology advance.

Determining Death in Jewish Law

While death has no sacramental significance in Judaism, its determination is essential for legal issues and rituals including mourning, burial, ritual impurity, inheritance, personal status (dissolution of marriage), criminal adjudication of murder and medical care. *Halakha* (Jewish law) is the normative structure undergirding traditional Jewish life, and provides normative prescriptions for behaviour in all areas of public and private activity. While *halakha* is often translated as 'Jewish law', its scope extends beyond the legal to encompass ethical and moral dimensions of behaviour [21]. *Halakha* is an ongoing creation of scholars and jurists who base their decisions on rabbinic commentary, codes and response literature. The ongoing relevance of *halakha* among its adherents is a testimony to the system's capacity to maintain its nomos while responding to the contingent and unforeseen cultural, social, technological, scientific and political changes that occur over time [22–26].

Contemporary halakhic discourse focuses on defining a particular moment of death based on the assessment of one or more clinical signs (cessation of cardiac, pulmonary or brain activity) [27–29]. This focus on definition parallels traditional categorical approaches to disease, as discussed above. This is not surprising since the rabbinic community is responsive to queries and accommodates itself to medical advances and contemporary theories.

Nonetheless, despite the detailed characterisation of many other life cycle events in Jewish codes and rabbinic literature, it is striking that no primary source in the Talmud or in subsequent halakhic codes provides a comprehensive listing of signs used to determine death or a detailed description of the procedure [30]. Several Talmudic references, however, mention different signs of death and are cited in nearly all halakhic discussions on the topic.

Primary Sources

Talmud Bavli Yoma

In Jewish tradition, the obligation to save another human being supersedes all other religious obligations except the prohibitions forbidding murder, serious sexual misconduct and idol worship (Talmud Bavli Sanhedrin 73a). For example, if someone holds a gun to Z's head and says, 'If you do not kill X, I will kill you', *halakha* states that Z is not permitted to shoot X to save himself. Rather, the tradition asks the rhetorical question, 'Who is to say that your blood is redder' than that of Mr X [31]?

The suspension of all other religious obligations when confronted with the opportunity to save a life only apply only to saving individuals who are alive. As such, in the discourse on this issue, the Talmud discusses how to determine whether an individual is dead. If he is dead, there is no longer conflict between activities forbidden on the Sabbath and the requirement to do those very same activities on the Sabbath if doing so might save the individual's life.

The Talmud Bavli Yoma 83a states:

> If debris falls on someone on the Sabbath and it is uncertain if he is alive or dead . . . one must probe the debris for him. If he is alive, one must remove debris for him and if he is dead, you must leave him.
>
> The rabbis learned: To what extent does one examine the person to determine if he is alive or dead? To his nose and others state to his heart [navel].
>
> If you searched and the individuals uncovered on top are dead, do not say the individuals below are dead . . .
>
> These *tannaim* [teachers] hold the same positions of other tannaim. As we have learned: How is the fetus formed? From his head . . . Abba Shaul says from the navel . . . Both of the tannaim may hold like Abba Shaul. Abba Shaul only takes his position with respect to fetal development, since all development starts in the middle.
>
> However, with respect to saving a life, even Abba Shaul agrees that essential life is located in the nostrils, as written in the verse: 'All in whose nostrils was the breath of the spirit of life' (Genesis 7).
>
> Rav Pappa said, 'The argument is when you initially uncover his feet and continue upward. But if you first examine his nose and find no signs of breathing, you do not have to examine any additional sites, since the verse says, "All in whose nostrils was the breath of the spirit of life"' (Genesis 7) (Talmud Bavli, Yoma 85a).

The simplest reading of the text suggests that all the parties cited agree that the presence or absence of respiratory function was sufficient for determining whether an individual was dead. The difference of opinion about nose/heart/navel is rooted in the question as to which body location was the most sensitive indicator of residual pulmonary function. Thus, the heart was mentioned not because cardiac function had to be assessed, but because it was considered the optimal anatomical location to assess breathing.

The use of the word 'heart' in this text means 'chest' rather than an internal organ. Based on alternate texts which have the word 'heart' rather than 'navel', a minority of scholars have suggested that the dispute in this text is whether cardiac or pulmonary functions are the primary determinants of death [32]. Nonetheless, even in the sources with alternate readings, i.e. 'heart', the Talmudic conclusion seems clearly to favour a pulmonary criterion.

This citation is important since it provides Talmudic evidence that the absence of breathing was used to determine death. However, in this text, there is no mention of any additional necessity to check for concomitant loss of consciousness, absence of cardiac activity or lack of movement. Furthermore, there is no evidence in this text that the Talmud is speaking of a *definition* of death rather than identifying a sensitive *indicator* that could be used to determine if the individual who had been buried under the debris was dead [33].

Because most of the legal prescriptions in the Talmudic texts are in the form of case law, one might argue that, given the extreme circumstances and contingencies of the case being discussed, it is unclear whether the procedure described should be generalised to standard circumstances. Furthermore, this text does not rule out the possibility that there are other signs that can or must be employed to determine death.

The most common reading of this text by commentators integrates all its segments by focusing the entire discussion on the optimal means to assess the presence or absence of breathing. Although other clinical signs are not mentioned in the text, many commentators like the Hatam Sofer (Yoreh Deah 336) presuppose that additional clinical signs must be ascertained (i.e. the individual must be unconscious, immobile and lack evidence of a heart beat) before an assessment of breathing can be employed to determine death.

The lack of details about other necessary clinical signs for determining death, in this primary text, underscores why many contemporary rabbinic authorities find it difficult to justify testing clinical signs other than respiratory function for determining death. This absence of such details in rabbinic literature has led some rabbinic authorities to suggest that some fact-dependent areas of halakhic practices were established on the basis of the best scientific knowledge available at the time [24]. However, because the sources do not explicitly state that this is the case, many rabbinic authorities resist modifying past halakhic decisions to the current state of scientific knowledge. Nonetheless, despite this resistance to change, halakha does accommodate to scientific knowledge though only gradually over a protracted period of time (i.e. treatment of premature infants on the Sabbath) [25, 34].

Mishna Oholot 1:6

According to halakha, contact with a corpse causes ritual impurity.

> The Rabbis taught: A man cannot defile [as a corpse] until his soul has departed. Even an individual who is '*meguyad*' or even a '*goses*' [is still alive] and therefore can still make levirate marriage obligatory or liberates from levirate marriage. Qualifies his mother for eating terumah [food offering] and disqualifies his mother from eating terumah. Similarly, cattle or wild animals, cannot defile until their soul has departed. If their heads have been cut off, even though they are moving convulsively, like a lizard's tail, which moves convulsively, they are unclean.
>
> (Mishna Oholot 1:6)

This text juxtaposes two categories of terminally ill individuals to illustrate that although their medical conditions are incompatible with survival, they are considered to be fully alive until they expire. While several possible explanations have been proposed for the term *meguyad*, most agree that the term is likely to refer to a penetrating traumatic injury which is incompatible with life such as a stabbing or knifing that causes irreparable injury to large vessels in the neck and results in the victim exsanguinating. The term *goses* usually refers to an individual in the throes of death.

The text does not explicitly characterise other clinical details. Nonetheless, several commentators note that despite their imminent death due to their underlying conditions, both individuals who are discussed in this text are conscious, with intact or impaired cognition. Thus, according to these commentators the text may imply consciousness is incompatible with an individual being considered dead even in the presence of a fatal injury or medical condition.

The end of the mishna states that when an animal is decapitated, it is considered dead even if it manifests movements in its extremities. This would suggest that in cases other than decapitation movement is a sign of life [35]. Taken together both portions of this mishna could lend support to the idea that in the absence of trauma, loss of consciousness and absence of movement are preconditions for determining that an individual has expired.

While one could read the rule about decapitation as applying only to animals, the Talmud Bavli Hulin 21B extends the decapitation rule to humans as well as extending it to severe traumatic spinal cord and trunk injuries. This source suggests that like individuals who are decapitated, victims of severe trauma that disrupts the anatomical integrity of the human body, may be considered dead even in the presence of other standard indicators of life such as cardiac or respiratory activity.

Each of the clinical indicators mentioned in these sources needs to be re-evaluated since many no longer serve as reliable indicators of inevitable death once modern medical facilities are available [36]. The overriding importance of updating the importance assigned to these sources in light of medical advances lends further support to the idea that a definition for the moment of death is not inherent in these sources [34]. Some contemporary rabbinic authorities have suggested a further conceptual expansion, positing that brain death represents 'physiologic decapitation'. If this analogy is accepted, then like physical decapitation, the continued beating of the heart would not be incompatible with a determination of death. The degree to which rabbinic sources in the mishna *Oholot* and talmud *Yoma* are based on a uniform definition of death is the subject of ongoing debate among contemporary rabbinic authorities.

The idea of physiologic decapitation is interesting. However, several issues have not been adequately addressed by its proponents. While respiration is absent in decapitation, complete dislocation and severance of the spinal cord below the C7 level will not affect breathing and cardiac function. The expansion of the decapitation category by Hulin 21a to include severe trauma to the entire extent of spinal cord and even the trunk suggest that the indicators for traumatic and non-traumatic death may be different. This underscores the need for a better conceptual framework that integrates the various indicators found in rabbinic sources before one can assess whether non-traumatic physiologic decapitation is included. Furthermore, with further medical advances the significance of the human body and its anatomical integrity in regulating death is likely to grow less compelling.

Other Talmudic Sources

Additional Talmudic sources presuppose a procedure for determination of death without describing its details, while still other sources express concerns about the sensitivity and specificity of extant procedures for determining death. For example, the Talmud Bavli Sanhedrin 46a discusses an uncontested biblical law that mandates burial on the day of death. The discussion in this text and its biblical proof text presuppose a procedure for determining death which is not described. Moreover, although the Rabbis (Semachot 8:1) recognised that their determination of death was not foolproof, the text in Sanhedrin mandated burial on the day an individual died, suggesting that these concerns were not sufficient to delay burial.

This source in Sanhedrin might be at variance with another Talmudic source (Bavli Nida 69B) which seems to suggest that until a corpse is observed to decompose there might be concern that breathing had ceased due to a 'faint'. Concerns about false positive assessments of absent respiration persisted and a mandated observation period following the determination of death was included in subsequent codes [33]. This observation period was generally for less than an hour after the cessation of respiration so that burial could occur within 24 hours from the time of death. This codification suggests that clinical signs in Talmudic sources were treated as indicators of death rather than as a definition of death.

Modern Rabbinic Controversy about Determining Death

Concerns about false positive determinations of death were not limited to the Jewish community. In seventeenth- and eighteenth-century European society, there were medical and social concerns that traditional cardiopulmonary criteria were not reliable indicators of death. Various legislative efforts delayed burials for up to three days until irrevocable signs of tissue decomposition were observed. This delay in burial beyond 24 hours was contested by the Jewish communities [37].

Some Jewish religious leaders believed that the traditional practice of same-day burial should be abandoned in light of then-contemporary medical opinion [38]. They argued that while there was no debate that burial was mandated on the day of death, the obligation to bury the dead and the prohibition of leaving them unburied was not considered absolute. Furthermore, the Jewish legal imperative that any potential life-saving action overrides all religious obligations was uniformly accepted. Thus, delaying burial because it might lead to saving a life by reducing the chances of mistakenly determining death should be embraced by rabbinic authorities, not just allowed.

This challenge to traditional orthodoxy is instructive as a counterpoint for the brain death controversy nearly 200 years later. In the seventeenth and eighteenth centuries, in contrast to the arguments put forth by rabbis and lay leaders (above), more senior and distinguished rabbinic leaders argued that the standard cardiopulmonary determination of death had been employed in the Jewish community since antiquity and that the medical community had not provided sufficient new information to justify its change. In his responsum, Rabbi Sofer in his decision (Yoreh Deah 338) states it is obvious based on laws described in the Bible, that there must have been a measure for death, despite his acknowledged inability to identify the origin of such a measure.

Rabbi Sofer suggests three possible sources for the standard employed for determining death. First, the rabbis may have based their decisions on a tradition received from the ancient 'naturalists' – a tradition that current doctors have forgotten. Second, they may have received an oral tradition which goes back to the time of revelation at Sinai and was received by Moses. Third, the rabbis may have derived or found support for common practice from the Biblical verse quoted from Genesis in Talmud Bavli Yoma 85 discussed above.

It is clear that with respect to the original query, Rabbi Sofer objected to delaying burials and had no qualms about determining death using the procedure that had been used for generations. Nonetheless, there has been much contemporary debate about whether his response can be used to support or oppose current clinical brain death criteria.

This responsum represents an important conceptual transition from a discussion about indicators of death to a position that a traditional definition of the moment of death exists in halakha. The difference is significant: if we are dealing with indicators or signs of death, then the salient question is what features characterise the underlying state we are trying to identify? Since indicators such as respiration, which were reliable indicators in the past, may lose their utility with advances in medical knowledge and technology, other indicators for the underlying state may be substituted. If on the other hand, there is a definition of death based on rabbinic tradition, it is more likely to be reified, suggesting its modification, even based on new information would be viewed as a challenge to the religious tradition.

Contemporary Rabbinic Controversy about Brain Death

The burial controversies in the seventeenth and eighteenth centuries did not arise from then-new medical data. By contrast, contemporary medical advances have challenged the rabbinic community with novel data and precipitated a need to reassess its reliance on the cardiopulmonary standard for determining death. In an interesting role reversal, it was the medical community in the seventeenth and eighteenth centuries which was unsure of when to establish death, and the rabbinic community simply held steadfast to their traditional practices. By contrast, at the time that the brain death controversy began in the late 1960s, the medical community perceived disease and diagnosis as well defined and demarcated. Brain death was like other scientific facts: it was rigorously defined and its biologic markers could be ascertained and identified like other diseases and diagnoses. The rabbinic community was called upon to respond to the medical community's claim of a biological definition for death [39].

As discussed above one could read the primary rabbinic sources as describing indicators rather than definitions of death. Nonetheless, since the same-day burial controversies in the eighteenth century, the predominant view within the rabbinic community has been that these sources delineate a biologic definition for the moment of death in halakha. The ongoing contemporary rabbinic controversy continues this focus on biologic definitions and revolves around whether brain death can be subsumed within the varying opinions about the biological-halachic definitions of death. Thus, all sides in the ongoing rabbinic controversy focus on the degree to which particular biologic markers and medical tests identify a precise moment of death.

Reconceptualising dying as a continuum obviates the expectation that biology can provide a clearly defined moment of death because there are no clear natural boundaries. This reconceptualisation challenges the rabbinic community as well as society at large to look beyond the biologic markers to indicators or signs that point to an underlying state. What are the human characteristics which must be absent when life irrevocably ends?

Challenges of Applying Rabbinic Sources for Determining Death with a Continuum Model

No rabbinic sources provide a conceptual framework for how or why the indicators which are mentioned in the Talmud were chosen. This makes it difficult to translate or anchor the indicators mentioned in the Talmud into cut-points consonant with a conceptualisation of the end of life as a biologic continuum. This challenge to the contemporary rabbinic community is further complicated by medical advances that can replace the functions of traditional indicators (circulation and respiration) [40–41].

Numerous paradigm shifts have occurred between pre-modern and contemporary medicine. Probability, induction and statistical inference were not formalised until after the seventeenth century and where applicable may provide new perspectives [42–44]. The conceptual framework for human physiology in classic rabbinic literature predates not only modern concepts of neuroscience but even William Harvey's (1578–1657) description of systemic circulation and the properties of blood being pumped to the brain and body by the heart.

Concepts of Galenic medicine dominated Western medicine until the seventeenth century and persisted in the rabbinic literature into the eighteenth century and in some cases even later [35]. How does one draw conclusions from sources formulated in a premodern context based on antiquated conceptions of the human body and apply them to our current reality [32]? Moreover, the persistent focus by both rabbinic advocates and opponents of brain death regarding which biological functions should be employed for determining death, underscores the absence of a conceptual consensus regarding the human characteristics that should define the presence of human life.

To some degree the purported gaps in the rabbinic literature discussed above are based on several assumptions about the nature of determining death based on rabbinic sources. First, many contemporary readers expect that the information we seek was always formulated systematically and should be found in rabbinic sources. They also assume that our contemporary formulation of the issues underlie and frame the recorded discussions. Furthermore, the contemporary discussion of determining death is predicated on a view in which the entire range of human experience is encompassed by a halakhic framework with which our behaviours must be aligned [45–47]. Additionally, apart from assumptions about halakha or rabbinic literature, the necessity to reassess traditional cardiopulmonary standard for determining death derives from medical and technological advances that have changed our current reality.

In pre-modern times, in the absence of any interventions, the experience of death did not need to be formalised since the procedure for determining death was recognised and employed universally. Thus, rabbinic literature did not dwell on defining a procedure for determining death. Rather, a central motif and recurrent theme in rabbinic literature is the obligation and importance of interventions whenever there was any chance for survival. In nearly every rabbinic responsum about determining death, a proviso is always added, stating that medical intervention is mandated if there is even the slightest chance of survival, even if usual indicators for death are present.

In our contemporary reality, this aggressive approach must be tempered by concerns about the life that will result if an intervention is successful. Rabbi Y. Reischer (Shevut Yaakov O.C. 1:13) notes that one of the several sources for the mandate to 'heal' in Jewish law was derived from the biblical injunction of returning a lost object to its owner. Rabbi Y. Reischer reasons that physicians are mandated to heal, but if they can't heal, they are not mandated to prolong dying. This principle has important consequences for decisions about the choice of treatments at the end of life.

Nonetheless, at the point in a person's life when no medical interventions are available, it must be determined when life has ended. Shifting the focus of the discussion to the obligation for aggressive medical interventions even if there is only a small chance of success does not free us from the difficult task of developing a conceptual consensus for a cut-off point for when life has irrevocably ceased [34, 48].

Conclusion

Recent changes in medical concepts of disease provide an opportunity to shape social discourse about a wide range of issues which are generally treated as distinct and unrelated domains. A growing body of evidence from studies of human disease indicates that human biology and physiology is best characterised by continua without clear natural boundaries. This conceptual shift distinguishes two inter-related processes, our advancing knowledge about human biology and concomitant technologic advances as distinct from decisions about how we translate these advancements into daily life.

Medical advances such as contraception, stem cell research, surrogacy, prenatal genetic testing, critical care medicine and transplantations have catalysed the resurgence of controversy about a wide range of issues by forcing a reassessment of how we define the beginning and end of life. Positions about when life begins or ends cannot be derived from our knowledge about their underlying biology, which has no natural boundaries. Rather, deciding when life begins or ends is a social construct which requires a consensus that balances diverse concerns and must accommodate changes as scientific knowledge and technology advance.

Innovative research in the neurosciences and rapid technological advancements will continue to enhance our daily lives. These enhancements will expand and challenge our notions of self-conception. Questions about 'brain transplants' or 'brain in the vat' are often dismissed as either science fiction or elements in philosophic thought experiments. However, they may provide helpful constructs for social discourse which seeks to develop consensus about what characterises personhood and human life.

The conceptualisation of life as a continuum has the potential to shape discourse about defining the beginning and end of life as well as stages across the entire life span. Efforts to incorporate new technologies and enhancements into our daily life may provide a richer lexicon that informs and facilitates efforts to develop conceptual consensus about the human characteristics which can be used to capture different stages across the continuum of life as well as its beginning and end.

References

1 Jackson, A., and J. B. Zimmermann. 2012. Neural interfaces for the brain and spinal cord – restoring motor function. *Nature Reviews Neurology* 8: 690–9.

2 Attiah, M. A., and M. J. Farah. 2014. Minds, motherboards, and money: futurism and realism in the neuroethics of BCI technologies. *Frontiers in Systems Neuroscience* 8: 86.

3 Rose, G. 1992. *The Strategy of Preventive Medicine*. Oxford: Oxford University Press.

4 Jack, C. R., Jr., M. Albert, D. S. Knopman, G. M. McKhann, R. A. Sperling, M. C. Carrillo et al. 2011. Introduction to revised criteria for the diagnosis of Alzheimer's disease: National Institute on Aging and the Alzheimer's Association workgroup. *Alzheimer's and Dementia* 7: 256–62.

5 Stern, M. B., A. Lang and W. Poewe. 2012. Toward a redefinition of Parkinson's disease. *Movement Disorders* 27: 54–60.

6 Gorelick, P. B., A. Scuteri, S. E. Black, C. DeCarli, S. M. Greenberg, C. Iadecola et al. 2011. Vascular contributions to cognitive impairment and dementia. *Stroke* 42: 2672–713.

7 Posner, J. B., C. B. Saper, N. D. Schiff and F. Plum. 2007. *Plum and Posner's Diagnosis of Stupor and Coma*. 4th edn. Ed. M. Sid Gilman. Oxford: Oxford University Press.

8 Kass, L. R. 1971. Death as an event: a commentary on Robert Morison. *Science* 173: 698–702.

9 Morison, R. S. 1971. Death: process or event? *Science* 173: 694–8.

10 Wijdicks, E. F. M. 2001. The diagnosis of brain death. *New England Journal of Medicine* 344: 1215–21.

11 de Jong, B. M. 2013. 'Complete motor locked-in' and consequences for the concept of minimally conscious state. *Journal of Head Trauma Rehabilitation* 28: 141–3.

12 Stender, J., O. Gosseries, M. A. Bruno, V. Charland-Verville, A. Vanhaudenhuyse, A. Demertzi et al. 2014. Diagnostic precision of PET imaging and functional

MRI in disorders of consciousness: a clinical validation study. *Lancet* 384: 476–7.

13 Controversies in the Determination of Death: A White Paper by the President's Council on Bioethics. 2008. The President's Council on Bioethics, Washington, DC.

14 Giacomini, M. 1997. A change of heart and a change of mind? Technology and the redefinition of death in 1968. *Social Science and Medicine* 44: 1465–82.

15 Bioethics PsCo. 2014. Controversies in the determination of death 2008. 8 April.

16 Wijdicks, E. F., P. N. Varelas, G. S. Gronseth and D. M. Greer. 2010. Evidence-based guideline update: determining brain death in adults: report of the Quality Standards Subcommittee of the American Academy of Neurology. *Neurology* 74: 1911–18.

17 Shewmon, D. A. 1998. Chronic 'brain death': meta-analysis and conceptual consequences. *Neurology* 51: 1538–45.

18 Luaute, J., D. Maucort-Boulch, L. Tell, F. Quelard, T. Sarraf, J. Iwaz et al. 2010. Long-term outcomes of chronic minimally conscious and vegetative states. *Neurology* 75: 246–52.

19 Halevy, A., and B. Brody. 1993. Brian death: reconciling definitions, criteria, and tests. *Annals of Internal Medicine* 119: 519.

20 Emanuel, L. L. 1995. Reexamining death: the asymptotic model and a bounded zone definition. *Hastings Center Report* 25, no. 4: 27–35.

21 Blidstein, G. J. 1996. Halakhah – the governing norm. *Jewish Political Studies Review* 8: 37–80.

22 Cover, R. 1983. The Supreme Court, 1982 term-foward: nomos and narrative. *Harvard Law Review* 4: 4–68.

23 Silman, Y. D. 1999. *The Voice Heard at Sinai: Once or Ongoing?* Jerusalem: Magnes Press, Hebrew University.

24 Sternberg, S. 1997. Review of 'Guide to Masechet Hullin and Masechet Bechorot' by I. M. Levinger. *Bekhol Derakhekha Daehu* 4: 81–102.

25 Gutel, N. 1998. *Changes in Reality in Jewish Law.* Jerusalem: Yachdov.

26 Soloveitchik, H. 2013. *Collected Essays.* Oxford: Littman Library of Jewish Civilization.

27 Steinberg, A. 1998. Moment of death. In *Medicine and Jewish Law*, ed. Fred Rosen, 18–68. Lanham, MD: Jason Aronson.

28 Shabtai, D. 2012. *Defining the Moment: Understanding Brain Death in Halakhah.* New York: Shoresh.

29 Halperin, M., ed. 2007. *Determining the Moment of Death.* 2nd edn. Jerusalem: Schleisinger Research Institute for Medicine and Jewish Law.

30 Jakobovits, I. 1975. *Jewish Medical Ethics.* 2nd edn. New York: Bloch.

31 Hershler, M. 1981. Obligation to save the sick and individuals in danger. In *Halakha and Medicine*, ed. M. Hershler, 2:27–70. Jerusalem: Regensberg Institute.

32 Reifman, D. 2012. Ancient sources, modern problems: a methodological analysis of Rashi's position on brainstem death. *Tradition* 45, no. 4: 9–23.

33 Rabinowitz, G. A., and M. Keningsberg. 1971. The definition and determining the time of death from the perspective of Halakha. *Hadarom* 32: 59–76.

34 Rabinovitz, N. A. 1998. *Scientific Assessment as the Basis for Halackhic Decisions: Investigations in the Works of the Rambam.* Jerusalem: Yeshovat Birakt Moshe.

35 Reichman, E. 1993. The Halakhic definition of death in light of medical history. *Torah U'Madda Journal* 4: 148–74.

36 Knutsdottir, S., H. Thorisdottir, K. Sigvaldason, H. Jonsson Jr., A. Bjornsson and P. Ingvarsson. 2012. Epidemiology of traumatic spinal cord injuries in Iceland from 1975 to 2009. *Spinal Cord* 50: 123–6.

37 Landes, D. J. 2010. *Traditional Struggles: Studying, Deciding and Performing the Law at the Rabbi Isaac Elchanan Theological Seminary.* Princeton, NJ: Princeton University Press.

38 Chajes, Z. H. 1958. *Darchai Horaah: Kol Kitvei Maharitz Chajes.* Jerusalem: Divrei Chachamim.

39 Moses, N. 2011. *Really Dead? The Israeli Brain-Death Controversy, 1967–1986.* Israel: Naftali Moses.

40 Stadlan, N. 2010. Conceptual and logical problems arising from defining life by the presence or absence of circulation. *Meorot* 8: 1–11.

41 Rosenfeld, A. 1970. The heart, the head and the halakhah. *New York State Journal of Medicine* 70: 2615–19.

42 Rabinovitch, N. L. 1973. *Probability and Statistical Inference in Ancient and Medieval Jewish Literature.* Toronto: University of Toronto Press.

43 Franklin, J. 2002. *The Science of Conjecture: Evidence and Probability before Pascal.* Baltimore: Johns Hopkins University Press.

44 Hacking, I. 2006. *The Emergence of Probability: A Philosophical Study of Early Ideas about Probability, Induction and Statistical Inference.* Cambridge: Cambridge University Press.

45 Lorberbaum, M. 2001. *Politics and the Limits of Law: Secularizing the Political in Medieval Jewish Thought.* Stanford, CA: Stanford University Press.

46 Elon, M. 2003. *Community Legislation.* Philadelphia: Jewish Publication Society.

47 Lichtenstein, A. 1975. Does Jewish tradition recognize an ethic independent of Halacha. In *Modern Jewish Ethics*, ed. M. Fox, 52–88. Columbus: University of Ohio.

48 Rabinowitz, G. A. 1983. Gosses and defining the time of death. In *Halakha and Medicine*, ed. M. Hersler, 3:102–14. Jerusalem: Machon Regensberg.

Chapter 19

II.III *Death and the Brain*

Near-Death and Out-of-Body Experiences

A Case for Dialogue between Scientist and Theologian?

Michael Marsh*

The underlying philosophy of this new volume aims to facilitate – even expand – dialogue between clinically orientated scientists, theologians and philosophers over questions posed by neurological disorders in relation to emergent 'spiritual/religious' outcomes, real or artefact. This chapter specifically engages with Near-Death and Out-of-Body Experiences (ND/OBE), examining how these events might contribute to such dialogue.

Phenomenologies of NDE/OBE

The question is how an objective purchase can be gained on the subjective recollections of ND/OBE subjects. One approach is to interview those who have undergone some kind of stressful event, whether medical or psychological, thus to identify those who have subsequently undergone these specific outcomes. But that is very time-consuming and, prospectively, not full of promise. Investigators therefore usually select post-intensive/cardiac-care patients, as these are the easiest cases to accumulate. But that almost certainly introduces selective bias due to the nature of the severe metabolic illnesses accompanying such cases, and the predominance of male subjects: these are points not always recognised within the public domain. Moreover, after several years of chasing these post-cardiac/resuscitation patients, ND/OBE totals may still be frustratingly small.

In my case, while writing a thesis on ND/OBE [1], I opted to critically evaluate eight key texts [2–9] which supported the notion that some form of non-bodily life is evidenced by these experiences: this approach gave me immediate access to ~800 recollected thoughts. While some books claimed to be 'scientific' writings, the selection was arbitrary, in that they represented the existing literature at the time of my writing. Nor did I necessarily distinguish between NDE and OBE even thought their aetiologies are different, since many accounts often contain aspects of both. Nevertheless, in all these books, physical or physiological factors as determinants of ND/OBE (such as brain-based aberrations) tended

* This chapter embodies material given as lectures at S. Mary's Theological Institute, Little Rock, Arkansas, USA (April 2013) and at the Antonianum Pontificia Università, Rome, Italy (May 2014), and since considerably updated. I am grateful both to Rev Dr Christof Keller and Rev Professor Lluis Oviedo, OFM, respectively, for their kind invitations to speak and generous hospitality given on each occasion.

to be played down in favour of metaphysical claims that souls, consciousness or mind, having escaped from the body, were now occupying some other-worldly, 'spiritual' realm. Interestingly, it would be enlightening to consider whether these same authors would adopt an identical approach today.

I give a brief outline of these phenomena below.

Aspects of NDE Phenomenology

Apart from those having undergone, or formally studied NDE, most casual impressions are shaped by media reports, the latter comprising out-of-focus pictures, bright lights with individuals floating through vacuous space, a great emphasis on tunnels and vague references to 'spiritual' [B]eings, with capitalised initials as if to imply their true, ontological basis. We also hear much of blue skies, white clouds, flowers and trees, although these seem to be representative more of the underlying dream-world which underpins the contours of these experiences. Yet from my analysis of ~800 published NDE [1], there emerged a clear pattern indicating that NDE are intensely personal, even idiosyncratically structured adventures, and in addition, contextually modulated – historically, culturally and geographically [5, 8, 10, 11].

Several features, often overlooked, point to the cerebral nature of ND/OBE. The most important concerns the abrupt termination of NDE as subjects' conscious awareness returns to normal: that is an objective time-point, as revealed here:

> The Angel [of Death] said my life was not as it should be, and that I was going back. The next thing was that I was back in the recovery room, back in my body. [12, pp. 116–17]

or

> He [Christ] embraced me. Then I felt this violent jolt. I started careering backwards. Then I felt this thud and I was back in my body with a lot of pain. [8, p. 86–7]

In other words, ND/OBE occur *not* when the brain is supposedly 'dead' and non-functional as frequently insisted [4, 5, 8, 11], *but* as cerebral tissues are returning to their normal, co-ordinated activities, thus precluding escapes of mind, soul or consciousness from the body [1].

Thus:

> [I came] rushing through a tunnel and snapped back into my body.
>
> When they put the shocks [electrical defibrillation] on me I fell back, down to my body, like a dead weight. And the next thing, I was in my body again.
>
> Then there was sudden confusion – I was upset and scared – something was wrong. I regained my body and felt tremendous pain all over.

These typically abrupt terminations to full conscious awareness were succinctly summarised by Ring [4, p. 101]:

> Once the individual has returned, painfully or otherwise to his body, the . . . experience is over . . . but . . . how exactly does one accomplish this return? – that is, re-unite with one's body?

But my response to that question is to ask *what* actually needs to be re-united? Because it logically follows that if NDE are reawakening phenomena, as I have indicated above, nothing needs to re-unite with the body. Ring's speculative baggage confuses the issue.

The second piece of corroborative evidence centres on the duality of conscious awareness as the NDE terminates. As these short periods elapse (seconds, or perhaps minutes)

NO MORAL QUALMS LEAVING FAMILY	'MORAL' FEELING TO COME BACK
CROSSING OF SOLID OBJECTS	UNWILLING TO CROSS BARRIERS
WEIGHTLESSNESS	HEARING REAL VOICES
SEEING LIGHT & DECEASED PEOPLE	BUMPY RETURN TO BODY
ABSENCE OF PAIN	INCREASED PAIN PERCEPTION

Figure 19.1 The 'core' and 'depth' aspects (Moody & Ring) of ND/OBE are descriptively invalid (see Figure 19.3). A more truthful portrayal of what subjects actually recall is briefly summarised here as early- and late-phase components. Contents of late-phase reactions indicate the return of full conscious awareness, sometimes accompanied by a short period of dualism, during which the 'other world' and the real world are simultaneously experienced. Such dualistic experiences indicate that subjects cannot have been either outside their bodies or their minds at the same time as experiencing a hospital bed.

during the return to normality, subjects inhabit both worlds – the hallucinatory 'other-world' as well as the looming real world, manifest concurrently by the prick of a needle, application of a face-mask, body manipulations by clinical staff or hearing their voices. Another further characteristic, late-phase component of NDE (Figure 19.1) involves subjects experiencing the growing urgency to return earthwards and resume hitherto unfulfilled responsibilities (spouse, family, household tasks):

> I don't know. I think it was because I had two young children: they needed me more than [me] up there. [4, p. 71]

and

> But I take my responsibilities very seriously, and I knew that I had a duty to my family. So I decided to try to get back. [2, p. 78]

These late-phase 'moral' concerns suggest returning top-down influences of dorso-lateral pre-frontal cortex (dlPFC) in suppressing irrelevant other-worldly hallucinations during that critical period when normal conscious awareness begins to supervene.

Third, 'dead' or seriously compromised brains cannot put down memories: if not, anterograde and retrograde amnesias following severe head trauma would not exist. NDE should therefore be envisaged as brain-derived, dream-like reminiscence occurring just as full conscious awareness dawns. As such, they are comparable to extremely vivid, hypnopompic dream-awakenings: the hallucinatory event ends rapidly as conscious awareness resumes. And, like hypnopompic awakenings, NDE are remembered as highly pictured adventures. This is not unique, as similar brain-based vivid hallucinations characterise peduncular hallucinosis, psychedelic drug usage and partial occlusions (including contrast angiography) of the midbrain vertebro-basilar arterial system [1, p. 183]. In this regard, subjects' remarks that NDE are not like dreams are incorrect: the vividness is conditioned by the *reawakening phenomenon*: that is quite different from ordinary dreaming.

The Out-of-Body Component

NDE phenomenology, in addition, involves either hallucinatory motion – flying, ascending, floating, accelerations, falling, weightlessness or of bumping back into the body with resumption of consciousness, and aberrant misperceptions of bodily location in peri-personal space:

> I was in a black tunnel . . . shooting through it incredibly fast: I was spinning – like water going down a plug.

or

> Then I was travelling in darkness in an unknown direction but at tremendous speed.
> [8, pp. 47, 122]

These motor accompaniments are usually perceived supine, given the relevant precipitating aetiologies (Figure 19.2) [13–14]. In that position, the sensors for gravity (otoliths within the saccule and utricle of the inner ear, and vestibular components of cranial nerve VIII) are largely inactive [15], thus encouraging sensations 'of non-corporeal floating in space'. As Figure 19.2 indicates, there are additional inputs from the joints and tendons (proprioception), the skin (touch), ears and nose, and turning of the head and eyes (opto-kinetic reflexes). Together, these neural messages find confluence in the temporoparietal junction (TPJ) of the right cerebral hemisphere, generating an internal sense both of body image and of the body's relationship to the environment. Disturbances (vascular for instance) in TPJ engender anomalous feelings of bodily displacements; non-ownership; or projection into local, peri-personal space. Blanke's extensive research [16] has demonstrated the neurological basis of OBE, involving key brain structures as illustrated below, making it unnecessary to explain these experiences as actual psychical intrusions [17]. However, that aspect of the experience, seen as an aberration in sensed bodily position, when also tied to an NDE severely undermines the whole notion that ND/OBE could be ventures beyond the body. So often, NDE and OBE form intertwined parts of the one recollected event: the literature does not specifically separate each process.

Clearly, it is possible to be out of one's body as an isolated event, as is seen with migraine [18], temporal lobe epilepsy [1, pp. 113–14, 19] or following ingestion of various pharmaceutical agents. Seen from this important perspective, an OBE as a brain-determined phenomenon thus brings doubt on the view that body displacements, or fictive movement, could actually be due to one's body floating loosely through 'space'.

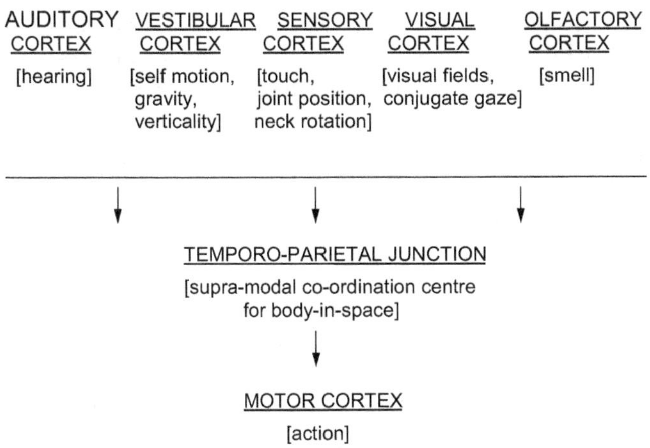

Figure 19.2 The main players contributing to egocentric and paracentric space, or body image: visual, haptic (touch), auditory, olfactory, proprioceptive and vestibular. Disturbances to the central representation of the latter, in the temporoparietal junctional cortex, give rise to weightlessness, spurious movements and hallucinatory body displacements. For simplicity, other important components of body imagery, such as cerebellum, limbic system, hippocampus and memory, are excluded.

Furthermore, it should be obvious that with mixed ND/OBE phenomenology, one cannot be partly undergoing a brain-induced reverie (OBE) while, at the same time, having some kind of 'other-worldly' experience (NDE) resulting supposedly from a 'dead' brain, as others continue to insist [4, 7, 11, 19].

Overview of ND/OBE Phenomenology

It might still be insisted that such accounts, as briefly summarised above, do not really prove a brain-based aetiology: but to insist otherwise poses many more problems. We know, for example, some subjects may have an NDE just as they are losing consciousness, analogous to that in normal persons on falling asleep, or while being put to sleep at the beginning of a general anaesthetic – the so-called hypnagogic hallucination. Such events are often remembered, but that presumption rests upon a brain which is still functioning – in other words not requiring life-restoring resuscitation due to some antecedent cause such as prolonged falls in blood pressure. Others may have an NDE but if they did not survive their precipitating catastrophe, we would be none the wiser.

What I am at pains to disaver is that ND/OBE are possible only when the brain is 'dead', or at least, in a moribund state. Of course, the problem with that idea, although asserted with such vigour, is that there would have to be an interval (involving the acute resuscitation procedure) between the occurrence of an NDE, and the (later) return to full conscious awareness. But punctuated reminiscence of that type has never been recorded. For most people, the event ends as they awaken. That can only mean that the phenomenology must be taking place during those moments leading up to the resumption of full conscious awareness: there is no alternative. But more importantly, dead or dying brains, as stated above cannot, and do not, put down memories: therefore, and this is another most critical part of my argument, what is remembered can only be set down as reawakening progresses.

Therefore, on balance, I maintain my original thesis [1, pp. 86–91] that NDE are awakening phenomena, based on the following empirically based conclusions:

1 NDE terminate as subjects regain full conscious awareness: the NDE never encroaches on, or continues into, conscious awareness. That was the problem with the NDE-like experiences caused by ketamine [20] – and which therefore rendered it ineffective as an explanation of NDE [21].

2 With the use of word counts, as employed by dream researchers, it seems that most NDE only last several seconds or minutes of real time, and that in the majority of instances, the experiences undergone must therefore occur before, *and immediately up to*, that point at which conscious awareness is fully regained. Although there are no neurophysiological techniques which indicate that subjects are experiencing an ND/OBE, there is no escape from this conclusion, and is a key issue which the NDE fraternity has still to come to terms with;

3 That (note 2) is also a rational conclusion, because memories can only be set down when the brain is not in a moribund state, a vital point that needs recognition. Surely it is more sensible, on those grounds, to conclude that ND/OBE occur, and are remembered, during those final moments while subjects are rapidly regaining conscious awareness. Therefore NDE are more than likely to be brain-generated phenomena, and not trips to 'Heaven', 'Hell' or other imagined cosmic spaces [22], neither events generated by external agencies.

4 Next, and allied to the preceding, is that during the reawakening process, subjects quite spontaneously recall the simultaneous occurrence of *other-worldly* fantasy with *this-worldly* action, including the sound of voices around the bedside; a painful injection; or the suffocating application of an oxygen mask. It is highly unlikely that a 'dead' person inhabiting a so-called *other-worldly* realm (as NDE authors continue to assert) would be able, at the same time, to experience the commerce of *this-worldly* action. Such a proposition is totally unintelligible. This duality of conscious experience is not, of course, exclusive to subjects awakening from NDE: it occurs with lucid dreaming, auras of temporal lobe epilepsy, drug-taking and experimental electrical brain stimulation. But this is *not* Cartesian duality, which most scientists and philosophers resist adamantly. On the other hand, the most logical explanation is that each facet of the ongoing experiences is brain-driven.

5 NDE accounts are non-identical, non-uniform and personally idiosyncratic, reflected in perceptions of 'light': 16 per cent [4]; 28 per cent [5]; 39 per cent [7]; 72 per cent [8]. Further disparate results are revealed in Figure 19.3 which is the first occasion on which the accumulated data have been collated: they reveal a marked lack of uniformity relative to each category of experiences undergone. In perusing this collection of data, we should note that the majority of percentages hardly exceeds 50–60 per cent, indicating how few of these items mentioned are, in reality, undergone by subjects. The results are hardly impressive and do not concur with in the smoothed accounts we are usually accustomed to reading about.

These collected results do not support the concept devised by Ring of a 'core' experience. Indeed, no so-called core would ever be discernible if this graphical figure were presented afresh to any unbiased observer. If that were the case, which features, from the data presented (Figure 19.3), would stand out to be specifically chosen as constituting this imaginary 'core'? If, on the other hand, three or four experiential

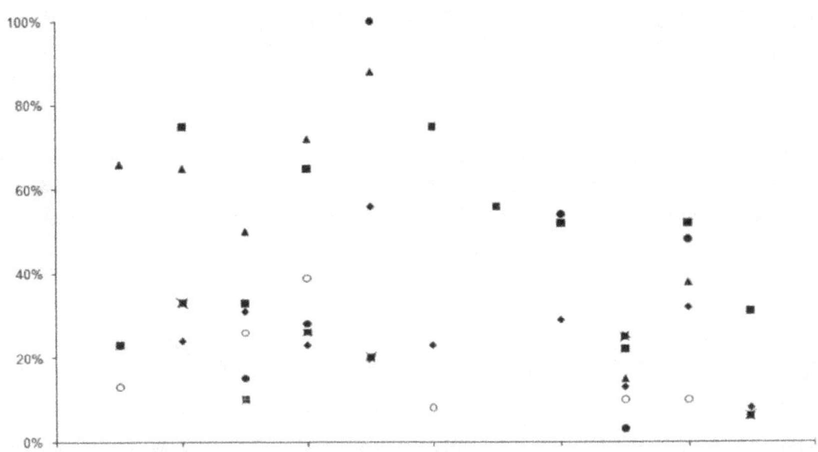

Figure 19.3 A plot-scattergram of percentages (vertical axis) of subjects experiencing components of ND/OBE (horizontal axis). The latter comprise (left to right) blackness, OBE, tunnel, light, love, senses, knowledge, heaven, life review, meetings with persons and barriers. This is the first occasion when results based on 800 published series referred to in the text accounts have been collated. Contrary to most views, there is no symmetry or uniformity among the experiences reported.

aspects were shown independently in all writers' accounts to exceed 95 per cent, then we could all take notice and be convinced. Moreover, Ring's equally vacuous concept of a 'deep' experience should more properly be related to duration: and indeed, if we look at his chart [4, p. 40], it reveals that only a dwindling minority have the privilege of sensing more of the options on offer. Ring fails to consider, or even exclude, the possibility that temporal factors could be at play here. In addition, how can one measure the 'depth' of any experience. I would suggest, only by its experiential impact, rather than by any empirical tool. Likewise, dreams do not have to be temporally extended to have impact: as we know from experience, a transient dream can have a most enduring impact.

6 NDE accounts are both historically and culturally biased as illustrated in the detailed account given by the Anglo-Saxon historian and theologian, Bede [23]. He describes a nobleman of high standing called Drycthelm who was led through mediaeval perceptions of Hell, where he was attacked by verminous creatures. But he was protected by his guide who ultimately led him towards Heaven, just down the road – literally – from Hell. From the account offered, it seems evident that the event happened during recovery from an attack of pneumococcal lobar pneumonia (the so-called vigil coma of pre-antibiotic times).

On the other hand, in Indian folklore, encounters with divine beings in NDE are not necessarily pleasant, involving confrontations with the (Hindu) god of death, Yam-raj [10]. One man had his legs amputated to prevent escape, but he was the wrong person called for interview, and so was allowed to retrieve his legs from a cupboard housing all previous amputees' limbs. Another man was pushed back to earth by someone with a hot arm: but this was seemingly a delirium-induced hallucination since the subject, on regaining consciousness, was febrile due to an abscess on his arm. These historic and geographic portrayals make sharp contrast with the anodyne, soft loci of beautiful vistas, lovely flowers and scented environments sampled by US and UK subjects. Surely, such culturally determined reports derive directly from brain-derived memories and, as noted above, these traces are recollected and embroidered in true dream-like fashion, as subjects return to full conscious awareness.

7 Finally, it is clear that two or more experiences undergone by the same person are rarely identical, despite the fact that recurrent episodes are not very often recounted. If everyone was going to the same 'place', or even driven by van Lommel's 'cosmic consciousness' [11], they would be expected to be identical. These examples, in revealing the non-conformity of successive NDEs, point powerfully to individualised experiences, and hence to cerebral origins. This is a grave problem for those asserting that NDE are representative of other-worldly locations, or influenced by (undefined) cosmic forces.

Further, Independent Empirical Corroboration That ND/OBE Are Brain Derived

There are other, independent studies offering empirical data which firmly substantiate my conclusions as just outlined above [1]:

1 concerning suicide survivors who, jumping from the Golden Gate Bridge [24–25], experience episodes of transcendence. A fall from the pedestrian parapet to the water 250 feet below takes ~4 seconds, occasioning impact speeds >70 mph [26]. Some

survivors do not remember the impact, so had probably been rendered unconscious before hitting the water.

2 from laboratory-controlled investigations of self-induced fainting attacks, lasting ~20 secs [27]. While undergoing these self-induced faints, 25/42 subjects (60 per cent) recalled darkness, greyness, coloured variegated patches to fully formed visual imagery including persons and objects. Likewise, auditory experiences ranged from uninterpretable noises, swishing or rushing sounds, screams, to human speech. Sixteen per cent experienced OBEs, and 8 per cent tunnels – the latter clearly not exclusive to NDE – despite persistent media claims. Note again how the progression of recalled experiences (ranging from uninterpretable to meaningful) parallels upward cortical processing of inputs leading to full conscious awareness and comprehension.

3 military pilots centrifuged to unconsciousness [28]. At the point when unconsciousness set in, pilots were inert and unable to continue with the tests prescribed for them while being rotated in the laboratory centrifuge. However, on gradually reawakening (after ~40secs), they underwent transcendental experiences of beautiful, extremely vivid, coloured surroundings, encountered deceased relatives, became deliriously happy and experienced such highly emotive feelings that made them reluctant to 'return to earth': 'I was floating in a blue ocean, on my back – the sun was up – and someone was trying to wake me. I did not want to wake up – I could see myself on the water and look at the sun'.

But the military investigators [28] were extraordinarily impressed by the possibility that 'such coherent visual illusions could be generated and remembered by the brain, within such *short periods of time*' (my emphasis): that is, as personnel recovered from their preceding episodes of unconsciousness. That is a highly significant comment pertinent to NDE, in that these (laboratory-timed) memories occurred and were set down during waking, and *NOT* when the pilots' brains were in demonstrably non-functional mode.

While neurophysiological explanation goes a long way in explaining NDE as hypnopompic dream-like awakenings, there are additional avenues through which NDE can be interrogated – but from the same perspective.

NDE Narratives: Critical Interrogations of Their Semantic Content

It is quite intriguing to observe that subjects' recollections over the years have never been critically assayed for semantic content. What, then, do we discover about the 'otherworld', about 'Heaven' or even about Jesus?

First, what is the descriptive geography of the 'otherworld'? For Sabom [5], subjects (see his Table XII) reported a miscellany of blue skies: clouds: parkland: mist: water: the Sea of Galilee: a road: a fence: a long corridor: mountain top: golden gates: geographic peoples undertaking cultural handicrafts. From Long's correspondents we get blue skies, rolling hills, flowers, colours, music, distant city vistas, and so on [15]. And from van Lommel, a miscellany of a perceived 'celestial landscape', meeting dead friends and relatives, seeing colours and getting a life review [11, p. 146]. Note how anthropomorphic all these otherworldly items are: we have no revelatory data on what 'heaven' might look like – even if there were a geo-cosmic 'beyond' – but based on those assumptions.

Second, let us analyse the actual content of messages brought back to earth. Following a heart attack, a son during an NDE meets his father deceased 15 years previously [7, p. 79], who was

> dressed just like he used to be . . . in grey trousers and a cardigan. He hadn't changed a bit. We chatted quite naturally [about the family] and he joked.

The rather obvious questions arising from this chance meeting with his father are: had his father ever undressed and showered – or his clothes been laundered in the interval?

Another woman following cardiac arrest [7, p. 54] explained,

> I found myself in front of a nice prefabricated building – and mother was visible inside.

The patient observes that, having brought some dress-making material, her mother took some scissors to begin cutting. That horrified the daughter knowing that she (mother) lacked dress-making skills. The mother replied that since arriving [there] she has been *taught* to be a seamstress. Then having been refused entry to the house, the daughter had to return home (? to earth, maybe), not a little disgruntled, perhaps.

A third woman, having endured a painful labour followed by caesarean section, agonised [8, p. 101]:

> I'm not staying here – [my husband] can't cope with the new baby, he's just got a new job and I've left a pile of shirts to be ironed and he doesn't know how to do them.

These are some of the most weird as well as banal accounts I could muster from the books I studied. Yet they were used, one must presume, by authors as serious contributions to NDE literature. We cannot therefore dismiss them, nor fail to notice their ego-centred, intensely anthropomorphic as well as bizarre content – just like dream-states.

Third, let us consider any descriptions of Jesus that are available from these sources: these would be of immense importance to Christian theology, since the gospels and cognate writings fail to give us those precise details. Have NDE reports provided the much sought-after, robust descriptions of him which scripture lacks?

> I can see that form now – it had blond-gold hair . . . and a beard – very light, and a moustache [and] a white garment on – there was a red spot here [points to image of a Sacred Heart on gown] – and a chalice in his hand.

or

> He was tall – had a white robe on – his face was beautiful – his skin was glowing and absolutely flawless.

and

> She [in reference to the subject's mother] was wearing a long sparkling silver gown – [as] did Christ – he had long hair – long beard.

Finally,

> There was Christ with a very long white robe – he had jet black hair – very short black beard – teeth extremely white – eyes blue, very blue.

As in most Christic visions experienced by healthy subjects [29], such descriptions owe more to inherited cultural depictions of Jesus derived from typical Sunday School images or more recent Hollywood productions, rather than the typical appearances of a Sephardi Jew in first-century Palestine. From contemporary illustrations, Jesus is likely to have had short hair, possibly a small beard, dark skin and dark brown eyes. With regard to clothing, in stark comparison with the reports given above, a more sober account [30] appeals to local custom, partly confirmed by the gospel accounts. At that time, men wore a knee-length cotton dress next to the skin, known as a *chitōn*, supplemented by one or two outer tunics, known as a *himation*.

To summarise so far, I have asserted that NDE/OBE occur as subjects are awakening, and not when deeply unconscious: these exclude NDE/OBE phenomenology occurring as people are going to sleep (hypnagogic dream-state experiences) or being induced for general anaesthesia. I make that claim because these experiences are remembered, and memories cannot be put down when a brain is non-functional – or 'dead' as widely asserted, consequential to a period of reduced blood flow subsequent to a cardiac arrest, shock due to haemorrhage or from some other episodic catastrophe that impairs conscious activity or blood flow. Despite what is repeatedly stated by the media, there is no idealised sequence to NDE/OBE phenomenology while, on the contrary, the diagram (Figure 19.3) reveals how so few subjects sample every aspect of the available collectivised experiential content.

In conclusion, NDE are personally idiosyncratic and are rarely duplicated should the subject happen to undergo a second NDE. Moreover, the experiential content of NDE recollections is strikingly tempered by historic, geographic and cultural influences, which strongly imply a brain-determined phenomenology to which past memories and contemporary cultural material make notably significant contributions.

The other-worldly domain, therefore, is clearly in the mind of the observer rather than a locus offering uniform content to all its visitors. Indeed, if 'heaven' has truly been visited, then its descriptive foundations are intensely earthbound and anthropomorphic, and from which no hitherto unknown facts about the terrain sampled have ever been derived, or elucidated. On those grounds, NDE/OBE have not provided additional 'other-worldly' facts with which we were not already acquainted.

Hellish Experiences

Hellish NDE are rarely reported, even denied. Jeffrey Long [31] suggests a figure of ~10 per cent but, if true, would imply 70 000 000 people (of 7 billion total) worldwide. But where are they and why are they denied opportunity to speak? Perhaps subjects resist revisiting extremely vivid, violent events. More likely, however, the portrayal of horrific events disrupts the edenic paradise so frequently and uncritically perpetuated in NDE/OBE literature, and by the media.

Most accounts relate occasions of intense blackness, associated with spurious vestibular-related movements (see below) or auditory accompaniments of unintelligible screams, sounds or noises. Frightening creatures, the colour red, fear, panic, anguish and desolation are typical, followed by either a conventional NDE or rapid resumption of conscious awareness. Here is an experience during general anaesthesia:

> I was above my body and [below there was] a black pit with hands trying to grab me and pull me down into it. A lion came out and jumped on me.

The lion, obviously, is entirely hallucinatory: probably the rest is, too. Similar experiences were described by the neurosurgeon Dr Eben Alexander [32] and the US art critic Howard Storm [33]. Storm was attacked by frighteningly horrible people poking and threatening him. There immediately followed a typical NDE.

Could darkness suggest incipient conscious awareness? Rather like the first moment of coming round from a faint. That proposal would be buttressed by the fact that many NDE subjects were suffering from infections (Drycthelm, Alexander) or in *toxic delirium* (Storm,

Drycthelm), which are associated with only moderately depressed levels of conscious awareness. Indeed, it is noticeable (but rarely observed) that they all felt being 'plucked at', reflecting perceptions of being handled by carers – turning and washing, bed-making, being prepared for X-rays etc. These examples indicate that the mode of precipitation, in differentially impacting on key brain centres, almost certainly conditions the repertoire of hallucinatory responses reported. If that is true, then we should be somewhat suspicious of published studies based solely on patients surviving an emergency admission to either cardiac, or intensive, care units: the experiential repertoire recollected by such patients may be subject to bias resulting from the mode of precipitation and to the influence of cerebral atherosclerosis.

The Out-of-Body Component

As we saw above briefly, much of the phenomenology of NDE/OBE – hellish and heavenly – involves illusory motion: flying, ascending, floating, spinning, falling and bumping back into one's body after a period of weightlessness, the latter due to reduced graviception (OBEs usually occur in recumbent positions, when the sensation of gravity may be markedly reduced). Similar experiences fill dream recollections. These are all referable to the temporoparietal junction creating a virtual image within conscious awareness of body-shape (egocentric), and of its relationship to the immediate environment (paracentric space) (Figure 19.2), including gravity. This virtual image of the external environment is created through the higher cortical amalgamation of multi-modal sensory inputs to the posterior parietal lobule (parietal lobe of brain), temporoparietal junction and a perceived 'vestibular' cortex associated with the insula within the depths of the Sylvian fissure [34–38]. The commonly reported illusion of floating beneath the ceiling represents misperceived bodily location as a false projection of conscious awareness, which is always short-range within paracentric space and never extending, it might be noticed, miles away to the true geographic horizon.

Neurophysiological investigations have demonstrated the origins of OBE, experiences of a 'tunnel' and of spiralling forwards or upwards into a light. Yet the tunnel illusion, although repeatedly enshrouded in 'mystical' overtones, only occurs in 10–20 per cent of all cases, and thus is not a particularly common accompaniment of OBE [39]. A closer reading of accounts reveals that a tunnel seems to be perceived *only* if the light is accompanied by vestibular-induced illusory movement. This association becomes more explicable in view of cerebral damage known to follow cardiorespiratory resuscitations. One particular form of damage [40] involves the optic radiation linking visual cortex to the temporoparietal region, resulting in a relative loss of peripheral vision, although central (macular) vision is spared. This observation could therefore account for the perception of a centrally located, expanding light as consciousness is progressively regained. We should recall that 8 per cent of 'laboratory fainters' experienced a tunnel, and 16 per cent OBE, these latter having no associated commerce with so-called heavenly vistas, nor even contact with 'cosmic consciousness': and likewise, with reference to reports from subjects with sleep paralysis.

Subjects sometimes have reported on things or events impossible to have been witnessed from their resuscitative viewpoint, thus encouraging associations of OBE with 'telepathic' qualities. Unfortunately, all such accounts lack hard, critical, empirical data obtained and recorded through independent third-party surveillance, *during the time of the resuscitation itself.* As far as is known, no writer or investigator has compared levels of increasing conscious awareness measured, for example, by EEG (for instance bispectral analysis as sometimes used by anaesthetists to gauge levels of surgical anaesthesia) with the events later narrated by the subject and extrapolated backwards from the objective time-point at which full conscious awareness re-emerged.

Is OBE Content Believable?

Conversely, OBE testimony is often inaccurate, as with (the late) Pam Reynolds. This American woman published worldwide her famous account of an OBE, through which she gained tremendous notoriety. She was treated by ultra low-temperature neurosurgery to remove a deeply located aneurysm on the basilar artery, lying beneath her medullary brainstem. This formidable procedure was effected by cooling her body using cardiopulmonary bypass, and by depleting her brain of blood. The anaesthetic lasted >6 hours. Her verbatim account of her experiences only comprises ~725 words, as reported by the cardiologist Michael Sabom [5, 9].

Elsewhere I have discussed this case in detail [1, pp. 19–27], from which account, some key remarks follow. Reynold's NDE/OBE occurred as her head was opened from the right side, but although she declared she was '*sitting on the neurosurgeon's shoulders with heightened visual acuity*', she made several significant errors, for instance (1) she did not report that her head was turned on its left and held there by a robust, three-pointed mechanical brace; (2) she did not seem to realise that her hair had not been completely shaved; (3) she was unable to state *where* the bone saw was used in cutting open her skull, despite her allegedly grandstand view; and (4) she mistakenly recalled that the use of the bone saw and femoral vein cannulation were *consecutive.* The surgical notes indicate that these procedures were *simultaneous,* since cardiopulmonary bypass had to be up-and-running once the surgeon had decided to continue. Obviously, she was not out of her body on that fateful morning. Her NDE abruptly stopped because '*her grandmother refused to accompany her to the tunnel*': consequently '*she jumped with her uncle*', thereby simultaneously and painfully re-occupying her body which '*felt like ice-cold water*'.

The crucial outcome here, so far unquestioned, concerns where her mind/consciousness actually were during the 6+ hour period of anaesthetic unconsciousness, given that the sparse 725-word report offered only contained a few unconnected events which, in real time, could only have lasted a few minutes [1, 5, 9]. Surely a free-wandering mind whether connected to cosmic consciousness [11] or merely acting as a conduit for consciousness [41, p. 116] could perform more effectively? Nevertheless, despite all those exultant proposals, a critical question remains. Where was Reynold's brain, and what exactly was it doing, when it was supposedly outside her body for that very long, 6-hour blank period?

In a more recently extended account of this controversial experience [42], I refer to the use of barbiturates as a brain protectant during the operative period, since her body had to be frozen to 60°F (normal body temperature: 98.4) to permit removal of the aneurysm [43]. That may be of considerable importance since barbiturates may be toxic to the upper midbrain, causing a particular form of hallucination, termed peduncular hallucinosis [44–45] (and see my extended discussion [1, pp. 182–6]). We cannot be certain, but I mention this important point because no other expert commentator has ever noted its possible contributory relevance. Moreover, because of the severe body cooling, metabolic functions through her body would have been stopped. In those circumstances, the dose of barbiturate initially given would have remained within the circulation, and not progressively excreted by her kidneys.

Finally, special ear-plugs containing thermometers were used to monitor the low body temperature, thereby blocking all air-conduction and rendering her deaf. Her distinct recall of hearing the bone saw has therefore been taken as indubitable evidence by the NDE community to her being out-of-body during the operation. But that position fails because bone conduction transmits sounds to the ears from *within* the skull: we have only to recollect memories of the dentist's drill to appreciate that possibility.

Reynold's case, unfortunately, provides no exemplary proof of authentic out-of-body visual, or auditory, awareness during resuscitation. Incidentally, the phenomenology described is rather odd, and certainly does not concur with Ring's 'core' basis.

In another telling example, a young girl *'imagined'* going through a *'momentary'* period of external heart massage. In reality, her chest was opened to permit (internal) cardiac massage by a thoracic surgeon, a process requiring *'several hours'* to secure her life [46].

And Are OBE Subjects Really Outside Their Bodies?

Attempts by hopeful investigators to expect subjects to report on marked cards, or look at devices placed near the ceilings of resuscitation units have failed dismally. Perhaps subjects were never out of their bodies and therefore did not float upwards to sample the experimental goods placed on high. That is more prosaic an explanation than Fenwick's rather weak response that they were drawn to their own resuscitations rather than go looking for specifically placed objects [8]. We might wonder, as with Reynolds above, what a free-wheeling 'mind' gets up to when freed from corporeal constraints: and why would such a free mind even know that it had to look at some weird coded message, or engage with a concealed TV screen?

Clearly, until we have some decent, properly collected data, contentious issues of this kind will always sadly persist to cloud and frustrate authentic understandings [47]. Even the long-awaited results of the so-called AWARE (*awa*reness during *re*suscitation) project have hardly provided triumphantly acclaimed results which dispel all prevailing uncertainties whether these patients are actually out of their bodies [48]. This much-hyped international study aimed to examine occurrences of mental activity during resuscitations from cardiac arrest. Across 15 specialised units 2060 patients were recruited, of whom only 330 survived and from whom only 140 were deemed able to be interrogated for any recollected mental activity.

Mental activity in this study was to be discovered from visual and auditory recollections. For the former, shelves were erected in appropriate places bearing symbols on their upper surfaces, and visible only from the ceiling. Conversely, triangles were attached to their under-surfaces being viewable from the recovery trolley. But only 22 per cent of acute resuscitations took place in these surroundings. And, in order to test for auditory reminiscence, staff were to use special words during each resuscitation: but personnel could not manage this extra workload so this idea was also abandoned. Indeed, one might have thought it unethical to expect busy resuscitation staff to additionally contribute to an ongoing experiment designed to collect data on conscious perception during an emergency procedure. Despite the shortcomings of this study, 46 had some kind of recall of unusual experiences around the time of their resuscitation. However, this was largely confined to hallucinatory material, such as lions and tigers; a bright light; violence, terror and scenes of horror; and seeing family members (their Table 3). Another nine had some kind of NDE, among whom was a single subject who recollected certain items and people associated with his resuscitation. No patient reported seeing the hidden symbols. So, this important study confirmed the phenomenon of NDE, but did not validate the external reality of the experience.

We should appreciate that state-boundary controls between consciousness and dream-states usually permit instantaneous switching, so the possible occurrence of episodes of consciousness in this single patient would cause no undue surprise. This is reminiscent of Rawling's patient with ventricular fibrillation [12, pp. 18–20] whose conscious awareness fluctuated with hallucinations of terrifyingly hellish proportions on each occasion when cardiac massage was stopped to allow heart catheterisation.

These AWARE results are, in my view, extremely disappointing since they fail signally to produce the results originally intended by the study – that recollections would be expected to include reports on all the shelved pictures placed for observation. But in order to observe this material, subjects had to be floating beneath the ceiling – and hence outside their bodies. Parnia, the originator of the study, nevertheless is 'intrigued' by apparent consciousness occurring during cardiac arrest, but he has produced no new data that subjects are actually undergoing some kind of conscious experience during the resuscitation process rather than later, as they recover. Despite all the hard work, time and hype, I am not convinced that this study has advanced our perceptions of the relationship between cardiac arrest and occurrences of conscious awareness to any significant degree.

Nevertheless, the neurological basis of OBE, occurring with NDE or in other non-death-related circumstances, is clear. At least, that's one outcome to be sure of [14, 36] due to centres around the temporoparietal junctional region of the (mainly) right hemisphere. Here there is a large 'multimodal' area which underpins one's sense of personhood, one's relationship to the near environment and to other minds, as well as a sense of verticality and gravity.

Moreover, it is most important that we should take into consideration, apart from OBE, the occurrence of associated aberrations of ego/paracentric space perception – that is, 'autoscopy', 'heautoscopy' and the 'sensing of invisible presences'. Defined, autoscopy is the reproduction, usually of the upper torso, in a static mirror-image of self. Heautoscopy, on the other hand, is of greater interest in respect of ND/OBE, since subjects' conscious awareness oscillates between their own body and its externally hallucinated image. Recently modified computerised technology that permits subjects to 'see' themselves in paracentric space [48] should deliver further understandings about the many types of spatial delusions to which the human body is subject. Moreover, those prone to OBE appear to have a deficit in posterior hippocampal processing of that crucial relationship between first-person perspective-taking, involving one's body and the relationship with paracentric space [49].

Summarising the Neurophysiological Options

My argument asserts that ND/OBE are neurophysiologically conditioned, for the reasons listed above. Such explanation also provides the basis for the bizarre, illusory juxtapositioning of 'Hell' and 'Heaven' as seen characteristically in mediaeval texts. ND/OBE occur during the final moments of a crisis when full conscious awareness is being resumed, thus resembling highly vivid, hypnopompic dream-awakenings. They are therefore analogous to the re-awakenings from other states of reduced consciousness. Too much emphasis is paid to 'dead' brains and speculative comments arising from that shaky basis.

So I return to perhaps the most pressing problem for the NDE fraternity to explain: how do these supposedly defunct brains memorise, either simultaneously or in tandem, the extremely complex sensory experiences later recalled in such detail? And so, precisely when does this memorised information, albeit crucially necessary for NDE subjects to later recall, become bound – if their brains are always asserted to be either non-functional, or alternatively, floating around in virtual space?

Another problem is that so much is sampled, or that the contents of vast libraries are instantly taken in: 'It seemed that all of a sudden all knowledge – of all that had been started from the very beginning, that would go on without end . . . that for a second I knew all the secrets of the universe, the stars, the moon – of everything . . . as the Bible says "to you all things will be revealed". For a minute, there wasn't any question that did not have an answer' [3, pp. 10–11]. Yet the answers to these big questions are never remembered once the subject returns to earth! All we get is banality, bizarreness but – depressingly – nothing new or revelatory beyond what we already knew.

Reports of surges in EEG activity in rats dying from experimentally induced cardiac arrest suggest that enhanced agonal brain activation could be taken as evidence of ND/OBE [45]. Similar surges (EEG processed by bispectral analysis) occurred in tissue-donor subjects at death following life-support withdrawal [46]. Unfortunately, rats or dead humans do not talk, so it is not possible to clarify any possible relationship between observed increases in EEG activity and NDE phenomenology: critically, EEGs do not monitor all regions and depths of brain activity. Clearly, greater in-depth work is required which, given the acute clinical situations during which ND/OBE occur, may be very difficult to correlate.

ND/OBE are more effectively, and truthfully, classified as either early, or late, phase events (see Figure 19.1). That all NDE are culturally conditioned (see my discussion in [1] through time, geography, religious beliefs, and subjects' culturally determined backgrounds), firmly argues for brain-conjured phenomenology. Furthermore, OBE phenomenology appears directly welded to brain mis-function at the TPJ location resulting in hallucinatory disturbances of body position in space.

In proceeding, I now consider the theologically based implications of NDE, their impact on subjects' subsequent lives, and particularly why so few subjects, having also survived either physiological or psychological crises, do not undergo subsequently changed-life patterns. Although rarely acknowledged, that needs some attention.

Spiritual Aspects of NDE/OBE

Several classical spiritual encounters are available for comparison with NDE.

> One day when I was at prayer . . . I saw . . . or was conscious of . . . Christ at my side . . . I saw nothing with my eyes (S Teresa of Avila). [50, p. 13]

or

> God surrounds me like the physical atmosphere. He is closer to me than my own breath. In him, literally, I live, move, and have my being. [51, p. 71]

and

> God sheds his sweetness . . . not his brightness . . . his beauty is not seen. He is surrounded by darkness . . . he does not appear in the light . . . [but] in the fire . . . the fire warms rather than illumines (S Richard of Victor). [50, p. 52]

These quiet, almost evasive and remarkably introspective reflections of divine encounter contrast sharply with typical NDE reportage:

> I could see my mother and Christ saying 'Come home', and waving their hands at me. She [wore] a long sparkling silver gown, and so did Christ – long hair, long beard – they were both smiling. [5, p. 169]

or

> I heard his voice say 'Go back!' I said 'Why me, Lord?' and whoever spoke said my work on earth wasn't over yet . . . all I heard was his voice: it was loud, thundering, just like a clap of thunder coming out of nowheres [*sic*]. [5, p. 54]

But these are intensely anthropomorphic, geo-centred reports. Here, one should distinguish between anthropomorphisms of the kind notably recorded of St. Paul who, following a flash of light, was commanded to enter Damascus (Acts 9:6), or St. John on Patmos to 'Write' (Rev 1:11). Obviously any call from God, however dramatic, must be received by the brain in earthly terms and location. But that requirement, obviously, differs radically from the accounts given of supposed visits by NDE subjects to other realms beyond the earth. The problem is that although these vistas are supposedly 'other-worldly', their descriptive content is entirely earthbound being related solely to worldly artefact. We receive no further revelatory knowledge about the afterlife which we did not know before. That is the difference. And that crucial difference recalls Moody's comment, who so pertinently and perhaps unwittingly encapsulated the stark gulf that clearly exists between NDE experiences and accounts of divine disclosure upon earth:

> Again and again, my NDE subjects have described to me a panoramic, wrap-around, full-colour, three-dimensional vision of these events in their lives. [3, pp. 31–5]

I think that sums up the position very well. Given the this-worldly content of NDE reports, one might be somewhat reluctant in crediting to them any serious value whether divine, or revelatory.

Despite that, Long in his book *Evidence of the Afterlife* [31] insists: 'There is the "spiritual" content of NDEs, namely answers to age-old questions: Why are we here? What is important about our earthly existence? Is there an afterlife?'

In other words, from Long's viewpoint, NDE reportage offers indisputable answers to these eternal questions. While evasively side-stepping an incisive definition of 'spiritual', he asserts:

> Now that I have reviewed thousands of NDE case studies, I can say that the content of NDE had substantial consistency in these answers.

Really? But not from the kind of banal case reports cited throughout this chapter, surely?

Yet, undeflated, Long [31] persists: 'I would emphasise that this consistency tells us that something real is taking place' – but what is that 'something' and how 'real' is it? – 'and that this remarkable consistency of spiritual messages suggests' – only suggests? – 'something extremely important, not only for subjects, but for all of us'. Dare we enquire about the kind of '*extreme importance*' he has in mind, and which might affect '*all of us*'?

Unfortunately, the problem questions set up have emphatically *not* been answered. That's the real flaw in a continued presentation of the psycho-phenomenological anecdotes with which Dr Long occupies his time and which, despite his titular claim, unfortunately fail miserably in offering any respectable 'proof of afterlife' or its detailed characteristics.

These 'spiritual' questions simply remain to taunt us.

What, then, are we being told by such NDE reports? Anything? Hardly anything, perhaps, other than the quest for cosmic consciousness [11, pp. 247–8] and that our brains are but mere receptors of a small slice of universal 'cosmic consciousness'. However, at certain times (e.g. during NDE) some people apparently find themselves beyond these cerebral restrictions thus being enabled to taste reality as it actually *should* be tasted – with the acquisition of greater and higher powers of thinking and knowing, and of seeing things in a more lucid light, beyond that which earthbound brain activity seemingly curtails. On van Lommel's account NDEs neither require added elaboration nor critical analysis, since they already constitute one certain, indubitable element as 'proof' of afterlife, albeit operative when subjects are ONLY 'clinically' dead – as they say: but, of course, by no means irreversibly dead, thus awaiting the undertaker.

Readers, however, should be made very aware that van Lommel [11], Ring [6] and Grey [7] have passed beyond any further need to question whether NDE are valid pointers to some kind of afterlife, and second, to understand the implications of such speculative adventures, of which 'Cosmic Consciousness' [11] or a 'Universalised Spirituality' [6] seems to be the ultimate end.

The Post-Experiential Subject

ND/OBE phenomenology involves cerebral mechanisms. But they also transform the lives of many subjects once they have returned to day-to-day life. One remarkable alteration is a reduced fear of death and a strengthened belief in the reality of afterlife – however conceived. In addition, there emerges increased personal motivation, self-respect and confidence, often translated into heightened concerns for others as expressed through compassion, tolerance and a strengthening of family ties. This is not a universal outcome, and it is difficult to put a precise figure on those who do manifest altered behaviour, throughout the post-NDE period.

Nevertheless, from this arises a critical question: are NDE occasions of true spiritual uplift arising out of divine action and from which a changed perspective on life becomes its notable fruit? But from my preceding text, I cast much doubt on the issue whether NDE could qualify as truly spiritual encounters, if they are merely generated from within the brain as hallucinatory dream-like sequences. The analogy is with the 'pseudo-religiosity' of temporal lobe epilepsy. However, if we consider the outcomes of Paul's Damascene light, or the voice heard by John on Patmos, specific commands were given to which notable responses were forthcoming.

Moreover, two further considerations need resolution. One concerns understandings of 'spiritual' and 'spirituality', both of which are tricky words especially when associated with NDE, yet needing precise definition. Second, we have to consider predisposition to NDE, on account of the very small numbers of susceptible people involved, compared with those who do not react to similar crises.

Here, I am drawn to John Cottingham's approach to 'spirituality' [52, pp. 3ff.]. Although he recognises fringe elements – magic crystals under the floorboards, scented candles and astrological wizardry, a richer spirituality offers an opportunity for deeper meaning in people's lives, thereby providing a satisfaction beyond the material world, or from science and technology. It concerns activities rather than theory, ways of living rather than doctrinal allegiances, and praxis rather than belief. On those grounds, if taken alone, the aftermath of NDE could be regarded as spiritual.

But before ratifying that acceptance, we must consider subjects' susceptibility to undergo NDE. It is noteworthy that first, the majority of subjects do not undergo NDE during a crisis and hence do not have later changed behavioural profiles [53]. That is contrary to van Lommel's pronouncement that such patients do, after eight years of follow-up, manifest changed outlooks [54, p. 151]. But the flaw here is due to his failure of incorporating an additional large, healthy age/gender-matched control group (and exterior to the cardiac setting), so to compare any changes in *their outlooks, beliefs and behaviours over the same time period* with his non-NDE, cardiac subjects. Obviously, van Lommel's study needs repeating with the extra controls which I have suggested.

Seen in this way, my hypothesis would be that the brains of the minority exhibiting propensity for NDE are different from those in the general populace, thus to conclude that an NDE is a reactive epiphenomenon [55], the principal outcome being a changed perspective on life and living. In other words, too much emphasis has been paid to NDE phenomenology itself, rather than to the more important behavioural outcomes apparent in the longer term, and dependent on a postulated subclinically damaged brain. An analogous occurrence is PTSD (post-traumatic stress disorder) where, following a severe, life-threatening crisis, long-term behavioural changes including genomic alterations occur. In many cases, however, there is a preceding history of childhood abuse [56–57], indicating such abuses can alter later life behavioural profiles in response to a specific crisis [58–59].

General enquiries show that NDE are unrelated to gender, ethnicity, social standing. Therefore, deeper mechanisms must be considered, including genetic polymorphisms of important brain neurotransmitters [60–61], serotonin and dopamine which although influenced by environmental cues, also contribute to traits like 'spirituality' and 'transcendence'. Loss of transcendence has been noted in patients interviewed before and after neurosurgery, especially involving either parietal lobe [62]. Other genes and their neural loci of operation will also be relevant. For example, we do not know whether ND/OBE occur frequently in twins, although there must be a sufficiently large sample for any possible genetic predispositions to be explored.

How might the brain itself be predisposed – other than through influences already discussed above (Figure 19.4)? In a sample of 1069 undergraduates, 45 per cent were adjudged through a questionnaire to have experienced latent temporal lobe symptoms, related to previous minor closed head injury or severe febrile infections [63], while in another group with similarly suggestive symptomatology, marked regression with carbamazepine was attributed to focal temporal lobe discharges [64].

It is on this highly relevant background that 23 NDE subjects were compared with age-/gender-matched 'controls' who gave no previous history [65] of early illness or stress. The NDE group revealed highly significant differences from the controls on the Complex Partial Epileptic Signs and the Temporal Lobe Symptoms inventories, and showed inter-ictal spiking on EEG. Clearly, the NDE group (~20 per cent) showed a proneness to subclinical seizures, without ictal development, who were evidently at risk for an ND/OBE.

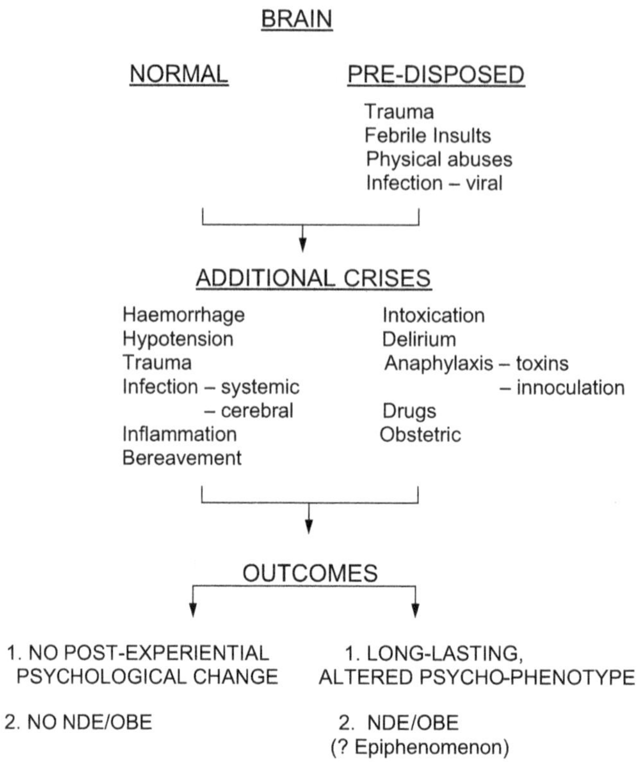

Figure 19.4 Data indicate that >90 per cent of subjects under stress do not experience ND/OBE. This suggests that those undergoing these events have pre-disposed brains, similar to post-traumatic stress disorder. On those grounds, the most important outcome is the changed psycho-phenotype which re-orientates subjects' viewpoints for the remainder of their lives. Consequently, ND/OBE phenomenology itself, although extremely vivid, could be viewed merely as a transient, reawakening epiphenomenon.

Given the thousands of subjects reporting an NDE, it would not be too difficult to reassess large cohorts for subclinical neurological disease of the types discussed here, so to establish some hard principles which might possibly be at work in this setting. Further cohorts could be watched prospectively, especially those with cardiac problems thereby making it possible to evaluate such people after a cardiac arrest, and to make comparisons (pre- and post-event) between those later reporting an NDE against those without this phenomenology. It is regrettable that such large groups are not being analysed for subclinical brain abnormalities. These suggestions are indicative of several new lines of neurophysiological study aimed at evincing deeper understandings of the underlying mechanisms of reactive ND/OBE.

Conclusion

ND/OBE phenomenology, considered from various viewpoints in the foregoing text, is dependent on neurophysiological process. It is probably true to assert that a variety of mechanisms plays a role, thus negating earlier views that one specific causal aetiology could universally explain the phenomenology (hypoxia, ischaemia, temporal lobe epilepsy, endorphins) [1, pp. 170–86]. Indeed, additional explanations might involve contributions from infections (cerebral or generalised), delirium, anaphylaxis and so on, while deep psychological factors are also clearly important, as with the bereaved (Figure 19.4).

If we consider other pathologies, outcomes reflecting NDE/OBE phenomenology may often be encountered. That these only reproduce certain aspects of an NDE does not diminish their explanatory role. That is because, as noted above, there is neither a specific global causative agent for these happenings, nor a demonstrably invariant blueprint for the experiences undergone. However, a greater awareness of multi-factorial influences needs to be held in mind when aetiological considerations are being reviewed. Furthermore, whatever the predisposing factors, a wide range of resultant effects may be felt and whose interpretation by the subjects concerned may have long-lasting effects and influences. Claimed 'spiritual' experiences are most difficult to decipher, from an objective, third-party stance. From the large repertoire of reports which I have perused, I was never convinced that I came across one that appeared to be revelatory in that respect. Many people are influenced by life events, including epileptics or schizophrenics, and following an intense nightmare, or febrile delirium. Prolonged starvation in the mediaeval era was a sure way of having 'mystical' experiences: perhaps these did influence the recipient – but to what end?

On page 160 of my book [1] I have listed a large number of references written throughout the twentieth century which describe many types of cerebral pathology resulting in hallucinatory transcendence of time, space, self and which, variously include life-reviews, vestibular kinetic aspects, joy, pleasure, ecstasy, euphoria and ineffability: of being in a light, meeting deceased relatives, seeing God or Jesus, experiencing 'presences', and so on. It should be realised, therefore, that any factor influencing brain physiology can give rise to the entire repertoire recorded by ND/OBE subjects. We no longer have need to espouse esoteric explanations in order to gain a simple explanation for these strange dream-like episodes – even though they are not as common as widely presupposed. From that latter perspective, influences about predisposed brains, from previous episodes of fever, closed injury or varied abuses, should occupy our thoughts more.

Factors other than the brain and its perturbed physiology also play a role. This refers in part to the activation of vagal (tenth cranial nerve) afferents arising from the heart and great vessels and projecting to the upper midbrain where changes in conscious levels may be altered. This would occur during prolonged episodes of hypotension, occasioned by many of the major aetiologies in NDE production (Figure 19.4), interfering with arousal through stimulation of REM sleep [66–69] by means of the ventrolateral peri-aqueductal grey matter. Nelson draws attention to the possible disturbances that could exist between being either awake, or in REM or non-REM sleep modes [64, pp. 185–218]. In anomalous circumstances with a predisposed brain of which the most obvious examples are lucid dreaming, sleep walking and sleep paralysis, subjects may not know where they are, giving rise to a spurious sense of belonging to Absolute Being, union with God, or existence in a 'mystical' state.

Through the ages people have tried to express this non-definable (religious) state of mind, which falls into James' category of ineffability [51]. Here now we have the glimmerings of a perfectly rational neurophysiological explanation for what has seemed to be a most difficult outcome to solve, and which the NDE fraternity still thinks is incapable of explanation.

While inhaling Davy's newly discovered gas, nitrous oxide, William James (with a shrewd eye to scientific business) conceived the bright idea of writing down all his cosmic insights for posterity's benefit [70]. Despite those transient moments of narcotic genius, it would nevertheless appear that 'to any sober reader, his written thoughts would seem but meaningless drivel – just pages and pages of isolated words: 'God', 'day', 'night', 'prayer', but which – at the moment inscribed – were fused in the fire of infinite rationality' [71].

And that's just with a whiff or two of nitrous oxide.

> In undergoing a loss of ego – I acquired a sense of unity. The cosmos is one and inter-related – giving a mystical state of consciousness. There is a certain point of the mind from which life and death; the real and imaginary; the past and future; the communicable and incommunicable; the high and low, cease being perceived as contradictions.

That insight followed from a modern nitrous oxide party [72].

For such reasons, readers may understand why I am hesitant to accept others' doubtful beliefs that NDEs are actual journeys beyond the physical body; constitute undeniable proof of life-after-death; provide evidential credentials for a so-called heaven or hell; or even less demonstratively, authenticate private viewings of God or Jesus. That is something which the NDE fraternity has yet to substantiate with firm, convincing empirical data. And if substantiated, what would they have achieved?

The human brain is susceptible to so many illusions and hallucinations that we need to be careful as to what we believe to be true, as opposed to falsehood [73]. Thus for me, at the moment, it seems as though there is little common ground across which scientists and theologians could usefully converse in discussing the subject of ND/OBE.

References

1 Marsh, M. N. 2010. *Out-of-Body and Near-Death Experiences: Brain-State Phenomena or Glimpses of Immortality?* Oxford: Oxford University Press.

2 Moody, R. 1976. *Life after Life.* New York: Bantam Books.

3 Moody, R. 1977. *Reflections on Life after Life.* New York: Bantam Books.

4 Ring, K. 1980. *Life at Death.* New York: Coward, McCann, and Geoghegan.

5 Sabom, M. 1982. *Recollections of Death.* New York: Harper Row.

6 Ring, K. 1985. *Heading towards Omega.* New York: Morrow.

7 Grey, M. 1985. *Return from Death.* Boston: Arkana.

8 Fenwick, P., and E. Fenwick. 1998. *Truth in the Light.* New York: Berkeley Books.

9 Sabom, M. 1998. *Light and Death.* Grand Rapids, MI: Zondervan.

10 Pasricha, S., and I. Stevenson. 1986. Near death experiences in India. *Journal of Nervous and Mental Disorders* 174: 165–70.

11 van Lommel, P. 2010. *Consciousness beyond Life: The Science of the Near-Death Experience.* New York: Harper One.

12 Rawlings, M. 1978. *Beyond Death's Door.* New York: Nelson.

13 Andersen, R. 1997. Multimodal intergration for the representation of space in the posterior parietal cortex. *Philosophical Transactions of the Royal Society of London* 352: 1421–8.

14 Blanke, O., and C. Mohr. 2005. Out-of-body experience, heautoscopy, and autoscopic hallucination of neurological origin: Implications for neurocognitive mechanisms of corporeal awareness and self-consciousness. *Brain Research Review* 50: 184–99.

15 Mittelstaedt, H. 1991. The role of the otoliths in the perception of the orientation of self and world to the vertical. *Zoologische Jahrbuch Physiol* 95: 419–25.

16 Blanke, O., and S. Dieguez. 2009. Leaving body and life behind: out-of-body and near-death experience. In *The Neurology of Consciousness*, ed. S. Laureys and G. Tonini, 303–25. San Diego CA: Academic Press.

17 Greyson, B. 1983. The Near-Death Experience Scale. *Journal of Nervous and Mental Disorders* 171: 369–75.

18 Lippman, C. 1953. Hallucinations of physical duality in migraine. *American Journal of Psychiatry* 117: 345–50.

19 Devinsky, O., E. Feldmann, K. Burrowes and E. Bromfield. 1989. Autoscopic phenomena with seizures. *Archives of Neurology* 46: 1080–8.

20 Jansen, K. 1990. Neuroscience and the near-death experience: roles for the NMDA-PCP receptor, the sigma receptor and the endopsychosins. *Medical Hypotheses* 31: 25–9.

21 Collier, B. 1972. Ketamine and the conscious mind. *Anaesthesia* 27: 120–34.

22 Marsh, M. N. 2018. The phenomenology of near-death and out-of-body experiences: no heavenly excursion for the soul? In *The Blackwell Companion to Substance Dualism*, ed. J. Loose, A. Mengue and J. P. Moreland, 247–66. Chichester, UK: Wiley-Blackwell.

23 Bede, the Venerable. 1968. *A History of the English Church and People*. Ed. L. Sherley-Price. London: Penguin Classics.

24 Seiden, R. 1968. Where are they now? A follow-up study of suicide attempters from the Golden Gate Bridge. *Suicide and Life-Threatening Behavior* 8: 203–16.

25 Rosen, D. 1975. Suicide survivors: a follow-up study of persons who survived jumping from the Golden Gate and San Francisco-Oakland bridges. *Western Journal of Medicine* 122: 289–94.

26 Snyder, R., and C. Snow. 1967. Fatal injuries resulting from extreme water impact. *Aerospace Medicine* 38: 779–83.

27 Lempert, T., M. Bauer and D. Schmidt. 1994. Syncope and near-death experience. *Lancet* 344: 829–30.

28 Forster, E., and J. Whinnery. 1988. Recovery from G_2-induced loss of consciousness: psychologic considerations. *Aviation, Space, and Environmental Medicine* 59: 2–5.

29 Wieber, P. 1998. *Visions of Jesus*. Oxford: Oxford University Press.

30 Taylor, J. 2015. What did Jesus really look like? *Ancient Near East Today* 6: 1–16.

31 Long, J. 2010. *Evidence of the Afterlife*. New York: Harper One.

32 Alexander, E. 2012. *Proof of Heaven*. London: Piatkus.

33 Wilson, I. 1997. *Life after Death*. London: Pan Books.

34 Blanke, O., S. Perrig, G. Thut, T. Landis and M. Seeck. 2000. Simple and complex vestibular responses induced by electrical cortical stimulation of the parietal cortex in humans. *Journal of Neurology, Neurosurgery, and Psychiaitry* 69: 553–6.

35 Blanke, O., C. Mohr, C. Michel, A. Pascual-Leone, P. Brugger, M. Seeck, T. Landis and G. Thut. 2005. Linking out-of-body experience and self-processing to mental own-body imagery at the temporoparietal junction. *Journal of Neuroscience* 25: 550–57.

36 Blanke, O., and C. Mohr. 2005. Out-of-body experience, heautoscopy, and autoscopic hallucination of neurological origin: Implications for neurocognitive mechanisms of corporeal awareness and self-consciousness. *Brain Research Review* 50: 184–99.

37 Borel, L., C. Lopez, P. Péruch and M. Lacour. 2008. Le syndrome vestibulaire: un changement de représentation interne de l'espace. *Neurophysiologie Clinique* 38: 375–89.

38 Cheyne, J., and T. Girard. 2009. The body unbound: vestibular-motor hallucinations and out-of-body experiences. *Cortex* 45: 210–15.

39 Drab, K. 1981. The tunnel experience: reality or hallucination? *Journal of Near-Death Studies* 1: 126–52.

40 Els, T., J. Kassubek, R. Kubalek and J. Klish. 2004. Diffusion-weighted MRI during early global cerebral hypoxia: a predictor of clinical outcome? *Acta Neurologica Scandinavica* 110: 361–7.

41 Sartori, P. 2014. *The Wisdom of Near-Death Experiences*. London: Watkins.

42 Marsh, M. N. 2015. The near-death experience: a reality check? *Humanities* 5: 1–25.

43 Spetzler, R., M. Hadley, D. Rigamonti, P. Carter, P. Raudnes, S. Shedd et al. 1988. Aneurysms of the basilar artery treated with circulatory arrest, hypothermia, and barbiturate cerebral protection. *Journal of Neurosurgery* 68: 868–79.

44 Trelles, J., and D. Lagache. 1932. Intoxication barbiturique recidivante s'accompagnant d'hallucinose pedoculaire. *Annales Médico-Psychologiques* 16: 565–72.

45 L'Hermitte, J. 1922. Syndrome de la calotte peduncle cerebral: Les troubles psycholo-sensoriels dans les lesions du mesocaphale. *Review of Neurology (Paris)* 38: 1359–65.

46 Morse, M., with P. Perry. 1990. *Closer to the Light: Learning from the Near-Death Experiences of Children.* New York: Ivy Books.

47 Marsh, M. N. 2013. Near-Death and Out-of-Body Experiences. In *The Springer Encyclopedia of Sciences and Religions*, ed. A. Runehov and L. Oviedo, 1422–33. Berlin: Springer.

48 Ehrsson, H. 2007. The experimental induction of out-of-body experience. *Science* 317: 1048.

49 Bergouignan, L., L. Nyberg and H. Ehrsson. 2014. Out-of-body-induced hippocampal amnesia. *Proceedings of the National Academy of Sciences of the United States of America* 111: 4421–6.

50 Alston, P. 1997. *Perceiving God: The Epistemology of Religious Experience.* Ithaca, NY: Cornell University Press.

51 James, W. 1902. *The Varieties of Religious Experience.* New York: Longmans, Green.

52 Cottingham, J. 2005. *The Spiritual Dimension.* Cambridge: Cambridge University Press.

53 Roewer, W., T. Kloss and K. Puschel. 1985. Long-term result and quality of life following preclinical cardiopulmonary resuscitation. *Anasthesie, Intensivtherapie, Notfallmedizin* 20: 244–50.

54 van Lommel, P., R. van Wees, V. Meyers and I. Elfferich. 2001. Near-death experience in survivors of cardiac arrest: a prospective study in the Netherlands. *Lancet* 358: 2039–45.

55 Thonnard, M., V. Charland-Verville, S. Bredart et al. 2013. Characteristics of near-death experience memories as compared to real and imagined events memories. *PLOS One* 8: e57620.

56 Mahta, D., T. Klengal, K. Conneely, A. Smith, A. Altman et al. 2013. Childhood maltreatment is associated with distinct genomic and epigenetic profiles in post-traumatic stress disorder. *Proceedings of the National Academy of Sciences of the United States of America* 110: 8302–7.

57 Teicher, M., and J. Samson. 2013. Childhood maltreatment and psychology: a case for ecophenotypic variants as clinically and neurobiologically distinct subtypes. *American Journal of Psychiatry* 170: 1124–33.

58 Meyer-Lindenberg, A., J. Buckholtz, B. Kolachana et al. 2006. Neural mechanisms of genetic risk for impulsivity and violence in humans. *Proceedings of the National Academy of Sciences of the United States of America* 103: 6269–74.

59 Craig, M., M. Catani and Q. Deeley. 2009. Altered connections on the road to psychopathy. *Molecular Psychology* 14: 946–53.

60 Comings, D., N. Gonzales, G. Saucier, P. Johnson and J. MacMurray. 2000. The DR4 gene and the spiritual transcendence scale of the character temperament scale. *Psychiatric Genetics* 10: 185–9.

61 Loprenzi, C., A. Serretti, L. Mandelli, V. Tubazio, C. Ploia and E. Smeraldi. 2005. 5-HT 1A polymorphisms and self-transcendence in mood disorders. *American Journal of Medical Genetics, Part B* 137: 33–5.

62 Urgesi, C., S. Aglioti, M. Skrap and F. Fabbro. 2010. The spiritual brain: selective cortical lesions modulate human self-transcendence. *Neuron* 65: 309–19.

63 Roberts, R., N. Varney and J. Hulbert. 1990. The neuropathology of everyday

life: the frequency of partial seizure symptoms among normals. *Neuropsychology* 4: 65–85.

64 Neppe, V., and C. Kaplan. 1988. Short-term treatment of atypical spells with carbamazepine. *Clinical Neuropharmacology* 11: 287–9.

65 Britton, W., and R. Bootzin. 2004. Near-death experiences and the temporal lobe. *Psychological Science* 15: 254–8.

66 Nelson, K. 2012. *The Spiritual Doorway into the Brain*. New York: Plume Books.

67 Puizillout, J., and A. Foutz. 1976. Vago-aortic nerves and REM sleep: evidence for a REM-triggering and a REM-maintenance factor. *Brain Research* 111: 181–4.

68 Lu, J., D. Sherman, M. Devor and C. Saper. 2006. A putative flip-flop switch for control of REM sleep. *Nature* 441: 589–94.

69 Vagg, D., R. Bandler and K. Keay. 2008. Hypovolemic shock: critical involvement of a projection from the ventro-lateral periaqueductal grey to the caudal midline. *Neuroscience* 152: 1099–109.

70 James, W. 1882. Subjective effects of nitrous oxide. *Mind* 7: 186–208.

71 Blum, D. 2007. *Ghost Hunters*. London: Century.

72 Sheldin, M., D. Wallechininsky and S. Saunia. 1973. *Laughing Gas (Nitrous Oxide)*. California: And/Or Press.

73 Marsh, M. N. 2015. Hey! What's that gorilla doing over there? The illusory-hallucinatory nature of everyday living. *European Review* 23: 455–72.

Bibliography

Aadil, N., A. Fassi-Fihri, I. Houti, B. Benaji, M. Ouhakki, S. Kotbi, B. Diquet and F. Hakkou. 2000. Influence of Ramadan on the pharmacokinetics of a single oral dose of valproic acid administered at two different times. *Methods and Findings in Experimental and Clinical Pharmacology* 22: 109–14.

Aadil, N., I. E. Houti and S. Moussamih. 2004. Drug intake during Ramadan. *British Medical Journal* 329: 778–82.

Abdeldayem, S. M., and A. H. Hossam Zyton. 2012. The effect of Ramadan fasting on multiple sclerosis. *Egyptian Journal of Neurology, Psychiatry, and Neurosurgery* 494: 341–5.

Abu-Salameh, I., Y. Plakht and G. Ifergane. 2010. Migraine exacerbation during Ramadan fasting. *Journal of Headache Pain* 11: 513–17.

Advocat, J., J. Enticott, B. Vandenberg, C. Hassed, J. Hester and G. Russell. 2016. The effects of a mindfulness-based lifestyle program for adults with Parkinson's disease: a mixed methods, wait list controlled randomised control study. *BMC Neurology* 16: 166.

Afrasiabi, A., S. Hassanzadeh, R. Sattarivand and S. Mahboob. 2003. Effects of Ramadan fasting on serum lipid profiles on 2 hyperlipidemic groups with or without diet pattern. *Saudi Medical Journal* 24: 23–6.

Aftanas, L. I., and S. A. Golocheikine. 2002. Non-linear dynamic complexity of the human EEG during meditation. *Neuroscience Letters* 330: 143–6.

Aggarwal, N. K. 2010. Diagnostic reasoning in Nizāmī 'Arūzī's *Four Discourses. Medical Humanities* 36: 88–92.

Aggarwal, N. K. 2010. Psychosis in the Firdaus al-Hikmat, the first major Arabic medical text. *British Journal of Psychiatry* 197: 447.

Aggarwal, N. K. 2013. 'On the Diseases of the Head' in the scale of medicine by Muhammad Akbar Arzānī [d. 1722]. *History of Psychiatry* 24: 106–17.

Aghabagheri, H., P. Mohammadkhani, S. Omrani and V. Farahmand. 2012. Mindfulness based group therapy on increase in subjective well-being and hope to MS patients. *Clinical Psychology* 4: 23–33.

Akhan, G., S. Kutluhan and H. R. Koyuncuoglu. 2000. Is there any change of stroke incidence during Ramadan? *Acta Neurologica Scandinavica* 101: 259–61.

Alajouanine, T. 1963. Dostoiewski's epilepsy. *Brain*, 86: 210–18.

Alexander, E. 2012. *Proof of Heaven*. London: Piatkus.

Allan, K., and J. Killick. 2010. Communication with people with dementia. In *Supportive Care for the Person with Dementia*, ed. J. C. Hughes, M. Lloyd-Williams and G. A. Sachs, 217–25. Oxford: Oxford University Press.

Allen, F. B., and P. G. Coleman. 2006. Spiritual perspectives on the person with dementia: identity and personhood. In *Dementia: Mind, Meaning, and the Person*, ed. J. C. Hughes, S. J. Louw and S. R. Sabat, 205–21. Oxford: Oxford University Press.

Al-Qattan, M. M. 2000. Burns in epileptics in Saudi Arabia. *Burns* 26: 561–3.

Alston, P. 1997. *Perceiving God: The Epistemology of Religious Experience*. Ithaca, NY: Cornell University Press.

Amancio, E. J., S. T. Zymberg and M. F. Pires. 1994. [Temporal lobe epilepsy and aura with happiness and pleasure: report of 2 cases and review of the literature]. *Arquivos de Neuro-Psiquiatria* 52: 252–9.

American Psychiatric Association. 2013. *Diagnostic and Statistic Manual of Mental Disorders*. 5th edn. Arlington, VA: American Psychiatric Publishing.

Ames, D., A. Burns and J. O'Brien, eds. 2010. *Dementia*. 4th edn. London: Hodder Arnold.

Aminoff, M. J., and R. P. Simon. 1980. Status epilepticus: causes, clinical features, and consequences in 98 patients. *American Journal of Medicine* 69: 657–66.

Andersen, R. 1997. Multimodal integration for the representation of space in the posterior parietal cortex. *Philosophical Transactions of the Royal Society of London* 352: 1421–8.

Anderson, M. 2014. *After Phrenology: Neural Reuse and the Interactive Brain*. Cambridge, MA: MIT Press.

Andrejč, G. 2012. Bridging the gap between social and existential-mystical interpretations of Schleiermacher's 'feeling'. *Religious Studies* 48: 377–401.

Argyle, M. 2002. State of the art: religion. *The Psychologist* 15: 22–6.

Armstrong, K. 1983. *Beginning the World*. New York: St Martin's Press.

Asheim Hansen, B., and E. Brodtkorb. 2003. Partial epilepsy with 'ecstatic' seizures. *Epilepsy and Behavior* 4: 667–73.

Aslam, M., and A. Assad. 1986. Drug regimens and fasting during Ramadan: a survey in Kuwait. *Public Health* 100: 49–53.

Aslam, M., and M. A. Healy. 1986. Compliance and drug therapy in fasting Moslem patients. *Journal of Clinical and Hospital Pharmacy* 11: 321–5.

Asp, E. W., and D. Tranel. 2013. False tagging theory: toward a unitary account of prefrontal cortex function. In *Principles of Frontal Lobe Function*, 2nd edn., ed. D. T. Stuss and R. T. Knight, 383–416. New York: Oxford University Press.

Asp, E. W., K. Manzel, B. Koestner, C. A. Cole, N. L. Denburg and D. Tranel. 2012a. A neuropsychological test of belief and doubt: damage to ventromedial prefrontal cortex increases credulity for misleading advertising. *Frontiers in Neuroscience* 6: 100–9.

Asp, E. W., K. Manzel, B. Koestner, N. L. Denburg and D. Tranel. 2013. Benefit of the doubt: a new view of the role of the prefrontal cortex in executive functioning and decision making. *Frontiers in Neuroscience* 7: 86.

Asp, E. W., K. Ramchandran and D. Tranel. 2012b. Authoritarianism, religious fundamentalism, and the human prefrontal cortex. *Neuropsychology* 26: 414–21.

Asp, E. W., K. A. Warner, N. L. Denburg and D. Tranel. N.d. Credulity and religious beliefs in patients with dorsolateral prefrontal cortex damage. Department of Neurology, University of Iowa.

Atran, S., and A. Norenzayan. 2004. Religion's evolutionary landscape: counterintuition, commitment, compassion, communion. *Behavioural and Brain Sciences* 27: 713–70.

Attiah, M. A., and M. J. Farah. 2014. Minds, motherboards, and money: futurism and realism in the neuroethics of BCI technologies. *Frontiers in Systems Neuroscience* 8: 86.

Attwood, T. 2007. *The Complete Guide to Asperger's Syndrome*. London: Jessica Kingsley.

Augustinack, J. C., A. J. van der Kouwe, D. H. Salat, T. Benner, A. A. Stevens, J. Annese, B. Fischl, M. P. Frosch and S. Corkin. 2014. H.M.'s contributions to neuroscience: a review and autopsy studies. *Hippocampus* 24: 1267–86.

Aull-Watschinger, S., E. Pataraia and C. Baumgartner. 2008. Sexual auras: predominance of epileptic activity within the mesial temporal lobe. *Epilepsy and Behavior* 12: 124–7.

Au-Yeung, S. S. Y., C. W. Y. Hui-Chan and J. C. S. Tang. 2009. Short-form Tai Chi improves standing balance of people with chronic stroke. *Neurorehabilitation and Neural Repair* 23: 515–22.

Azari, N. P., J. Nickel, G. Wunderlich, M. Niedeggen, H. Hefter, L. Tellman, H. Herzog, P. Stoerig, D. Birnbacher and R. J. Seitz. 2001. Neural correlates of religious experience. *European Journal of Neuroscience* 13: 1649–52.

Baddeley, A., and B. Wilson. 1994. When implicit learning fails: amnesia and the problem of error elimination. *Neuropsychologia* 32: 53–68.

Bahammam, A. S., K. Almushailhi, S. R. Pandi-Perumal and M. M. Sharif. 2014. Intermittent fasting during Ramadan: does it affect sleep? *Journal of Sleep Research* 23: 35–43.

Bahammam, A., M. Alrajeh, M. Albabtain, S. Bahammam and M. Sharif. 2010. Circadian pattern of sleep, energy expenditure, and body temperature of young healthy men during the intermittent fasting of Ramadan. *Appetite* 54: 426–9.

Bahammam, A. S., S. Nashwan, O. Hammad, M. M. Sharif and S. R. Pandi-Perumal. 2013. Objective assessment of drowsiness and reaction time during intermittent Ramadan fasting in young men: a case-crossover study. *Behavioral and Brain Functions* 9: 32.

Ball, A. 2006. Ellen's prayer. In *Palliative Care in Severe Dementia*, ed. J. C. Hughes, 134. London: Quay Books.

Barbey, A. K., and S. A. Sloman. 2007. Base-rate respect: from ecological rationality to dual processes. *Behavioural and Brain Sciences* 30: 241–56.

Bargh, J. A., M. Chen and L. Burrows. 1996. Automaticity of social behavior: direct effects of trait construct and stereotype-activation on action. *Journal of Personality and Social Psychology* 71: 230–44.

Barker, A. T., R. Jalinous and I. L. Freeston. 1985. Non-invasive magnetic stimulation of human motor cortex. *The Lancet* 325: 1106–7.

Baron-Cohen, S. 1995. *Mindblindness: An Essay on Autism and Theory of Mind.* Cambridge, MA: MIT Press.

Barrett, J. 1999. Theological correctness: Cognitive constraint and the study of religion. *Method and Theory in the Study of Religion* 11: 325–39.

Barrett, J. 2004. *Why Would Anyone Believe in God?* Lanham, MD: AltaMira.

Barrett, J. 2012. *Born Believers: The Science of Children's Religious Beliefs.* New York: Free Press.

Barrett, J., and E. Burdett. 2011. The cognitive science of religion. *The Psychologist* 24: 252–5.

Barrett, J. L., and F. C. Keil. 1996. Conceptualizing a nonnatural entity: anthropomorphism in god concepts. *Cognitive Psychology* 31: 219–47.

Barsalou, L. W. 2008. Grounded cognition. *Annual Review of Psychology* 59: 617–45.

Bastille, J. V., and K. M. Gill-Body. 2004. A yoga-based exercise program for people with post-stroke chronic hemiparesis. *Physical Therapy* 84: 33–48.

Baumeister, R. 1992. *Meanings of Life.* New York: Guilford Press.

Baylor Institute for Studies of Religion. 2006. *American Piety in the 21st Century: New Insights to the Depth and Complexity of Religion in the US.* Houston, TX: Baylor Institute for Studies of Religion.

Bear, D. M., and P. Fedio. 1977. Quantitative analysis of interictal behavior in temporal lobe epilepsy. *Archives of Neurology* 34: 454–67.

Beaumont, M. I. 2005. Early Muslim interpretation of the Gospels. *Transformation: An International Journal of Holistic Mission Studies* 22: 20–7.

Beauregard, M., and V. Paquette. 2006. Neural correlates of a mystical experience in Carmelite nuns. *Neuroscience Letters* 405: 186–90.

Beauregard, M., and V. Paquette. 2008. EEG activity in Carmelite nuns during a mystical experience. *Neuroscience Letters* 444: 1–4.

Bechtel, W. 2008. *Mental Mechanisms Philosophical Perspectives on Cognitive Neuroscience.* New York: Routledge.

Beck, A., C. Ward, M. Mendelson, J. Mock and J. Erbaugh. 1961. An inventory for measuring depression. *Archives of General Psychiatry* 4: 561–71.

Bedard, M., M. Felteau, C. Gibbons, R. Klein, D. Mazmanian, K. Fedyk and G. Mack. 2005. A mindfulness-based intervention to improve quality of life among individuals who sustained traumatic brain injuries: one-year follow-up. *Journal of Cognitive Rehabilitation*, Spring, 2–7.

Bedard, M., M. Felteau, S. Marshall, S. Dubois, C. Gibbons, R. Klein and B. Weaver. 2012. Mindfulness-based cognitive therapy: benefits in reducing depression following a traumatic brain injury. *Advances in Mind–Body Medicine* 26: 14–20.

Bedard, M., M. Felteau, D. Mazmanian, K. Fedyk, R. Klein, J. Richardson, W. Parkinson and M. B. Minthorn-Biggs. 2003. Pilot evaluation of a mindfulness-based intervention to improve quality of life among individuals who sustained traumatic brain injuries. *Disability and Rehabilitation* 25: 722–31.

Bede, the Venerable. 1968. *A History of the English Church and People.* Ed. L. Sherley-Price. London: Penguin Classics.

Behbehani, A. 1984. Rhazes: the original portrayer of smallpox. *JAMA* 252: 3156–9.

Bellah, R. 2011. *Religion in Human Evolution.* Cambridge, MA: Harvard University Press.

Ben Yishay, Y. 1996. Reflections on the evolution of the therapeutic milieu concept. *Neuropsychological Rehabilitation* 6: 327–43.

Bener, A., A. Hamad, A. Fares, H. M. Al-Sayed and J. Al-Suwaidi. 2006. Is there any effect of Ramadan fasting on stroke incidence? *Singapore Medical Journal* 47: 404–8.

Bennett, C. M., G. L. Wolford and M. B. Miller. 2009. The principled control of false positives in neuroimaging. *Social Cognitive and*

Affective Neuroscience 4: 417–22. doi:10.1093/scan/nsp053.

Bennett, M. and P. M. S. Hacker. 2003. *Philosophical Foundations of Neuroscience.* London: John Wiley.

Bennett, M. R. and P. M. S. Hacker. 2008. *History of Cognitive Neuroscience.* Hoboken, NJ: Wiley-Blackwell.

Benson, D. F. 1991. The Geschwind syndrome. *Advances in Neurology* 55: 411–21.

Benson, H., et al. 1990. Three case reports of the metabolic and electroencephalographic changes during advanced Buddhist meditation techniques. *Journal of Behavioral Medicine* 16: 90–95.

Bergouignan, L., L. Nyberg and H. Ehrsson. 2014. Out-of-body-induced hippocampal amnesia. *Proceedings of the National Academy of Sciences of the United States of America* 111: 4421–6.

Bering, J. 2002. The existential theory of mind. *Review of General Psychology* 6: 3–24.

Biesterfeldt, H. H. 2011. Medicine in the Arab world. In *Encyclopedia of Medieval Philosophy*, ed. H. Lagerlund, 742–6. Dordrecht: Springer Netherlands.

Bioethics PsCo. 2014. Controversies in the determination of death 2008. 8 April.

Bird, G., and R. Cook. 2013. Mixed emotions: the contribution of alexithymia to emotional symptoms of autism. *Translational Psychiatry* 3: 1–8.

Blake, H., and M. Batson. 2006. Exercise intervention in brain injury: a pilot randomized study of Tai Chi Qigong. *Clinical Rehabilitation* 23: 589–98.

Blanke, O., and S. Dieguez. 2009. Leaving body and life behind: out-of-body and near-death experience. In *The Neurology of Consciousness*, ed. S. Laureys and G. Tonini, 303–25. San Diego CA: Academic Press.

Blanke, O., and C. Mohr. 2005. Out-of-body experience, heautoscopy, and autoscopic hallucination of neurological origin: Implications for neurocognitive mechanisms of corporeal awareness and self-consciousness. *Brain Research Review* 50: 184–99.

Blanke, O., C. Mohr, C. Michel, A. Pascual-Leone, P. Brugger, M. Seeck, T. Landis and G. Thut. 2005. Linking out-of-body experience and self-processing to mental own-body imagery at the temporoparietal junction. *Journal of Neuroscience* 25: 550–7.

Blanke, O., S. Ortigue, T. Landis and M. Seeck. 2002. Stimulating illusory own-body perceptions. *Nature* 419: 269–70.

Blanke, O., S. Perrig, G. Thut, T. Landis and M. Seeck. 2000. Simple and complex vestibular responses induced by electrical cortical stimulation of the parietal cortex in humans. *Journal of Neurology, Neurosurgery, and Psychiaitry* 69: 553–6.

Blankespoor, R. J., M. P. J. Schellekens, S. H. Vos, A. E. M. Speckens and B. A. de Jong. 2017. The effectiveness of mindfulness-based stress reduction on psychological distress and cognitive functioning in patients with multiple sclerosis: a pilot study. *Mindfulness*. Published online. doi:10.1007/s12671-017-0701-6.

Blidstein, G. J. 1996. Halakhah – the governing norm. *Jewish Political Studies Review* 8: 37–80.

Block, N. 1995. On a confusion about a function of consciousness. *Behavioral and Brain Sciences* 18: 227–87.

Block, N. R., D. C. Perry, V. E. Sturm, Z. A. Miller and B. L. Miller. 2013. *Religious Dogmatism in Neurodegenerative Disease.* Boston: Alzheimer's Association International Conference.

Bloom, P. 2007. Religion is natural. *Developmental Science* 10: 147–51.

Blum, D. 2007. *Ghost Hunters.* London: Century.

Bogosian A., P. Chadwick, S. Windgassen, S. Norton, P. McCrone, I. Mosweu, E. Silber and R. Moss-Morris. 2015. Distress improves after mindfulness training for progressive MS: a pilot randomised trial. *Multiple Sclerosis Journal* 21: 1184–94.

Bogosian, A., A. Hughes, S. Norton, E. Silber and R. Moss-Morris. 2016. Potential treatment mechanisms in a mindfulness based intervention for people with progressive multiple sclerosis. *British Journal of Health Psychology* 21: 859–80.

Borel, L., C. Lopez, P. Péruch and M. Lacour. 2008. Le syndrome vestibulaire: un changement de représentation interne de l'espace. *Neurophysiologie Clinique* 38: 375–89.

Bornstein, M. H., C. Hahn and T. D. Suwalsky. 2013. Physically developed and exploratory young infants contribute to their own long-term academic achievement. *Psychological Science* 24: 1906–10.

Botvinick, M. M., T. S. Braver, D. M. Barch, C. S. Carter and J. D. Cohen. 2001. Conflict monitoring and cognitive control. *Psychological Review* 108: 624–52.

Botvinick, M. M., J. D. Cohen and C. S. Carter. 2004. Conflict monitoring and anterior cingulate cortex: an update. *Trends in Cognitive Sciences* 8: 539–46.

Bowen, C., G. Yeates and S. Palmer. 2010. *A Relational Approach to Rehabilitation: Thinking about Relationships after Brain Injury*. London: Karnac.

Brady, M. J., A. H. Peterman, G. Fitchett, M. Mo and D. Cella. 1999. A case for including spirituality in quality of life measurement in oncology. *Psycho-oncology* 8: 417–18.

Bramley, N., and V. Eatough. 2005. The experience of living with Parkinson's disease: an interpretative phenomenological analysis case study. *Psychology and Health* 20: 223–35.

Brewer, H. 2004. Early Arabic medicine. *Journal of the Royal Society for the Promotion of Health* 124: 184–7.

Britton, W., and R. Bootzin. 2004. Near-death experiences and the temporal lobe. *Psychological Science* 15: 254–8.

Brock, J., C. B. Brown, J. Boucher and G. Rippon. 2002. The temporal binding deficit hypothesis of autism. *Development and Psychopathology* 14: 209–24.

Brooks, D. N., and A. Baddeley. 1976. What can amnesic patients learn? *Neuropsychologia* 14: 111–22.

Browne, E. G. 1921. *Arabian Medicine: The FitzPatrick Lectures Delivered at the College of Physicians in November 1919 and November 1920*. Cambridge: Cambridge University Press.

Browne, M., G. Pennycook, B. Goodwin and M. McHenry. 2014. Reflective minds and open hearts: cognitive style and personality predict religious and spiritual thinking in a community sample. *European Journal of Social Psychology* 44: 736–42.

Burazeri, G., A. Goda and J. D. Kark. 2008. Religious observance and acute coronary syndrome in predominantly Muslim Albania: a population-based case-control study in Tirana. *Annals of Epidemiology* 18: 937–45.

Bürgel, J. C. 1998. Secular and religious features of medieval Arabic medicine. In *Asian Medical Systems: A Comparative Study*, ed. C. Leslie, 44–62. Delhi: Motilal Banarsidass.

Burschka, J. M., P. M. Keune, U. Oy, P. Oschman and P. Kuhn. 2014. Mindfulness-based interventions in multiple sclerosis: beneficial effects of Tai Chi on balance, coordination, fatigue and depression. *BioMedCentral Neurology* 14: 165–174.

Bussing, A., A. Michalsen, H. J. Balzat et al. 2009. Are spirituality and religiosity resources for patients with chronic pain conditions? *Pain Medicine* 10: 327–39.

Butler, P. M., P. McNamara and R. Durso. 2010. Deficits in the automatic activation of religious concepts in patients with Parkinson's disease. *Journal of the International Neuropsychological Society* 16: 252–61. doi:10.1017/S1355617709991202.

Butler, P. M., P. McNamara and R. Durso. 2011. Side of onset in Parkinson's disease and alterations in religiosity: novel behavioral phenotypes. *Behavioral Neurology* 24: 133–41.

Butler, P. M., P. McNamara, J. Ghofrani and R. Durso. 2011a. Disease-associated differences in religious cognition in patients with Parkinson's disease. *Journal of Clinical and Experimental Neuropsychology* 33: 917–28.

Caap-Ahlgren, M., L. Lannerheim and O. Dehlin. 2002. Older Swedish women's experiences of living with symptoms related to Parkinson's disease. *Journal of Advanced Nursing* 39: 87–95.

Cahill, L., N. Weinberger, B. Roozendaal and J. McGaugh. 1999. Is the amygdala a locus of 'conditioned fear'? Some questions and caveats. *Neuron* 23: 227–8.

Cahn, B. R., and J. Polich. 2006. Meditation states and traits: EEG, ERP and neuroimaging studies. *Psychological Bulletin* 132: 180–211.

Caldwell-Harris, C. 2012. Understanding atheism/non-belief as an expected individual-differences variable. *Religion, Brain, and Behavior* 2: 4–47.

Calhoun, L. G., A. Cann, R. G. Tedeschi et al. 2000. A correlational test of the relationship between posttraumatic growth, religion, and cognitive processing. *Journal of Trauma and Stress* 13: 521–7.

Call, J., and M. Tomasello. 2008. Does the chimpanzee have a theory of mind? 30 years later. *Trends in Cognitive Science* 12: 187–92. www.ncbi.nlm.nih.gov/pubmed/18424224.

Calver, A. 2009. The unicorn who came to stay and other stories: mothers' experiences of having a child with autism with an imaginary friend. Doctoral dissertation, University of London.

Carhart-Harris, R. L., D. Erritzoe, T. Williams, J. M. Stone, L. J. Reed, A. Colasanti et al. 2012. Neural correlates of the psychedelic state as determined by fMRI studies with psilocybin. *Proceedings of the National Academy of Sciences of the United States of America* 109: 2138–43. doi:10.1073/pnas.1119598109.

Carhart-Harris, R. L., R. Leech, D. Erritzoe, T. M. Williams, J. M. Stone, J. Evans et al. 2013. Functional connectivity measures after psilocybin inform a novel hypothesis of early psychosis. *Schizophrenia Bulletin* 39: 1343–51. doi:10.1093/schbul/sbs117.

Carhart-Harris, R. L., S. Muthukumaraswamy, L. Roseman, M. Kaelen, W. Droog, K. Murphy et al. 2016. Neural correlates of the LSD experience revealed by multimodal neuroimaging. *Proceedings of the National Academy of Sciences of the United States of America* 113: 4853–8. doi:10.1073/pnas.1518377113.

Carrazana, E., et al. 1999. Epilepsy and religious experiences: Voodoo possession. *Epilepsia* 40: 239–41.

Carrette, J. 2004. *William James and 'The Varieties of Religious Experience'*. London: Routledge.

Carver, C., and M. Scheier. 1990. Origins and function of positive and negative affect: a control process view. *Psychological Review* 97: 19–36.

Cash, T., V. Ekouevi, C. Kilbourn and S. Lageman. 2015. Pilot study of a mindfulness-based group intervention for individuals with Parkinson's disease and their caregivers. *Mindfulness* 7: 361–71.

Cavaco, S., S. Anderson, J. Allen, A. Castro-Caldas and H. Damasio. 2004. The scope of preserved procedural memory in amnesia. *Brain* 127: 1853–67.

Cavanna, A. E., S. Cavanna and A. Cavanna. 2010. Epileptic seizures and spirit possession in Haitian culture: report of four cases and review of the literature. *Epilepsy and Behavior* 19: 89–91.

Central Council of Indian Medicine. 2014. *Syllabus of Kamil-E-Tib-Wa-Jarahat (BUMS) Course*. New Delhi: Government of India. https://ccimindia.org/pdf/UG-1st-2nd-3rd-yr-Syllabus-BUMS-Unani.pdf.

Chajes, Z. H. 1958. *Darchai Horaah: Kol Kitvei Maharitz Chajes*. Jerusalem: Divrei Chachamim.

Chalmers, D. 1995. Facing up to the problem of consciousness. *Journal of Consciousness Studies* 2: 200–219.

Chalmers, D. 1996. *The Conscious Mind.* Oxford: Oxford University Press.

Chan, A. W., J. W. Sit and S. Y. Chair. 2017. Tai Chi exercise reduces stroke risk factors: a randomized controlled trial. *Stroke* 48: AWP416.

Chan, D., V. Anderson, Y. Pijnenburg, J. Whitwell, J. Barnes, R. Scahill, J. M. Stevens, F. Barkhof, P. Scheltens, M. N. Rossor and N. C. Fox. 2009. The clinical profile of right temporal lobe atrophy. *Brain* 132: 1287–9.

Chappell, S. G. 2011. On the very idea of criteria for personhood. *Southern Journal of Philosophy* 49(1).

Chappell, S. G. 2013. Knowledge of persons. *European Journal for Philosophy of Religion* 5 (4): 3–28.

Chappell, S. G. 2014. *Knowing What to Do.* Oxford: Oxford University Press.

Charlton, G. S., and C. J. Barrow. 2002. Coping and self-help group membership in Parkinson's disease: an exploratory qualitative study. *Health and Social Care in the Community* 10: 472–8.

Chaves, M. 2010. Rain dances in the dry season: overcoming the religious congruence fallacy. *Journal for the Scientific Study of Religion* 49: 1–14.

Chemero, A. 2011. *Radical Embodied Cognitive Science*. Cambridge, MA: MIT Press.

Cheyne, J., and T. Girard. 2009. The body unbound: vestibular-motor hallucinations and out-of-body experiences. *Cortex* 45: 210–15.

Cheyne, J. A., and G. Pennycook. 2013. Sleep paralysis postepisode distress: modeling potential effects of episode characteristics, general psychological distress, beliefs, and cognitive style. *Clinical Psychological Science* 1: 135–48.

Churchland, P. 2013. *Matter and Consciousness*. 3rd edn. Cambridge, MA: MIT Press.

Cicerone, K., C. Dahlberg, J. Malec, D. Langenbahn, T. Felicetti, S. Kneipp, W. Ellmo, K. Kalmar, J. Giacino, J. P. Harley, L. Laatsch, P. Morse and J. Catanese. 2005. Evidence-based cognitive rehabilitation: updated review of the literature from 1998 through 2002. *Archives of Physical Medicine and Rehabilitation* 86: 1681–92.

Clark, A. 1997. *Being There: Putting Brain, Body, and World Together Again*. Cambridge, MA: MIT Press.

Clark, K. J. 2019. *God and the Brain*. Grand Rapids, MI: Eerdmans.

Clark, K. J., and J. Barrett. 2010. Reformed epistemology and the cognitive science of religion. *Faith and Philosophy* 27: 174–89.

Clifford Rose, F., ed. 1999. *A Short History of Neurology*. Oxford: Butterworth-Heinemann.

Cloninger, C. R. 1994. Temperament and personality. *Current Opinion in Neurobiology* 4: 266–73.

Cloninger, C. R., T. R. Przybeck, D. M. Svrakic and R. D. Wetzel. 1994. *The Temperament and Character Inventory (TCI): A Guide to Its Development and Use*. St. Louis, MO: Center for Psychobiology of Personality, Washington University.

Cohen, N., and L. Squire. 1980. Preserved learning and retention of pattern analysing skill in amnesia: dissociation of knowing how and knowing that. *Science* 210: 207–9.

Collicutt, J. 2012. Some ethical issues in dementia care: re-membering the person. *Crucible*, October–December, 7–17.

Collicutt McGrath, J. 2007. *Ethical Practice in Brain Injury Rehabilitation*. Oxford: Oxford University Press.

Collicutt McGrath, J. 2008. Post acute rehabilitation following traumatic brain injury. In *Psychological Approaches to Rehabilitation after Traumatic Brain Injury*, ed. A. Tyerman and N. King, 39–64. Oxford: BPS-Blackwell.

Collicutt McGrath, J. 2011. Posttraumatic growth and spirituality after brain injury. *Brain Impairment* 12: 82–92.

Collier, B. 1972. Ketamine and the conscious mind. *Anaesthesia* 27: 120–34.

Comings, D., N. Gonzales, G. Saucier, P. Johnson and J. MacMurray. 2000. The DR4 gene and the spiritual transcendence scale of the character temperament scale. *Psychiatric Genetics* 10: 185–9.

Conklin, H. W. 1922. Cause and treatment of epilepsy. *American Journal of the Osteopathic Association* 26: 11–14.

Cook, C. M., and M. A. Persinger. 2001. Geophysical variables and behavior: XCII. Experimental elicitation of the experience of a sentient being by right hemispheric, weak magnetic fields: interaction with temporal lobe sensitivity. Percept. *Motor Skills* 92: 447–8.

Cools, R. 2011. Dopaminergic control of the striatum for high-level cognition. *Current Opinion in Neurobiology* 21: 402–7.

Cooper, D. E. 2002. *The Measure of Things: Humanism, Humility, and Mystery*. Oxford: Clarendon.

Cottingham, J. 2005. *The Spiritual Dimension*. Cambridge: Cambridge University Press.

Cottingham, J. 2009. *Why Believe?* London: Continuum.

Cover, R. 1983. The Supreme Court, 1982 term-foward: nomos and narrative. *Harvard Law Review* 4: 4–68.

Coyle, A., and J. Lochner. 2011. Religion, spirituality and therapeutic practice. *The Psychologist* 24: 264–6.

Craig, M., M. Catani and Q. Deeley. 2009. Altered connections on the road to psychopathy. *Molecular Psychology* 14: 946–53.

Cramer, H., R. Lauche, H. Azizi, G. Dobos and J. Langhorst. 2014. Yoga for multiple sclerosis: a systematic review and meta-analysis. *PLoS One* 9: e112414.

Craver, C. 2007. *Explaining the Brain: Mechanisms and the Mosaic Unity of Neuroscience*. Oxford: Oxford University Press.

Crescentini, C., S. M. Aglioti, F. Fabbro and C. Urgesi. 2014. Virtual lesions of the inferior parietal cortex induce fast changes of implicit religiousness/spirituality. *Cortex* 54: 1–15. doi:10.1016/j.cortex.2014.01.023.

Crescentini, C., M. Di Buccahinacio, F. Fabbro and C. Urgesi. 2015. Excitatory stimulation of the right inferior parietal cortex lessens implicit religiousness/spirituality. *Neuropsychologia* 70: 71–9. doi:10.1016/j.neuropsychologia.2015.02.016.

Crielesi, M., G. Monopoli, G. N. Yeates and S. Monte. Forthcoming. A mindfulness group intervention for people with aphasia: a pilot study. In *Neuro-disability and Psychotherapy, Specialist Topics: Vol. 2. Psychotherapy and Aphasia: Supporting Emotions and Relationships*, ed. G. N. Yeates and K. Meredith. Oxford: Routledge.

Csikszentmihalyi, M. 1990. *Flow: The Psychology of Optimal Experience*. New York: Harper and Row.

Csikszentmihalyi, M. 1997. *Finding Flow: The Psychology of Engagement with Everyday Life*. New York: Basic Books.

Csikszentmihalyi, M., S. Abuhamdeh and J. Nakamura. 2005. Flow. In *Handbook of Competence and Motivation*, ed. A. Elliot, 598–698. New York: Guilford Press.

Cullen, B., J. Pownall, J. Cummings, S. Baylan, N. Broomfield, C. Haig, D. Kersel, H. Murray and J. Evans. 2018. Positive PsychoTherapy in ABI rehab (PoPsTAR): a pilot randomised controlled trial. *Neuropsychological Rehabilitation* 28: 17–33.

Cummins, G. 2012. Social cognition in Parkinson's disease and other movement disorders. Unpublished PhD dissertation, University of Cambridge.

Curriculum Division, Higher Education Commission. 2004. *Curriculum of Eastern Medicine for BEMS & M.Phil*. Islamabad: Government of Pakistan. http://hec.gov.pk/english/services/universities/RevisedCurricula/Documents/2004-2005/Eastern%20Medicine%202004.pdf.

Dalley, J., B. Everitt and T. Robbins. 2011. Impulsivity, compulsivity, and top-down cognitive control. *Neuron* 69: 680–94.

Dalton, K. 1975. Food intake prior to a migraine attack-study of 2313 spontaneous attack. *Headache* 15: 188–93.

Damasio, A. 1999. *The Feeling of What Happens*. San Diego, CA: Harcourt.

David, O., I. Guillemain, S. Saillet, S. Reyr, C. Deransart et al. 2008. Identifying neural drivers with functional MRI: an electrophysiological validation. *PloS Biology* 6: 2683–97. doi:10.1371/journal.pbio.0060315.

Davidson, J., and M. Orsini. 2013. The shifting horizons of autism online. In *Worlds of Autism: Across the Spectrum of Neurological Difference*, ed. Davidson Joyce Orsini Michael, 285–303. Minneapolis: University of Minnesota Press.

Davis, B. 2004. *The Taijiquan Classics: An Annotated Translation*. Berkeley: North Atlantic.

Davis, P. E., H. Simon, E. Meins and D. L. Robin. 2018. Imaginary companions in children with autism spectrum disorder. *Journal of Autism and Developmental Disorders* 48: 1–10. http://csjarchive.cogsci.rpi.edu/proceedings/2011/papers/0782/paper0782.pdf.

Davis, R., and B. Davis. 1989. *My Journey into Alzheimer's Disease*. Wheaton, IL: Tyndale House.

Dawkins, R. 2006. *The God Delusion*. London: Random House.

Dean, S., R. Siegert and W. Taylor. 2012. *Interprofessional Rehabilitation: A Person-Centred Approach*. Oxford: Wiley-Blackwell.

De Haan, D. 2017. Hylomorphic animalism, emergentism, and the challenge of new mechanisms in neuroscience. *Scientia et Fides* 5(2): 9–38.

De Haan, D. 2018. The interaction of noetic and psychosomatic operations in a Thomist hylomorphic personalism. *Scientia et Fides* 6(2): 55–83.

Dein, S., and R. Littlewood. 2011. Religion and psychosis: a common evolutionary trajectory? *Transcultural Psychiatry* 48: 318–35. www.ncbi.nlm.nih.gov/pubmed/21742955

de Jong, B. M. 2013. 'Complete motor locked-in' and consequences for the concept of minimally conscious state. *Journal of Head Trauma Rehabilitation* 28: 141–3.

Del Tredici, K., U. Rub, R. A. De Vos et al. 2002. Where does Parkinson disease pathology begin in the brain? *Journal of Neuropathology and Experimental Neurology* 61: 413–26.

De Neys, W. 2014. Conflict detection, dual processes, and logical intuitions: Some clarifications. *Thinking and Reasoning* 20: 167–87.

De Neys, W., O. Vartanian and V. Goel. 2008. When our brains detect that we are biased. *Psychological Science* 19: 483–9.

Dennett, D. C. 1991. *Consciousness Explained*. Boston: Little, Brown.

Desrochers, P., D. Kairy, S. Pan, H. Corriveau and M. Tousignant. 2016. Tai Chi for upper limb rehabilitation in stroke patients: the patient's perspective. *Disability and Rehabilitation* 39: 1313–19.

Detert, N., and L. Douglas. 2014. Mindfulness MBSR/MBCT improves general psychiatric symptom severity, depression, anxiety and perceived stress in neurological disorders in an NHS clinical setting. *Neuro-disability and Psychotherapy* 2: 137–156.

Detert, V. Forthcoming. Mindfulness in neurological conditions. In *Psychological Therapies in Neuropsychological Rehabilitation*, ed. G. N. Yeates and F. Ashworth. Hove, UK: Psychology Press.

Devinsky, O., and G. Lai. 2008. Spirituality and religion in epilepsy. *Epilepsy and Behavior* 12: 636–43.

Devinsky, O., E. Feldmann, K. Burrowes and E. Bromfield. 1989. Autoscopic phenomena with seizures. *Archives of Neurology* 46: 1080–8.

de Vito, S., N. Gamboz, M. A. Brandimonte et al. 2012. Future thinking in Parkinson's disease: an executive function? *Neuropsychologia* 50: 1494–1501.

Dewhurst, K., and A. W. Beard. 1970. Sudden religious conversions in temporal lobe epilepsy. *British Journal of Psychiatry* 117: 497–507.

Dewhurst, K., and A. W. Beard. 2003. Sudden religious conversions in temporal lobe epilepsy. *Epilepsy and Behavior* 4: 78–87.

Dezutter, J., A. Wachholtz and J. Corveleyn. 2011. Prayer and pain: the mediating role of positive re-appraisal. *Journal of Behavioral Medicine* 34: 542–9.

Dickinson, J., P. Friary and C. M. McCann. 2016. The influence of mindfulness meditation on communication and anxiety: a case study of a person with aphasia. *Aphasiology* 31: 1044–58.

Ding, M. 2012. Tai Chi for stroke rehabilitation: a focused review. *American Journal of Physical Medicine and Rehabilitation* 91: 1091–6.

Dissanayaka, N. N., F. Idu Jion, N. A. Pachana, J. D. O'Sullivan, R. Marsh, G. J. Byrne et al. 2016. Mindfulness for motor and nonmotor dysfunctions in Parkinson's disease. *Parkinson's Disease*. Published online. doi:10.1155/2016/7109052.

Dodrill, C. B., and C. G. Matthews. 1992. The role of neuropsychology in the assessment and treatment of persons with epilepsy. *American Psychologist* 47: 1139–42.

Dolgoff-Kaspar, R., et al. 2011. Numinous-like auras and spirituality in persons with partial seizures. *Epilepsia* 52: 640–4.

Dolu, N., A. Yüksek, A. Sizer and M. Alay. 2007. Arousal and continuous attention during Ramadan intermittent fasting. *Journal of Basic and Clinical Physiology and Pharmacology* 18: 315–22.

Donald, M. 2004. *How Culture and Brain Mechanisms Interact in Decision Making*. Cambridge, MA: MIT Press.

Donnelly, K. Z., K. Linnea, D. A. Grant and J. Lichtenstein. 2014. The feasibility and impact of a yoga pilot programme on the quality-of-life of adults with acquired brain injury. *Brain Injury* 31: 208–14.

Dostoyevsky, F. 1869. *The Idiot*. London: Vizetelly.

Drab, K. 1981. The tunnel experience: reality or hallucination? *Journal of Near-Death Studies* 1: 126–52.

Drescher, M. J., Z. Wimpfheimer, S. Abu Khalef, A. Gammaitoni, N. Shehadeh and R. Torgovicky. 2012. Prophylactic etoricoxib is effective in preventing 'first of Ramadan' headache: a placebo-controlled double-blind and randomized trial of prophylactic etoricoxib for ritual fasting headache. *Headache* 52: 573–81.

Dubin, N., and J. E. Graetz. 2009. Through a different lens: spirituality in the lives of individuals with Asperger's syndrome. *Journal of Religion, Disability, and Health* 13: 29–39.

Duncan, J., and E. K. Miller. 2002. Cognitive focus through adaptive neural coding in the primate prefrontal cortex. In *Principles of Frontal Lobe Function*, ed. D. T. Stuss and R. T. Knight, 278–91. New York: Oxford University Press.

Ebrahimnejad, H. 2011. What is 'Islamic' in Islamic medicine? An overview. In *Science between Europe and Asia: Historical Studies on the Transmission, Adoption and Adaptation of Knowledge*, ed. F. Günergun and D. Raina, 259–70. Dordrecht: Springer Netherlands.

Edwards-Lee, T., B. L. Miller, D. F. Benson, J. L. Cummings, G. L. Russell, K. Boone et al. 1997. The temporal variant of frontotemporal dementia. *Brain* 120: 1027–40.

Egan, A. 2008. Seeing and believing: perception, belief formation and the divided mind. *Philosophical Studies* 140: 47–63.

Ehrsson, H. 2007. The experimental induction of out-of-body experience. *Science* 317: 1048.

Elliot, B. 2011. Arts-based and narrative inquiry in liminal experience reveal platforming as basic social psychological process. *The Arts in Psychotherapy* 38: 96–103.

Ellison, C. W. 1983. Spiritual well-being: conceptualization and measurement. *Journal of Psychology and Theology* 11: 330–40.

El-Mitwalli, A., A. A. Zaher and E. El Menshawi. 2010. Circadian rhythm of stroke onset during the month of Ramadan. *Acta Neurologica Scandinavica* 122: 97–101.

El-Mitwalli, A., A. A. Zaher, M. A. Mohamed and E. Elmenshawi. 2009. The effect of Ramadan fasting on cerebral stroke: a prospective hospital-based study. *European Journal of Neurology* 16, no. 4: e80.

Elon, M. 2003. *Community Legislation.* Philadelphia: Jewish Publication Society.

Els, T., J. Kassubek, R. Kubalek and J. Klish. 2004. Diffusion-weighted MRI during early global cerebral hypoxia: a predictor of clinical outcome? *Acta Neurologica Scandinavica* 110: 361–7.

Elsass, L. and G. Kinsella. 1987. Social interaction following severe closed head injury. *Psychological Medicine* 17(1): 67–78.

Emanuel, L. L. 1995. Reexamining death: the asymptotic model and a bounded zone definition. *Hastings Center Report* 25, no. 4: 27–35.

Emmons, R. 1999. *The Psychology of Ultimate Concerns: Motivation and Spirituality in Personality.* New York: Guilford Press.

Emmons, R. A., and R. F. Paloutzian. 2003. The psychology of religion. *Annual Review of Psychology* 54: 377–402.

Evans, J. J. 2011. Positive psychology and brain injury rehabilitation. *Brain Impairment* 12: 117–27.

Evans, J. J., and B. Cullen. Forthcoming. Positive psychotherapy for neurological conditions. In *Psychological Therapies in Neuropsychological Rehabilitation*, ed. G. N. Yeates and F. Ashworth. Hove, UK: Psychology Press.

Evans, J. St. B. T., and K. E. Stanovich. 2013. Dual-process theories of higher cognition: Advancing the debate. *Perspectives in Psychological Science* 8: 223–41.

Exline, J., C. Park, J. Smyth and M. Carey. 2011. Anger toward God: socialcognitive predictors, prevalence, and links with adjustment to bereavement and cancer. *Journal of Personality and Social Psychology* 100: 129–48.

Exline, J., M. Prince-Paul, B. Root, K. Peereboom and E. Worthington Jr. 2012. Forgiveness issues at the end of life: a study with family members of hospice patients. *Journal of Palliative Medicine* 15: 1113–19.

Faris, M. A., S. Kacimi, R. A. Al-Kurd, M. A. Fararjeh, Y. K. Bustanji, M. K. Mohammad and M. L. Salem. 2012. Intermittent fasting during Ramadan attenuates proinflammatory cytokines and immune cells in healthy subjects. *Nutrition Research* 32: 947–55.

Farmer, R. F., and L. R. Goldberg. 2008. A psychometric evaluation of the Revised Temperament and Character Inventory (TCI-R) and the TCi-140. *Psychological Assessment* 20: 281–91.

Feil, N. 1993. *The Validation Breakthrough: Simple Techniques for Communicating with People with 'Alzheimer's Type Dementia'.* Baltimore: Health Professions Press.

Fenwick, P., and E. Fenwick. 1998. *Truth in the Light.* New York: Berkeley Books.

Fingelkurts, A. A. 2009. Is our brain hardwired to produce God, or is our brain hardwired to perceive God? A systematic review on the role of the brain in mediating religious experience. *Cognitive Processing* 10: 293–326.

Fisk, J. D., P. G. Ritvo, L. Ross, D. A. Haasem, T. J. Marrie and W. F. Schlech. 1994. Measuring the functional impact of fatigue: initial validation of the fatigure impact scale. *Clinical Infectious Disease* 18(Suppl. 1): s79–83.

Fitzpatrick, L., J. Simpson and A. Smith. 2010. A qualitative analysis of mindfulness-based cognitive therapy (MBCT) in Parkinson's disease. *Psychology and Psychotherapy: Theory, Research, and Practice* 83: 179–92.

Fodor, J. 1983. *The Modularity of Mind.* Cambridge, MA: MIT Press.

Foltynie, T., C. E. G. Brayne, T. W. Robbins et al. 2004. The cognitive ability of an incident cohort of Parkinson's patients in the UK: The CamPaIGN study. *Brain* 127: 550–60.

Forster, E., and J. Whinnery. 1988. Recovery from G_2-induced loss of consciousness: psychologic considerations. *Aviation, Space, and Environmental Medicine* 59: 2–5.

Foss-Feig, J. H., L. D. Kwakye, C. J. Cascio, C. P. Burnette, H. Kadivar, W. L. Stone and M. T. Wallace. 2010. An extended multisensory temporal binding window in autism spectrum disorders. *Experimental Brain Research* 203: 381–9.

Fox, K. C. R., M. L. Dixon, S. Nijeboer, M. Girna, J. L. Floman, M. Lifshitz, M. Ellamild, P. Sedlmeier and K. Christoff. 2016. Functional neuroanatomy of meditation: a review and meta-analysis of 78 functional neuroimaging investigations. *Neuroscience and Biobehavioral Reviews* 65: 208–28. doi:10.1016/j.neubiorev.2016.03.021.

Frank, J. 2010. *Dostoevsky: A Writer in His Time.* Princeton, NJ: Princeton University Press.

Franklin, J. 2002. *The Science of Conjecture: Evidence and Probability before Pascal.* Baltimore: Johns Hopkins University Press.

Franzen, J. 2001. My father's brain: what Alzheimer's takes away. *New Yorker*, 10 September, 81–91.

Franzen, J. 2001. The long slow slide into the abyss. *Guardian Weekend*, 15 December, 15–29.

Frazer, J. 1890. *The Golden Bough: A Study in Comparative Religion.* London: Macmillan.

Freud, S. 1928. *The Future of an Illusion.* Trans. James Strachey. London: Hogarth Press.

Friston, K. 2009. Causal modelling and brain connectivity in functional magnetic resonance imaging. *PLoS Biology* 7: e1000033. doi:10.1371/journal.pbio.1000033.

Friston, K. J. and R. J. Dolan. 2010. Computational and dynamic models in neuroimaging. *Neuroimage* 52: 752–65.

Frith, C. 1992. *The Cognitive Neuropsychology of Schizophrenia.* Ed. L. Erlbaum. Hove, UK: Psychology Press.

Gallagher, S. and D. Zahavi. 2008. *The Phenomenological Mind: An Introduction to Philosophy of Mind and Cognitive Science.* London: Routledge.

Gallup. 2011. U.S. political ideology stable with conservatives leading. August 1. www.gallup.com/poll/148745/political-ideology-stable-conservatives-leading.aspx.

Gao, Q., A. Leung, Y. Yang et al. 2014. Effects of tai chi on balance and fall prevention in Parkinson's disease: a randomized controlled trial. *Clinical Rehabilitation* 28: 748–53.

Gehring, W. J., and R. T. Knight. 2000. Prefrontal-cingulate interations in action monitoring. *Nature Neuroscience* 3: 516–20.

Gemmell, C., and J. M. Leathem. 2006. A study investigating the effects of Tai Chi Chuan: individuals with traumatic brain injury compared to controls. *Brain Injury* 20: 151–6.

Gervais, W. M., and A. Norenzayan. 2012. Analytic thinking promotes religious disbelief. *Science* 336: 493–6.

Geschwind, N. 1979. Behavioural changes in temporal lobe epilepsy. *Psychological Medicine* 9: 217–19.

Geschwind, N. 1983. Pathogenesis of behavior change in temporal lobe epilepsy. *Research Publications – Association for Research in Nervous and Mental Disorders* 61: 355–70.

Geyelin, H. R. 1921. Fasting as a method for treating epilepsy. *Medical Record* 99: 1037–9.

Giacomini, M. 1997. A change of heart and a change of mind? Technology and the redefinition of death in 1968. *Social Science and Medicine* 44: 1465–82.

Giaquinto, S., L. Bruti, V. Dall'Armi et al. 2011. Religious and spiritual beliefs in outpatients suffering from Parkinson disease. *International Journal of Geriatric Psychiatry* 26: 916–22.

Gibson, J. J. 1979. *The Ecological Approach to Visual Perception.* Boston: Houghton Mifflin.

Gilbert, D. T. 1991. How mental systems believe. *American Psychologist* 46: 107–19.

Gilbert, D. T. 1993. The assent of man: mental representation and the control of belief. In *Handbook of Mental Control*, ed. D. M. Wegner and J. W. Pennebaker, 57–87. Engelwood Cliffs, NJ: Prentice Hall.

Gilbert, D. T., R. W. Tafarodi and P. S. Malone. 1993. You can't not believe everything you read. *Journal of Personality and Social Psychology* 65: 221–33.

Glascher, J., R. Adolphs, H. Damasio, A. Bechara, D. Rudrauf, M. Calamia et al. 2012. Lesion mapping of cognitive control and value-based decision making in the prefrontal cortex. *Proceedings of the National Academy of Sciences* 109: 14681–6.

Glisky, E., D. Scahcter and E. Tulving. 1986. Computer learning by memory impaired patients: acquisition and retention of complex knowledge. *Neuropsychologia* 24: 313–28.

Glock, C., and R. Stark. 1965. *Religion and Society in Tension*. Chicago: Rand McNally.

Goldie, P., ed. 2010. *The Oxford Handbook of Philosophy of Emotion*. Oxford: Oxford University Press.

Goldin-Meadow, Susan. 2003. *Hearing Gesture: How Our Hands Help Us Think*. Cambridge, MA: Harvard University Press.

Goldstein, K. 1959. Notes on the development of my concepts. *Journal of Individual Psychology* 15: 5–14.

Gomceli, Y. B., G. Kutlu, L. Cavdar and L. E. Inan. 2008. Does the seizure frequency increase in Ramadan? *Seizure* 17: 671–6.

Good, B., and M. J. D. Good. 1992. The comparative study of Greco-Islamic medicine: the integration of knowledge into local symbolic contexts. In *Paths to Asian Medical Knowledge*, ed. C. Leslie and A. Young, 257–71. Berkeley: University of California Press.

Goodall, M. A. 2009. The evaluation of spiritual care in a dementia care setting. *Dementia* 8: 167–83.

Gorelick, P. B., A. Scuteri, S. E. Black, C. DeCarli, S. M. Greenberg, C. Iadecola et al. 2011. Vascular contributions to cognitive impairment and dementia. *Stroke* 42: 2672–713.

Gorji, A., and M. K. Ghadiri. 2001. History of epilepsy in medieval Iranian medicine. *Neuroscience and Biobehavioral Reviews* 25: 455–61.

Gorji, A., and M. K. Ghadiri. 2002. History of headache in medieval Persian medicine. *Lancet Neurology* 1: 510–15.

Gowers, W. R. 1881. *Epilepsy and Other Chronic Convulsive Diseases*. London: Churchill.

Grabowski, T. J., H. Damasio and A. Damasio. 1998. Premotor and prefrontal correlates of category-related lexical retrieval. *Neuroimage* 7: 232–43.

Gracey, F., C. Ford and K. Psaila. 2015. A provisional transdiagnostic cognitive behavioural model of post brain injury emotional adjustment. *NeuroDisability and Psychotherapy* 3: 154–85.

Gracey, F., and T. Onsworth, eds. 2008. Self and identity changes in neuropsycholgical rehabilitation. *Neuropsychological Rehabilitation* 18: 5–6.

Graf, P., and D. Schacter. 1985. Implicit and explicit memory for new associations in normal and amnesic patients. *Journal of Experimental Psychology: Learning, Memory, and Cognition* 11: 501–18.

Granqvist, P., M. Fredrikson, P. Unge, A. Hagenfeldt, S. Valind, D. Larhammar and M. Larsson. 2005. Sensed presence and mystical experiences are predicted by suggestibility, not by the application of transcranial weak complex magnetic fields. *Neuroscience Letters* 379: 1–6.

Green, J. 2003. Science, religion and the mind–brain problem: the case of Thomas Willis (1621–1675). *Science and Christian Belief* 15: 165–85.

Grey, M. 1985. *Return from Death*. Boston: Arkana.

Greyson, B. 1983. The Near-Death Experience Scale. *Journal of Nervous and Mental Disorders* 171: 369–75.

Greyson, B. B., L. L. Derr and N. Fountain. 2015. Mystical experiences associated with seizures. *Religion, Brain and Behaviour* 5: 182–96.

Grèzes, J., C. D. Frith and R. E. Passingham. 2004. Inferring false beliefs from the actions of oneself and others: an fMRI study. *Neuroimage* 21: 744–50. www.sciencedirect.com/science/article/pii/S1053811903006657.

Griffiths, R. R., et al. 2011. Psilocybin occasioned mystical-type experiences: immediate and persisting dose-related effects. *Psychopharmacology* 218: 649–65.

Griffiths, R.R., et al. 2006. Psilocybin can occasion mystical-type experiences having substantial and sustained personal meaning and spiritual significance. *Psychopharmacology* 187: 268–83; discussion 284–92.

Grossman, P., L. Kappos, H. Gensicke, M. D'Souza, D. Mohr, I. Penner and C. Steiner. 2010. MS quality of life, depression and fatigue improve after mindfulness training. *Neurology* 75: 1141–9.

Guelpa, G. M. A. 1911. La lutte contre l'epilepsie par la desintoxication et par la reducation alimentaire. *Revue Therapeutique Medica-Chirugie* 78: 8–13.

Gutas, D. 1998. *Greek Thought, Arabic Culture: The Graeco-Arabic Translation Movement in Baghdad and Early 'Abbāsid Society (2nd–4th/8th–10th Centuries)*. London: Routledge.

Gutel, N. 1998. *Changes in Reality in Jewish Law*. Jerusalem: Yachdov.

Guthrie, S. E. 1993. *Faces in the Clouds: A New Theory of Religion*. Oxford: Oxford University Press.

Hacker, P. M. S. 2007. *Human Nature: The Categorial Framework*. Hoboken, NJ: Blackwell.

Hacker, P. M. S. 2013. *The Intellectual Powers: A Study of Human Nature*. Hoboken, NJ: Wiley-Blackwell.

Hacker, P. M. S. 2018. *The Passions: A Study of Human Nature*. Hoboken, NJ: Blackwell.

Hacking, I. 2006. *The Emergence of Probability: A Philosophical Study of Early Ideas about Probability, Induction and Statistical Inference*. Cambridge: Cambridge University Press.

Hackney, M. E. and G. M. Earhart. 2008. Tai Chi improves balance and mobility in people with Parkinson disease. *Gait and Posture* 28: 456–60.

Halevy, A., and B. Brody. 1993. Brian death: reconciling definitions, criteria, and tests. *Annals of Internal Medicine* 119: 519.

Halperin, M., ed. 2007. *Determining the Moment of Death*. 2nd edn. Jerusalem: Schleisinger Research Institute for Medicine and Jewish Law.

Hamarneh, S. K. 1997. Al-Tabarī. In *Encyclopaedia of the History of Science, Technology, and Medicine in Non-Western Cultures*, ed. H. Selin, 930. Dordrecht: Springer Netherlands.

Han, S., L. Mao, X. Gu, Y. Zhu, J. Ge and Y. Ma. 2008. Neural consequences of religious belief on self-referential processing. *Social Neuroscience* 3: 1–15. doi:10.1080/17470910701469681.

Harlow, J. M. 1868. Recovery from the passage of an iron bar through the head. *Publications of the Massachusetts Medical Society* 2: 327–47.

Hart, D. B. 2013. *The Experience of God: Being, Consciousness, Bliss*. Providence, RI: Yale University Press.

Hart, J., H. Kanner, R. Gilboa-Mayo, O. Haroeh-Peer, N. Rozenthul-Sorokin and R. Eldar. 2004. Tai Chi Chuan practice in community-dwelling persons after stroke. *International Journal of Rehabilitation Research* 27: 303–4.

Hartman, A. L., J. E. Rubenstein and E. H. Kossoff. 2013. Intermittent fasting: a 'new' historical strategy for controlling seizures? *Epilepsy Research* 104: 275–9.

Haslam, C., A. Holme, S. A. Haslam, A. Lyer, J. Jetten and W. H. Williams. 2008. Maintaining group memberships: social identity continuity predicts well-being after stroke. *Neuropsychological Rehabilitation* 18: 671–91.

Hasson, U., J. P. Simmons and A. Todorov. 2005. Believe it or not. *Psychological Science* 16: 566–71.

Hayton, S., L. S. Boylan, S. C. Jackson, and O. Devinsky. 2002. Religion and epilepsy. Paper presented at the annual meeting of the American Academy of Neurology, Denver, CO.

Hayward, R. D., A. D. Owen, H. G. Koenig, D. C. Steffens and M. E. Payne. 2011. Associations of religious behavior and experience with extent of regional atrophy in the orbitofrontal cortex during older adulthood. *Religion, Brain and Behavior* 1: 103–18.

Headache Classification Committee of the International Headache Classification. 1988. Classification and diagnostic criteria for headache disorders, cranial neuralgias and facial pain. *Cephalalgia* 8, Suppl. 7: 1–96.

Headache Classification Committee of the International Headache Society. 2013. The International Classification of Headache Disorders, 3rd edition (beta version). *Cephalalgia* 33, no. 9: 629–808.

Headache Classification Subcommittee of the International Headache Society. 2004. The International Classification of Headache Disorders. *Cephalalgia* 24, Suppl. 1: 1–160.

Heidegger, M. 1980. *Being and Time*. Trans. J. Macquarrie and E. Robinson. Oxford: Blackwell.

Herrag, M., S. Lahmiti and A. A. Yazidi. 2010. Ramadan: a different side of the emergencies? *African Health Sciences* 10: 215–16.

Hershler, M. 1981. Obligation to save the sick and individuals in danger. In *Halakha and Medicine*, ed. M. Hershler, 2:27–70. Jerusalem: Regensberg Institute.

Heywood, B. T. 2010. Meant to be: how religious beliefs, cultural religiosity, and impaired theory of mind affect the implicit bias to think teleologically. Doctoral dissertation, Queens University, Belfast.

Heywood, B. T., and J. M. Bering. 2013. Meant to be: how religious beliefs and cultural religiosity affect the implicit bias to think teleologically. *Religion, Brain, and Behavior* 41: 183–201.

Hill, D. R., and M. A. Persinger. 2003. Application of transcerebral, weak (1 microT) complex magnetic fields and mystical experiences: are they generated by field-induced dimethyltryptamine release from the pineal organ? Percept. *Motor Skills* 97: 1049–50.

Hill, P. C., and R. W. Hood Jr. 1999. *Measures of Religiosity*. Birmingham, AL: Religious Education Press.

Hill, P., and N. Gibson. 2008. Whither the roots? Achieving conceptual depth in psychology of religion. *Archive for the Psychology of Religion* 30: 19–35.

Hill, P., and R. Hood Jr. 1999. *Measures of Religiosity*. Birmingham, AL: Religious Education Press.

Hodges, J., and S. Oxbury. 1990. Persistent memory impairment following transient global amnesia. *Journal of Clinical and Experimental Neuropsychology* 12: 904–20.

Holmes, G. 1945. The organization of the visual cortex in man. *Proceedings of the Royal Society, Series B* 132: 348–61.

Hoogerwerf, A. E. W., Y. Bol, J. Lobbestael, R. Hupperts and C. M. van Heugten. 2017. Mindfulness-based cognitive therapy for severely fatigued multiple sclerosis patients: a waiting list controlled study. *Journal of Rehabilitation Medicine* 49: 497–504.

Hornsby, J. 2000. Personal and sub-personal: a defence of Dennett's early distinction. *Philosophical Explorations* 3(1): 6–24.

Hornstein, G. A. 2009. *Agnes's Jacket: A Psychologist's Search for the Meanings of Madness*. Emmaus, PA: Rodale Books.

Howden, J. C. 1873. The religious sentiment in epileptics. *Journal of Mental Science* 18: 482–97.

Hughes, J. C. 2001. Views of the person with dementia. *Journal of Medical Ethics* 27: 86–91.

Hughes, J. C. 2011. A situated embodied view of the person with dementia: where does the spiritual come in? In *Spirituality and Personhood in Dementia*, ed. A. Jewell, 198–206. London: Jessica Kingsley.

Hughes, J. C. 2011. *Alzheimer's and Other Dementias: The Facts*. Oxford: Oxford University Press.

Hughes, J. C. 2011. *Thinking through Dementia*. Oxford: Oxford University Press.

Hughes, J. C. 2013. Dementia is dead, long live ageing: philosophy and practice in connection with 'dementia'. In *Oxford Handbook of Philosophy and Psychiatry*, eds. K. W. M. Fulford, M. Davies, R. G. T. Gipps, G. Graham, J. Z. Sadler, G. Stanghellini and T. Thornton, 835–50. Oxford: Oxford University Press.

Hughes, J. R. 2005. The idiosyncratic aspects of the epilepsy of Fyodor Dostoevsky. *Epilepsy and Behavior* 7: 531–8.

Hunkin, N., and A. Parkin. 1995. The method of vanishing cues: an evaluation of its effectiveness in teaching memory-impaired individuals. *Neuropsychologia* 33: 1255–79.

Hunsberger, B., B. McKenzie, M. Pratt and S. M. Pancer. 1993. Religious doubt: a social-psychological analysis. *Research in the Social Scientific Study of Religion* 5: 27–51.

Hutto, D. 2007. *Folk Psychological Narratives*. Cambridge, MA: MIT Press.

Hutto, D. and E. Myin. 2012. *Radicalizing Enactivism: Basic Minds without Content*. Cambridge, MA: MIT Press.

Hwang, I., R. Song, S. Ahn, M. Lee, P. Wayne and M. K. Sohn. 2017. Exploring the adaptability of Tai Chi to stroke rehabilitation. *Rehabilitation Nursing*. Published online. doi:10.1097/rnj.0000000000000110.

Inzlicht, M., I. McGregor, J. B. Hirsh and K. Nash. 2009. Neural markers of religious conviction. *Psychological Science* 20: 385–92.

Inzlicht, M., A. M. Tullett and M. Good. 2011. The need to believe: a neuroscience account of religion as a motivated process. *Religion, Brain, and Behavior* 1: 192–212.

IPDGC. 2011. A two-stage meta-analysis identifies several new loci for Parkinson's disease. *PLoS Genetics* 7.

Irish, M., O. Piguet and J. R. Hodges. 2011. Self-projection and the default network in frontotemporal dementia. *Nature Reviews Neurology* 8: 152–61. www.ncbi.nlm.nih.gov/pubmed/22331029.

Ishihara, L., and C. Brayne. 2006. What is the evidence for a premorbid parkinsonian personality: a systematic review. *Movement Disorders* 21: 1066–72.

Jack, A. I., J. P. Friedman, R. E. Boyatzis and S. N. Taylor. 2016. Why do you believe in God? Relationships between religious belief, analytic thinking, mentalizing and moral concern. *PloS ONE* 11, no. 3: e0149989.

Jack, C. R., Jr., M. Albert, D. S. Knopman, G. M. McKhann, R. A. Sperling, M. C. Carrillo et al. 2011. Introduction to revised criteria for the diagnosis of Alzheimer's disease: National Institute on Aging and the Alzheimer's Association workgroup. *Alzheimer's and Dementia* 7: 256–62.

Jackson, A., and J. B. Zimmermann. 2012. Neural interfaces for the brain and spinal cord – restoring motor function. *Nature Reviews Neurology* 8: 690–9.

Jacobson, N. S. and P. Truax. 1991. Clinical significance: A statistical approach to defining meaningful change in psychotherapy research. *Journal of Consulting and Clinical Psychology* 59: 12–19.

Jahnke, R., L. Larkey, C. Rogers, J. Etnier and F. Lin. 2012. A comprehensive review of health benefits of Qi Gong and Tai Chi. *American Journal of Health Promotion* 24: e1–e25.

Jahromi, S. R., M. A. Sahraian, F. Ashtari, H. Ayromlou, M. Etemadifar, M. Ghaffarpour, E. Mohammadianinejad, S. Nafissi, A. Nickseresht, V. Shaygannejad, M. Togha, H. R. Torabi and S. Ziaie. 2014. Islamic fasting and multiple sclerosis. *BMC Neurology* 14: 56.

Jakobovits, I. 1975. *Jewish Medical Ethics*. 2nd edn. New York: Bloch.

James, W. 1882. Subjective effects of nitrous oxide. *Mind* 7: 186–208.

James, W. 1902. *The Varieties of Religious Experience*. New York: Longmans, Green.

Jankovic, J., and W. Poewe. 2012. Therapies in Parkinson's disease. *Current Opinion in Neurology* 25: 433–47.

Jansen, K. 1990. Neuroscience and the near-death experience: roles for the NMDA-PCP receptor, the sigma receptor and the endopsychosins. *Medical Hypotheses* 31: 25–9.

Jaworski, W. 2011. *Philosophy of Mind: A Comprehensive Introduction*. Hoboken, NJ: Wiley-Blackwell.

Jaynes, J. 1976. *The Origin of Consciousness in the Breakdown of the Bicameral Mind*. Boston: Houghton Mifflin.

Jeeves, M. B., and W. S. Brown. 2009. *Neuroscience, Psychology and Religion: Illusions, Delusions, and Realities about Human Nature*. West Conshohocken, PA: Templeton Foundation Press.

Jilek-Aall, L. 1999. Morbus sacer in Africa: some religious aspects of epilepsy in traditional cultures. *Epilepsia* 40: 382–6.

Johansson, B., H. Bjhur and L. Rönnbäck. 2012. Mindfulness-based stress reduction (MBSR) improves long-term mental fatigue after stroke and traumatic brain injury. *Brain Injury* 26: 1621–8.

Johnson, M. and M. de Haan. 2015. *Developmental Cognitive Neuroscience: An Introduction*. 4th edn. Hoboken, NJ: Wiley-Blackwell.

Johnson, M. L. 2007. *The Meaning of the Body: Aesthetics of Human Understanding*. Chicago: University of Chicago Press.

Johnson, M. W., R. A. Sewell and R. R. Griffiths. 2012. Psilocybin dose-dependently causes delayed, transient headaches in healthy volunteers. *Drug and Alcohol Dependency* 123: 132–40.

Johnstone, B., A. Bodling, D. Cohen, S. E. Christ and A. Wegrzyn. 2012. Right parietal lobe-related 'selflessness' as the neurophysiological basis of spiritual transcendence. *International Journal for the Psychology of Religion* 22: 267–84. doi:10.1080/10508619.2011.657524.

Johnstone, B., and B. A. Glass. 2008. Support for a neuropsychological model of spirituality in persons with traumatic brain injury. *Zygon* 43: 861–74. doi:10.1111/j.1467-9744.2008.00964.x.

Johnstone, B., D. P. Yoon, K. L. Franklin, L. Schopp and J. Hinkebein. 2009. Re-conceptualizing the Factor Structure of the Brief Multidimensional Measure of Religiousness/Spirituality. *Journal of Religion and Health* 48: 146–63. doi:10.1007/s10943-008-9179-9.

Jolley, D., S. M. Benbow, M. Grizzell, S. Willmott, S. Bawn and P. Kingston. 2010. Spirituality and faith in dementia. *Dementia* 9: 311–25.

Jolley, D., and N. Moreland. 2011. Dementia care: spiritual and faith perspectives. *Nursing and Residential Care* 13: 388–91.

Joseph, R. 2001. The limbic system and the soul: evolution and neuroanatomy of religious experience. *Zygon* 36: 105–36.

Kabat-Zinn, J. 2003. Mindfulness-based interventions in context: past, present and future. *Clinical Psychology: Science and Practice* 10: 144–56.

Kahneman, D., and A. Tversky. 1973. On the psychology of prediction. *Psychological Review* 80: 237–51.

Kaltenmark, M. 1969. *Lao Tzu and Taoism.* Trans. Roger Greaves. Stanford, CA: Stanford University Press.

Kaplan-Solms, K. and M. Solms. 2000. *Clinical Studies in Neuro-Psychoanalysis: An Introduction to a Depth Neuropsychology.* London: Karnac.

Kapogiannis, D., A. K. Barbey, M. Su et al. 2009. Neuroanatomical variability of religiosity. *PLoS One* 4, no. 9: e7180. doi:10.1371/journal.pone.0007180.

Kapogiannis, D., A. K. Barbey, M. Su, F. Krueger and J. Grafman. 2009a. Neuroanatomical variability religiosity. *PLoS One* 4(9): e7180.

Kapogiannis, D., A. K. Barbey, M. Su, G. Zamboni, F. Krueger and J. Grafman. 2009b. Cognitive and neural foundations of religious belief. *Proceedings of the National Academy of Sciences of the United States of America* 106: 4876–81. doi:10.1073/pnas.0811717106.

Kapogiannis, D., G. Deshpande, F. Krueger, M. P. Thornburg and J. H. Grafman. 2014. Brain networks shaping religious belief. *Brain Connectivity* 4: 70– 79. doi:10.1089/brain.2013.0172.

Kapuscinski, A., and K. Masters. 2010. The current status of measures of spirituality: a critical review of scale development. *Psychology of Religion and Spirituality* 2: 191–205.

Kass, L. R. 1971. Death as an event: a commentary on Robert Morison. *Science* 173: 698–702.

Keast, K., C. Leskovar and R. Brohm. 2010. A systematic review of spirituality and dementia in LTC. *Annals of Long-Term Care* 18: 41–7.

Kelemen, D. 2004. Are children 'intuitive theists'? *Psychological Science* 15: 295–301.

Kelemen, D., and E. Rosset. 2009. The human function compunction: teleological explanation in adults. *Cognition* 111: 138–43.

Kenuk, S., and H. Porter. 2017. The outcomes for mindfulness-based interventions for adults who have experienced a traumatic brain injury: a systematic review of the literature. *American Journal of Recreation Therapy* 16.

Kerndt, P. R., J. L. Naughton, C. E. Driscoll and D. A. Loxterkamp. 1982. Fasting: the history, pathophysiology and complications. *Western Journal of Medicine* 137: 379–99.

Kerns, J. G., J. D. Cohen, A. W. MacDonald, R. Y. Cho, V. A. Stenger and C. S. Carter. 2004. Anterior cingulate conflict monitoring and adjustments in control. *Science* 303: 1023–6.

Khattab, E., I. H. Mahmood and E. T. Abdul-Jabbar. 2007. Can epileptic patients on carbamazepine safely fast Ramadan? *JIMA* 38486: 156–60.

Khwaja, G. A. S., and N. Chadhury. 2007. Epilepsy and religion. *Annals of the Indian Academy of Neurology* 10: 165–8.

Kidd, I. J. 2013. A phenomenological challenge to 'enlightened secularism'. *Religious Studies* 49: 377–98.

Kidd, I. J. 2013. Is naturalism bleak? *Environmental Values* 22: 689–702.

Kidd, I. J. 2014. Emotion, religious practice, and cosmopolitan secularism. *Religious Studies* 50: 139–56.

Kidd, I. J. 2018. Spiritual exemplars. *International Journal of Philosophy and Theology* 79: 420–4.

Kirkpatrick, L. A. 2013. Evolutionary psychology as a foundation for the psychology of religion. In *The Psychology of Religion: A Multidisciplinary Approach*, ed. R. Paloutzian and C. Park, 118–37. New York: Guilford Press.

Kitwood, T. 1997. *Dementia Reconsidered: The Person Comes First.* Buckingham, UK: Open University Press.

Knutsdottir, S., H. Thorisdottir, K. Sigvaldason, H. Jonsson Jr., A. Bjornsson and P. Ingvarsson. 2012. Epidemiology of traumatic spinal cord injuries in Iceland from 1975 to 2009. *Spinal Cord* 50: 123–6.

Kolahkaj, B., and F. Zargar. 2015. Effect of mindfulness-based stress reduction on anxiety, depression and stress in women with multiple sclerosis. *Nursing and Midwifery Studies* 4: e29655.

Koons, R. and G. Bealer. 2010. *The Waning of Materialism.* Oxford: Oxford University Press.

Kordower, J. H., C. W. Olanow, H. B. Dodiya et al. 2013. Disease duration and the integrity of the nigrostriatal system in Parkinson's disease. *Brain* 136: 2419–31.

Koushali, A. N., Z. Hajiamini, A. Ebadi, N. Bayat and F. Khamseh. 2013. Effect of Ramadan fasting on emotional reactions in nurses. *Iranian Journal of Nursing and Midwifery Research* 18: 232–6.

Kousta, S. T., G. Vigliocco, D. P. Vinson et al. 2011. The representation of abstract words: why emotion matters. *Journal of Experimental Psychology – General* 140: 14–34.

Kumar, N., and S. Jivan. 2007. Ramadan and eyedrops: the Muslim perspective. *Ophthalmology* 114: 2356–60.

Kumar, N., S. Jivan and J. Buchan. 2008. Compliance with prescribed treatment during Ramadan. *Clinical and Experimental Ophthalmology* 36: 699.

Landes, D. J. 2010. *Traditional Struggles: Studying, Deciding and Performing the Law at the Rabbi Isaac Elchanan Theological Seminary*. Princeton, NJ: Princeton University Press.

Lang, A. E., and J. A. Obeso. 2004. Challenges in Parkinson's disease: restoration of the nigrostriatal dopamine system is not enough. *The Lancet Neurology* 3: 309–16.

Latifynia, A., M. Vojgani, T. Abofazeli and H. Jafarieh. 2007. Circulating immune complex during Ramadan. *Journal of Ayub Medical College Abbottabad* 19, no. 2: 15–18.

Latifynia, A., M. Vojgani, M. J. Gharagozlou and R. Sharifian. 2009. Neutrophil function (innate immunity) during Ramadan. *Journal of Ayub Medical College Abbottabad* 21, no. 4: 111–15.

Laures-Gore, J. and R. Shisler Marshall. 2016. Mindfulness meditation in aphasia: a case report. *NeuroRehabilitation* 38: 321–9.

Lawrence, R. M. 2003. Aspects of spirituality in dementia care: when clinicians tune into silence. *Dementia* 2: 393–402.

Lawrence, R. M. 2007. Dementia: a personal legacy beyond word. *Mental Health Religion and Culture* 10: 553–62.

Lazaridou, A., P. Philbrook and A. A. Tzika. 2013. Yoga and mindfulness as therapeutic interventions for stroke rehabilitation: a systematic review. *Evidence-Based Complementary and Alternative Medicine* 2013: 357108.

Le, C., and D. H. Silverman. 2011. Neuroimaging and EEG-based explorations of cerebral substrates for suprapentasensory perception: a critical appraisal of recent experimental literature. *Psychiatry Research* 194: 105–10.

LeDoux, J. 2003. The emotional brain, fear, and the amygdalea. *Cellular and Molecular Neurobiology* 23: 727–38.

LeDoux, J. 2014. Coming to terms with fear. *PNAS* 111: 2876.

Lee, B. 2000. *Striking Thoughts: Bruce Lee's Wisdom for Daily Living*. New York: Tuttle.

Lehmann, D., et al. 2001. Brain sources of EEG gamma frequency during volitionally meditation-induced, altered states of consciousness, and experience of the self. *Psychiatry Research* 108: 111–21.

Leigh, R. J., and D. Zee. 2015. *The Neurology of Eye Movements*. 5th edn. Oxford: Oxford University Press.

Lempert, T., M. Bauer and D. Schmidt. 1994. Syncope and near-death experience. *Lancet* 344: 829–30.

Leuba, J. H. 1925. *The Psychology of Religious Mysticism*. London: Kegan Paul, Trench, Trubner.

L'Hermitte, J. 1922. Syndrome de la calotte peduncle cerebral: Les troubles psycholo-sensoriels dans les lesions du mesocaphale. *Review of Neurology (Paris)* 38: 1359–65.

Li, F., P. Harmer, K. J. Fitzgerald, E. Eckstrom, R. Stock, J. Galver, G. Maddalozzo and S. S. Batya. 2012. Tai Chi and postural stability in patients with Parkinson's disease. *New England Journal of Medicine* 366: 511–19.

Lichtenstein, A. 1975. Does Jewish tradition recognize an ethic independent of Halacha. In *Modern Jewish Ethics*, ed. M. Fox, 52–88. Columbus: University of Ohio.

Liddle, P. F., K. J. Friston, C. D. Frith et al. 1992. Patterns of cerebral blood flow in schizophrenia. *British Journal of Psychiatry* 160: 179–86.

Lindeman, M., and J. Lipsanen. 2016. Diverse cognitive profiles of religious believers and nonbelievers. *International Journal for the Psychology of Religion* 26, no. 3: 1–8.

Lippman, C. 1953. Hallucinations of physical duality in migraine. *American Journal of Psychiatry* 117: 345–50.

Little, J., and B. Lee. 2000. *Bruce Lee: A Warrior's Journey*. TV documentary. CA, USA: Warner Home Video.

Logothetis, N. K. 2003. The underpinnings of the BOLD functional magnetic resonance imaging signal. *Journal of Neuroscience* 23: 3963–71.

Logothetis, N. K. 2008. What we can do and what we cannot do with fMRI. *Nature* 453: 869–78. doi:10.1038/nature06976.

Lombrozo, T., D. Kelemen and D. Zaitchik. 2007. Inferring design: evidence of a preference for teleological explanations in patients with Alzheimer's disease. *Psychological Science* 18: 999–1006.

Long, J. 2010. *Evidence of the Afterlife*. New York: Harper One.

Loprenzi, C., A. Serretti, L. Mandelli, V. Tubazio, C. Ploia and E. Smeraldi. 2005. 5-HT 1A polymorphisms and self-transcendence in mood disorders. *American Journal of Medical Genetics, Part B* 137: 33–5.

Lorberbaum, M. 2001. *Politics and the Limits of Law: Secularizing the Political in Medieval Jewish Thought*. Stanford, CA: Stanford University Press.

Lowe, E. J. 1995. There are no easy problems of consciousness. *Journal of Consciousness Studies* 2: 266–71.

Lu, J., D. Sherman, M. Devor and C. Saper. 2006. A putative flip-flop switch for control of REM sleep. *Nature* 441: 589–94.

Luaute, J., D. Maucort-Boulch, L. Tell, F. Quelard, T. Sarraf, J. Iwaz et al. 2010. Long-term outcomes of chronic minimally conscious and vegetative states. *Neurology* 75: 246–52.

Luhrmann, T. 2012. *When God Talks Back: Understanding the American, Evangelical Relationship with God*. New York: Vintage Books.

Lundgren, T., J. Dahl, N. Yardi and L. Melin. 2008. Acceptance and commitment therapy and yoga for drug-refractory epilepsy: a randomized controlled trial. *Epilepsy and Behaviour* 13: 102–8.

Luria, A. R. 1975. *The Man with a Shattered World*. Harmondsworth, UK: Penguin Books.

Lynton, H., B. Kligler and S. Shiflett. 2007. Yoga in stroke rehabilitation: a systematic review and results of a pilot study. *Topics in Stroke Rehabilitation* 14, no. 4: 1–8.

Lyu, D., X. Lyu, Y. Zhang, Y. Ren, F. Yang, L. Zhou, Y. Zou and Z. Li. 2018. Tai Chi for stroke rehabilitation: a systematic review and meta-analysis of randomized controlled trials. *Frontiers in Physiology* 9: 983. doi:10.3389/fphys.2018.00983.

MacDonald, D. A. 2000. Spirituality: description, measurement and relation to the five factor theory of personality. *Journal of Personality* 68: 153–97.

Macintyre, A. 1999. *Dependent Rational Animals*. Chicago: Open Court.

MacKay, D. M. 1991. *Behind the Eye*. Hoboken, NJ: Basil Blackwell.

MacLean, K. A., M. W. Johnson and R. R. Griffiths. 2011. Mystical experiences occasioned by the hallucinogen psilocybin lead to increases in the personality domain of openness. *Journal of Psychopharmacology* 25: 1453–61.

Mahta, D., T. Klengal, K. Conneely, A. Smith, A. Altman et al. 2013. Childhood maltreatment is associated with distinct genomic and epigenetic profiles in post-traumatic stress disorder. *Proceedings of the National Academy of Sciences of the United States of America* 110: 8302–7.

Maij, D. L. R., F. van Harreveld, W. Gervais, Y. Schrag, C. Mohr and M. van Elk. 2017. Mentalizing skills do not differentiate believers from non-believers but credibility enhancing displays do. *PLoS ONE* 12, no. 8: e0182764.

Mandelbaum, E. 2014. Thinking is believing. *Inquiry* 57: 55–96.

Margolis, S. A., and R. L. Reed. 2004. Effect of religious practices of Ramadan on sleep and perceived sleepiness of medical students. *Teaching and Learning in Medicine* 16: 145–9.

Marsh, M. N. 2010. *Out-of-Body and Near-Death Experiences: Brain-State Phenomena or Glimpses of Immortality?* Oxford: Oxford University Press.

Marsh, M. N. 2013. Near-Death and Out-of-Body Experiences. In *The Springer Encyclopedia of Sciences and Religions*, ed. A. Runehov and L. Oviedo, 1422–33. Berlin: Springer.

Marsh, M. N. 2015. Hey! What's that gorilla doing over there? The illusory-hallucinatory nature of everyday living. *European Review* 23: 455–72.

Marsh, M. N. 2015. The near-death experience: a reality check? *Humanities* 5: 1–25.

Marsh, M. N. 2018. The phenomenology of near-death and out-of-body experiences: no heavenly excursion for the soul? In *The Blackwell Companion to Substance Dualism*, ed. J. Loose, A. Mengue and J. P. Moreland, 247–66. Chichester, UK: Wiley-Blackwell.

Martin, R. C. 1980. The role of the Mu'tazilah in formulating the doctrine of the apologetic miracle. *Journal of Near Eastern Studies* 39: 175–89.

Mazzarella, E., R. Ramsey, M. Conson and A. Hamilton. 2013. Brain systems for visual perspective taking and action perception. *Social Neuroscience* 8: 248–67. www.ncbi.nlm.nih.gov/pubmed/23350907.

Mazzarin, C. M., S. R. Valderramas, F. M. de Paula, E. Tiepolo, L. Guérios, D. Parisotto and V. L. Israel. 2017. Effects of dance and of Tai Chi on functional mobility, balance, and agility in Parkinson disease. *Topics in Geriatric Rehabilitation* 33: 262–72.

McCabe, H. 1987. *God Matters*. London: Continuum.

McCauley, R. N. 2012. *Why Religion Is Natural and Science Is Not*. Oxford: Oxford University Press.

McCauley, R. 2013. *Why Religion Is Natural and Science Is Not*. Oxford: Oxford University Press.

McGrath, J. 1998. Fear following brain injury. Unpublished doctoral thesis, Oxford Brookes University.

McGrath, J. 2004. Beyond restoration to transformation: positive outcomes in the rehabilitation of acquired brain injury. *Clinical Rehabilitation* 18: 767–75.

McGrath, J., and L. Adams. 1999. Patient-centred goal planning: a systemic psychological therapy? *Topics in Stroke Rehabilitation* 6: 43–50.

McGrath, J., and A. Davis. 1992. Rehabilitation: where are we going and how do we get there? *Clinical Rehabilitation* 6: 255–335.

McGrath, J., J. Marks and A. Davis. 1995. Towards interdisciplinary rehabilitation: further developments at Rivermead Rehabilitation Centre. *Clinical Rehabilitation* 9: 320–6.

McHugh, L. and R. Wood. 2013. Stimulus over-selectivity in temporal brain injury: mindfulness as a potential intervention. *Brain Injury* 27: 1595–9.

Mcmillan, T., I. H. Robertson, D. Brock and L. Chorlton. 2002. Brief mindfulness training for attentional problems after traumatic brain injury: a randomised control treatment trial. *Neuropsychological Rehabilitation* 12: 117–25.

McNamara, P., ed. 2006. *Where God and Science Meet: How Brain and Evolutionary Studies Alter Our Understanding of Religion*. Westport, CT: Praeger.

McNamara, P. 2009. *The Neuroscience of Religious Experience*. Cambridge: Cambridge University Press.

McNamara, P. N.d. The god effect. *Aeon*. http://aeon.co/magazine/world-views/dopamine-marks-the-line-between-religious-believer-and-fanatic/.

McNamara, P., R. Durso and A. Brown. 2006. Religiosity in patients with Parkinson's disease. *Neuropsychiatric Disease and Treatment* 2: 341–8.

Merton, T. 1969. *The Way of Chuang Tzu*. New York: New Directions.

Meyerhof, M. 1931. `Alî at-Tabarî's 'Paradise of Wisdom', one of the oldest Arabic compendiums of medicine. *Isis* 16: 6–54.

Meyer-Lindenberg, A., J. Buckholtz, B. Kolachana et al. 2006. Neural mechanisms of genetic risk for impulsivity and violence in humans. *Proceedings of the National Academy of Sciences of the United States of America* 103: 6269–74.

Middleton, E., and M. Schwartz. 2012. Errorless learning in cognitive rehabilitation: a critical review. *Neuropsychological Rehabilitation* 22: 138–68.

Miller, B. L., J. Cummings, F. Mishkin, K. Boone, F. Prince, M. Ponton and C. Cotman. 1998. Emergence of artistic talent in frontotemporal dementia. *Neurology* 51: 978–82.

Miller, B. L., W. W. Seeley, P. Mychack, H. J. Rosen, I. Mena and K. Boone. 2001. Neuroanatomy of the self: evidence from patients with frontotemporal dementia. *Neurology* 57: 817–21. www.ncbi.nlm.nih.gov/pubmed/11552010.

Mills, N., and J. Allen. 2000. Mindfulness of movement as a coping strategy in multiple sclerosis: a pilot study. *General Hospital Psychiatry* 22: 425–31.

Mills, N., J. Allen and S. Carey-Morgan. 2000. Does Tai Chi/Qi Gong help patients with multiple sclerosis? *Journal of Bodywork and Movement Therapies* 4: 39–48.

Mittelstaedt, H. 1991. The role of the otoliths in the perception of the orientation of self and world to the vertical. *Zoologische Jahrbuch Physiol* 95: 419–25.

Moberg, D. 2002. Assessing and measuring spirituality: confronting dilemmas of universal and particular evaluative criteria. *Journal of Adult Development* 9: 47–60.

Moberg, D. O. 2005. Research in spirituality, religion, and aging. *Journal of Gerontology and Social Work* 45: 11–40.

Modestino, E. J., P. O'Toole and A. Reinhofer. 2016. Experiential and doctrinal religious knowledge categorization in Parkinson's disease: behavioral and brain correlates. *Frontiers in Human Neuroscience* 10: 113. doi:10.3389/fnhum.2016.00113.

Monod, S., M. Brennan, E. Rochat, E. Martin, S. Rochat and C. J. Büla. 2011. Instruments measuring spirituality in clinical research: a systematic review. *Journal of General Internal Medicine* 26: 1345–57. doi:10.1007/s11606-011-1769-7.

Moody, R. 1976. *Life after Life*. New York: Bantam Books.

Moody, R. 1977. *Reflections on Life after Life*. New York: Bantam Books.

Morison, R. S. 1971. Death: process or event? *Science* 173: 694–8.

Morse, M., with P. Perry. 1990. *Closer to the Light: Learning from the Near-Death Experiences of Children*. New York: Ivy Books.

Moscovitch, M. 1984. The sufficient conditions for demonstrating preserved memory in amnesia: a task analysis. In *The Neuropsychology of Memory*, ed. N. Butters and R. Squire, 104–14. New York: Guilford Press.

Mosek, A., and A. D. Korczyn. 1995. The Yom Kippur headache. *Neurology* 45: 1953–5.

Mosek, A., and A. D. Korczyn. 1999. Fasting headache, weight loss, and dehydration. *Headache* 39: 225–7.

Moser, P. 2010. *The Evidence for God: Religious Knowledge Reexamined*. Cambridge: Cambridge University Press.

Moses, N. 2011. *Really Dead? The Israeli Brain-Death Controversy, 1967–1986*. Israel: Naftali Moses.

Moustgaard, A., M. Bedard and M. Felteau. 2007. Mindfulness-based cognitive therapy (MBCT) for individuals who had a stroke: results from a pilot 90 study. *Journal of Cognitive Rehabilitation* 25: 4–10.

Mungas, D. 1982. Interictal behavior abnormality in temporal lobe epilepsy: a specific syndrome or nonspecific psychopathology? *Archives of General Psychiatry* 39: 108–11.

Muramoto, O. 2004. The role of the medial prefrontal cortex in human religious activity. *Medical Hypotheses* 62: 479–85.

Nachev, P. and P. Hacker. 2014. The neural antecedents to voluntary action: a conceptual analysis. *Cognitive Neuroscience* 5: 194.

Nadarevic, L., and E. Erdfelder. 2013. Spinoza's error: memory for truth and falsity. *Memory and Cognition* 41: 176–86.

Nagel, T. 2012. *Mind and Cosmos: Why the Materialist Neo-Darwinian Conception of Nature Is Almost Certainly False*. Oxford: Oxford University Press.

Nakhaee, N., K. Divsalar and N. Jadidi. 2009. Religious involvement and cigarette smoking among Iranian university students. *International Journal of Psychiatry and Medicine* 39: 189–98.

Nelson, K. 2012. *The Spiritual Doorway into the Brain*. New York: Plume Books.

Nematy, M., M. Alinezhad-Namaghi, M. M. Rashed, M. Mozhdehifard, S. S. Sajjadi, S. Akhlaghi, M. Sabery, S. A. Mohajeri, N. Shalaey, M. Moohebati and A. Norouzy. 2012. Effects of Ramadan fasting on cardiovascular risk factors: a prospective observational study. *Nutrition Journal* 11: 69.

Neppe, V., and C. Kaplan. 1988. Short-term treatment of atypical spells with carbamazepine. *Clinical Neuropharmacology* 11: 287–9.

Newberg, A., A. Alavi, M. Baime, M. Pourdehnad, J. Santanna and E. d'Aquili. 2001. The measurement of regional cerebral blood flow during the complex cognitive task of meditation: a preliminary SPECT study. *Psychiatry Research: Neuroimaging* 106: 113–22. www.sciencedirect.com/science/article/pii/S0925492701000749.

Newberg, A., M. Pourdehnad, A. Alavi and E. G. d'Aquili. 2003. Cerebral blood flow during meditative prayer: preliminary findings and methodological issues. *Perceptual and Motor Skills* 97: 625–30. www.amsciepub.com/doi/abs/10.2466/pms.2003.97.2.625.

Ni, X., S. Liu, F. Lu, X. Shi and X. Guo. 2014. Efficacy and safety of Tai Chi for Parkinson's disease: a systematic review and meta-analysis of randomized controlled trials. *PloS One*, June 13. https://doi.org/10.1371/journal.pone.0099377.

Nitsche, M. A., L. G. Cohen, E. M. Wassermann, A. Priori, N. Lang, A. Antal, W. Paulus, F. Hummel, P. S. Boggio, F. Fregni and A. Pascual-Leone. 2008. Transcranial direct current stimulation: state of the art 2008. *Brain Stimulation* 1: 206–23. doi:10.1016/j.brs.2008.06.004.

Nitsche, M. A., and W. Paulus. 2000. Excitability changes induced in the human motor cortex by weak transcranial direct current stimulation. *Journal of Physiology* 527: 633–9.

Nochi, M. 1997. Dealing with the 'void': traumatic brain injury as a story. *Disability and Society* 12: 533–55.

Nochi, M. 1998a. Struggling with the labelled self: people with traumatic brain injuries in social settings. *Qualitative Health Research* 8: 665–81.

Nochi, M. 1998b. 'Loss of self' in the narratives of people with traumatic brain injuries: a qualitative analysis. *Social Science and Medicine* 7: 869–78.

Nochi, M. 2000. Reconstructing self-narratives in coping with traumatic brain injury. *Social Science and Medicine* 51: 1795–1804.

Noë, A. 2009. *Out of Our Heads: Why You Are Not Your Brain, and Other Lessons from the Biology of Consciousness*. New York: Hill and Wang.

Nombela, C., P. J. Bustillo, P. F. Castell et al. 2011. Cognitive rehabilitation in Parkinson's disease: evidence from neuroimaging. *Frontiers in Neurology* 2: 82.

Nombela, C., T. Rittman and T. W. Robbins et al. 2011. Multiple modes of impulsivity in Parkinson's disease. *PLoS ONE* 9, no. 1: 0085747. doi:10.1371/journal.pone.0085747.

Noranzayan, A., and W. M. Gervais. 2013. The origins of religious disbelief. *Trends in Cognitive Sciences* 17: 20–5.

Normann, H. K., K. Asplund and A. Norberg. 1998. Episodes of lucidity in people with severe dementia as narrated by formal carers. *Journal of Advanced Nursing* 28: 1295–300.

Norouzy, A., M. Salehi, E. Philippou, H. Arabi, F. Shiva, S. Mehrnoosh, S. M. Mohajeri, S. A. Mohajeri, A. Motaghedi Larijani and M. Nematy. 2013. Effect of fasting in Ramadan on body composition and nutritional intake: a prospective study. *Journal of Human Nutrition and Diet* 26, Suppl. 1: 97–104.

Northoff, G., and F. Bermpohl. 2004. Cortical midline structures and the self. *Trends in Cognitive Sciences* 8: 102–7.

Northoff, G., A. Heinzel, M. de Greck, F. Bermpohl, H. Dobrowolny and J. Panksepp. 2006. Self-referential processing in our brain – a meta-analysis of imaging studies on the self. *Neuroimage* 31: 440–57.

Nuffield Council on Bioethics. 2009. *Dementia: Ethical Issues*. London: Nuffield Council on Bioethics. www.nuffieldbioethics.org/dementia.

O'Connell, K., J. Keaveney and R. Paul. 2013. A novel study of comorbidity between schizoaffective disorder and Geschwind syndrome. *Case Reports in Psychiatry* 2013: 486064.

Ogata, A., and T. Miyakawa. 1998. Religious experiences in epileptic patients with a focus on ictus-related episodes. *Psychiatry and Clinical Neuroscience* 52: 321–5.

Olanow, C. W., and J. A. Obeso. 2012. The significance of defining preclinical or prodromal Parkinson's disease. *Movement Disorders* 27: 666–9.

Oohashi, T., et al. 2002. Electroencephalographic measurement of possession trance in the field. *Clinical Neurophysiology* 113: 435–45.

Orenstein, E., A. Basilakos and R. Shisler Marshall. 2012. Effects of mindfulness meditation on three individuals with aphasia. *International Journal of Language and Communication Disorders* 47: 673–84.

Otto, R. 1917/1958. *Das Heliege/The Idea of the Holy*. Trans. J. W. Harvey. Oxford: Oxford University Press.

Otto, R. 1923. *The Idea of the Holy: An Inquiry into the Non-rational Factor in the Idea of the Divine and Its Relation to the Rational*. Trans. J. W. Harvey. London: H. Milford/Oxford University Press.

Owen, A. D., R. D. Hayward, H. G. Koenig, D. C. Steffens and M. E. Payne. 2011.

Religious factors and hippocampal atrophy in late life. *PLoS One* 6, no. 3: e17006. www.pubmedcentral.nih.gov/articlerender.fcgi?artid=3068149.

Pahnke, W. N. 1963. Drugs and mysticism: an analysis of the relationship between psychedelic drugs and the mystical consciousness. Doctoral dissertation, Harvard Univeristy.

Pahnke, W. N., and W. A. Richards. 1969/1990. Implications of LSD and experimental nysticism. In *Altered States of Consciousness*, ed. C. T. Tart, 399–428. New York: John Wiley.

Palhano-Fontes, F., K. C. Andrade, L. F. Tofoli, A. C. Santos, J. A. S. Crippa and J. E. C. Hallak et al. (2015). The psychedelic state induced by ayahuasca modulates the activity and connectivity of the default mode network. *PLoS One* 10: e0118143. doi:10.1371/journal.pone.0118143.

Pargament, K. 1997. *The Psychology of Religion and Coping: Theory, Research, Practice*. New York: Guilford Press.

Pargament, K. I., H. G. Koenig, N. Tarakeshwar et al. 2004. Religious coping methods as predictors of psychological, physical and spiritual outcomes among medically ill elderly patients: a two-year longitudinal study. *Journal of Health Psychology* 9: 713–30.

Park, C. L. 2005. Religion as a meaning making framework in coping with life stress. *Journal of Social Issues* 61: 707–29.

Park, C. L. 2013. The meaning making model: a framework for understanding meaning, spirituality, and stress-related growth in health psychology. *The European Health Psychologist* 15: 40–7.

Parkin, A., and N. Leng. 1993. *Neuropsychology of the Amnesic Syndrome*. Hove, UK: Erlbaum.

Pascual-Leone, A., V. Walsh and J. Rothwell. 2000. Transcranial magnetic stimulation in cognitive neuroscience – virtual lesion, chronometry, and functional connectivity. *Current Opinion in Neurobiology* 10: 232–7.

Pasricha, S., and I. Stevenson. 1986. Near death experiences in India. *Journal of Nervous and Mental Disorders* 174: 165–70.

Patel, T., A. Magdum and V. Ghura. 2012. Does fasting during Ramadan affect the use of topical dermatological treatment by Muslim patients in the UK? *Clinical and Experimental Dermatology* 37: 718–21.

Paterson, K. 2012. *It's about Time! Understanding the Experience of Speech Impairment*. Abingdon, UK: Routledge.

Penfield, W. 1955. The twenty-ninth Maudsley Lecture: the role of the temporal cortex in certain psychical phenomena. *Journal of Mental Science* 101: 451–65.

Penfield, W. 1958. Some mechanisms of consciousness discovered during electrical stimulation of the brain. *Proceedings of the National Academy of Sciences of the United States of America* 44: 51–66.

Penfield, W., and T. C. Erickson. 1941. *Epilepsy and Cerebral Localization*. Oxford: Charles C. Thomas.

Pennycook, G. 2014. Evidence that analytic cognitive style influences religious belief: comment on Razmyar and Reeve (2013). *Intelligence* 43: 21–6.

Pennycook, G., J. A. Cheyne, N. Barr, D. J. Koehler and J. A. Fugelsang. 2014a. Cognitive style and religiosity: the role of conflict detection. *Memory and Cognition* 42: 1–10.

Pennycook, G., J. A. Cheyne, N. Barr, D. J. Koehler and J. A. Fugelsang. 2014b. The role of analytic thinking in moral judgements and values. *Thinking and Reasoning* 20: 188–214.

Pennycook, G., J. A. Cheyne, D. J. Koehler and J. A. Fugelsang. 2013. Belief bias during reasoning among religious believers and skeptics. *Psychonomic Bulletin and Review* 20: 806–11.

Pennycook, G., J. A. Cheyne, P. Seli, D. J. Koehler and J. A. Fugelsang. 2012. Analytic cognitive style predicts religious and paranormal belief. *Cognition* 123: 335–46.

Pennycook, G., J. A. Fugelsang and D. J. Koehler. 2015. What makes us think? A three-stage dual-process model of analytic engagement. *Cognitive Psychology* 80: 34–72.

Pennycook, G., R. Ross, D. J. Koehler and J. A. Fugelsang. 2016. Atheists and agnostics are more reflective than religious believers: four empirical studies and a meta-analysis. *PLoS One* 11: e0153039.

Pennycook, G., D. Trippas, S. J. Handley and V. A. Thompson. 2014c. Base-rates: both neglected and intuitive. *Journal of*

Experimental Psychology: Learning, Memory, and Cognition 40: 544–54.

Persinger, M. A. 1984. People who report religious experiences may also display enhanced temporal-lobe signs. *Perceptual and Motor Skills* 58: 963–75.

Persinger, M. A. 1991. Preadolescent religious experience enhances temporal lobe signs in normal young adults. *Perceptual and Motor Skills* 72: 453–4.

Persinger, A. M., S. A. Koren and R. P. O'Connor. 2001. Geophysical variables and behavior: CIV. Power-frequency magnetic field transients (5 microtesla) and reports of haunt experiences within an electronically dense house. *Perceptual and Motor Skills* 92: 673–4.

Picard, F. 2013. State of belief, subjective certainty and bliss as a product of cortical dysfunction. *Cortex* 49: 2494–500.

Picard, F., and A. D. Craig. 2009. Ecstatic epileptic seizures: a potential window on the neural basis for human self-awareness. *Epilepsy and Behavior* 16: 539–46.

Picard, F., and F. Kurth. 2014. Ictal alterations of consciousness during ecstatic seizures. *Epilepsy and Behavior* 30: 58–61.

Picard, F., D. Scavarda and F. Bartolomei. 2013. Induction of a sense of bliss by electrical stimulation of the anterior insula. *Cortex* 49: 2935–7.

Pickut, B. A., W. Van Hecke, E. Kerckhofs, P. Mariën, S. Vanneste, P. Cras and P. M. Parizel. 2013. Mindfulness based intervention in Parkinson's disease leads to structural brain changes on MRI: a randomized controlled longitudinal trial. *Clinical Neurology and Neurosurgery* 115: 2419–25.

Pickut, B., S. Vanneste, M. A. Hirsch, W. Van Hecke, E. Kerckhofs, P. Marien et al. 2015. Mindfulness training among individuals with Parkinson's disease: neurobehavioral effects. *Parkinson's Disease*. Published online. doi:10.1155/2015/816404.

Plantinga, A. 2013. *Where the Conflict Really Lies: Science, Religion, and Naturalism*. Oxford: Oxford University Press.

Pointon, B. 2007. 'Who am I? – The search for spirituality in dementia. A family carer's perspective. In *Spirituality, Values and Mental Health: Jewels for the Journey*, ed. M. E. Coyte, P. Gilbert and V. Nicholls, 114–20. London: Jessica Kingsley.

Poletti, M., and U. Bonuccelli. 2012. Personality traits in patients with Parkinson's disease: assessment and clinical implications. *Journal of Neurology* 259: 1029–38.

Poletti, M, I. Enrici and M. Adenzato. 2012. Cognitive and affective theory of mind in neurodegenerative diseases: neuropsychological, neuroanatomical and neurochemical levels. *Neuroscience and Biobehavioral Reviews* 36: 2147–64.

Pormann, P. E., and E. Savage-Smith. 2007. *Medieval Islamic Medicine*. Washington, DC: Georgetown University Press.

Posner, J. B., C. B. Saper, N. D. Schiff and F. Plum. 2007. *Plum and Posner's Diagnosis of Stupor and Coma*. 4th edn. Ed. M. Sid Gilman. Oxford: Oxford University Press.

Postiglione, A., G. Milan, S. Pappatà, C. De Falco, F. Lamenza, V. Schiattarella, G. Gallotta, P. Sorrentino and S. Striano. 2008. Fronto-temporal dementia presenting as Geschwind's syndrome. *Neurocase* 14: 264–70.

Previc, F. H. 2006. The role of the extrapersonal brain systems in religious activity. *Consciousness and Cognition* 15: 500–39.

Prigatano, G. 1991. Disordered mind, wounded soul: the emerging role of psychotherapy in rehabilitation after brain injury. *Journal of Head Trauma Rehabilitation* 6: 1–10.

Puizillout, J., and A. Foutz. 1976. Vago-aortic nerves and REM sleep: evidence for a REM-triggering and a REM-maintenance factor. *Brain Research* 111: 181–4.

Qadeer, A. 2005. *History of Medicine and Medical Ethics*. Delhi: Rabbani.

Quinn, D., and K. Jones. 2012. Tai chi movement (TMW) and embodied mindfulness in mental and physical health. Inservice presentation for Herefordshire Primary Care Trust, UK.

Qujeq, D., K. Bijani, K. Kalavi, J. Mohiti and H. Aliakbarpour. 2002. Effects of Ramadan fasting on serum low-density and high-density lipoprotein-cholesterol concentrations. *Annals of Saudi Medicine* 22: 297–9.

Rabinovitch, N. L. 1973. *Probability and Statistical Inference in Ancient and Medieval Jewish Literature*. Toronto: University of Toronto Press.

Rabinovitz, N. A. 1998. *Scientific Assessment as the Basis for Halackhic Decisions:*

Investigations in the Works of the Rambam. Jerusalem: Yeshovat Birakt Moshe.

Rabinowitz, G. A. 1983. Gosses and defining the time of death. In *Halakha and Medicine*, ed. M. Hersler, 3:102–14. Jerusalem: Machon Regensberg.

Rabinowitz, G. A., and M. Keningsberg. 1971. The definition and determining the time of death from the perspective of Halakha. *Hadarom* 32: 59–76.

Radder, D. L., I. H. Sturkenboom, M. van Nimwegen, S. H. Keus, B. R. Bloem and N. M. de Vries. 2017. Physical therapy and occupational therapy in Parkinson's disease. *International Journal of Neuroscience* 1e14.

Rahman, F. 1987. *Health and Medicine in Islamic Tradition: Change and Identity*. New York: Crossroad.

Rajesh, B., D. Jayachandran, G. Mohandas and K. Radhakrishnan. 2006. A pilot study of a yoga meditation protocol for patients with medically refractory epilepsy. *Journal of Alternative and Complementary Medicine* 12: 367–71.

Ramachandran, V. S., et al. 1997. The neural basis of religious experiences. In *Society for Neuroscience Conference Abstracts*, 1316. New York.

Ramsey, W. M. 2007. *Representation Reconsidered*. Cambridge: Cambridge University Press.

Ratcliffe, M. 2004. Interpreting delusion. *Phenomenology and the Cognitive Sciences* 3 (1): 25–48.

Ratcliffe, M. 2005. The feeling of being. *Journal of Consciousness Studies* 12: 43–60.

Ratcliffe, M. 2006. Phenomenology, neuroscience and intersubjectivity. In *The Blackwell Companion to Phenomenology and Existentialism*, ed. H. Dreyfus and M. Wrathall, 327–43. Oxford: Blackwell.

Ratcliffe, M. 2007. *Rethinking Commonsense Psychology: A Critique of Folk Psychology, Theory of Mind and Simulation*. London: Palgrave.

Ratcliffe, M. 2008. *Feelings of Being: Phenomenology, Psychiatry, and the Sense of Reality*. Oxford: Oxford University Press.

Ratcliffe, M. 2009. Understanding existential changes in psychiatric illness: the indispensability of phenomenology. In *Psychiatry as Cognitive Neuroscience: Philosophical Perspectives*, ed. M. Broome and L. Bortolotti. New York: Oxford University Press.

Ratcliffe, M. 2012. The phenomenology of existential feeling. In *The Feeling of Being Alive*, ed. S. Marienberg and J. Fingerhut, 23–54. Berlin: de Gruyter.

Ratcliffe, M. 2013. Why mood matters. In *The Cambridge Companion to Heidegger's 'Being and Time'*, ed. M. Wrathall, 157–75. Cambridge: Cambridge University Press.

Ratcliffe, M. 2014. Evaluating existential despair. In *Emotion and Value*, ed. S. Roeser and C. Todd, 229–46. Oxford: Oxford University Press.

Ratcliffe, M. 2015. *Experiences of Depression: A Study in Phenomenology*. Oxford: Oxford University Press.

Rawlings, M. 1978. *Beyond Death's Door*. New York: Nelson.

Razmyar, S., and C. L. Reeve. 2013. Individual differences in religiosity as a function of cognitive ability and style. *Intelligence* 41: 667–73.

Reddish, P., P. Tok and R. Kundt. 2016. Religious cognition and behaviour in autism: the role of mentalizing. *International Journal for the Psychology of Religion* 26: 95–112.

Redgrave, P., M. Rodriguez, Y. Smith et al. 2010. Goal-directed and habitual control in the basal ganglia: implications for Parkinson's disease. *Nature Reviews Neuroscience* 11: 760–72.

Reeves, R. R., S. Kose and A. Abubakr. 2013. Temporal lobe discharges and glossolalia. *Neurocase* 20: 236–40.

Reichman, E. 1993. The Halakhic definition of death in light of medical history. *Torah U'Madda Journal* 4: 148–74.

Reifman, D. 2012. Ancient sources, modern problems: a methodological analysis of Rashi's position on brainstem death. *Tradition* 45, no. 4: 9–23.

Reynolds, E. H., and J. V. Kinnier Wilson. 2008. Psychoses of epilepsy in Babylon: the oldest account of the disorder. *Epilepsia* 49: 1488–90.

Richardson, R. 2007. *Evolutionary Psychology as Maladapted Psychology*. Cambridge, MA: MIT Press.

Ring, K. 1980. *Life at Death*. New York: Coward, McCann, and Geoghegan.

Ring, K. 1985. *Heading towards Omega*. New York: Morrow.

Rizvi, S. J., D. A. Pizzagalli, B. A. Sproule and S. H. Kennedy. 2016. Assessing anhedonia in depression: potentials and pitfalls. *Neuroscience and Biobehavioural Reviews* 65: 21–35.

Roberts, J. K., M. M. Robertson and M. R. Trimble. 1982. The lateralising significance of hypergraphia in temporal lobe epilepsy. *Journal of Neurology, Neurosurgery, and Psychiatry* 45: 131–8.

Roberts, R., N. Varney and J. Hulbert. 1990. The neuropathology of everyday life: the frequency of partial seizure symptoms among normals. *Neuropsychology* 4: 65–85.

Robinson, D., ed. 2014. *Scientism: The New Orthodoxy*. New York: Bloomsbury.

Robinson, R., K. Kubos, L. Starr, K. Rao and T. Price. 1984. Mood disorders in stroke patients: importance of lesion location. *Brain* 107: 81–93.

Rodin, E., and S. Schmaltz. 1984. The Bear–Fedio personality inventory and temporal lobe epilepsy. *Neurology* 34: 591–6.

Roewer, W., T. Kloss and K. Puschel. 1985. Long-term result and quality of life following preclinical cardiopulmonary resuscitation. *Anasthesie, Intensivtherapie, Notfallmedizin* 20: 244–50.

Roland, K. P. 2014. Applications of yoga in Parkinson's disease: a systematic literature review. *Journal of Parkinsonism and Restless Legs Syndrome* 4: 1–8.

Rose, G. 1992. *The Strategy of Preventive Medicine*. Oxford: Oxford University Press.

Rose, H. and S. Rose, eds. 2000. *Alas Poor Darwin: Arguments against Evolutionary Psychology*. New York: Crown.

Roseman, L., R. Leech, A. Feilding, D. J. Nutt and R. L. Carhart-Harris. 2014. The effects of psilocybin and MDMA on between-network resting state functional connectivity in healthy volunteers. *Frontiers in Human Neuroscience* 8: 204. doi:10.3389/fnhum.2014.00204.

Rosen, D. 1975. Suicide survivors: a follow-up study of persons who survived jumping from the Golden Gate and San Francisco-Oakland bridges. *Western Journal of Medicine* 122: 289–94.

Rosenfeld, A. 1970. The heart, the head and the halakhah. *New York State Journal of Medicine* 70: 2615–19.

Rowe, D. 1978. *The Experience of Depression*. London: Wiley.

Ruff, C. C., G. Ugazio and E. Fehr. 2013. Changing social norm compliance with noninvasive brain stimulation. *Science* 342: 482–4. doi:10.1126/science.1241399.

Russell, T. A. 2011. Body in mind training: mindful movement for severe and enduring mental illness. *British Journal of Wellbeing* 2, no. 4: 13–16.

Russell, T. A., and T. Tatton-Ramos. 2014. Body in mind training: mindful movement for the clinical setting. *Neuro-disability and Psychotherapy* 2: 108–36.

Saad, B., H. Azaizeh and O. Said. 2005. Tradition and perspectives of Arab herbal medicine: a review. *eCAM* 2: 475–9.

Saad, B., and O. Said. 2011. *Greco-Arab and Islamic Herbal Medicine: Traditional System, Ethics, Safety, Efficacy, and Regulatory Issues*. Hoboken, NJ: John Wiley.

Saadatnia, M., M. Etemadifar, F. Fatehi, F. Ashtari, V. Shaygannejad, A. Chitsaz and A. H. Maghzi. 2009. Short-term effects of prolonged fasting on multiple sclerosis. *European Neurology* 61: 230–2.

Saadatnia, M., M. Zare, F. Fatehi and A. Ahmadi. 2009. The effect of fasting on cerebral venous and dural sinus thrombosis. *Neurology Research* 31: 794–8.

Sa'adi, L. M. 1958. Glimpses into the history of Arabic medicine. *Bulletin of the Medical Library Association* 46: 206–18.

Sabat, S. R., and R. Harré. 1994. The Alzheimer's disease sufferer as a semiotic subject. *Philosophy, Psychiatry, and Psychology* 1: 145–60.

Sabom, M. 1982. *Recollections of Death*. New York: Harper Row.

Sabom, M. 1998. *Light and Death*. Grand Rapids, MI: Zondervan.

Sachdev, P. S. 2013. The DSM-5 approach to dementia. In *Oxford Textbook of Old Age Psychiatry*, 2nd edn., ed. T. Dening and A. Thomas, 377–81. Oxford: Oxford University Press.

Sacks, O. 1973. *Awakenings*. New York: Random House.

Sakr, A. H. 1975. Fasting in Islam. *Journal of the American Dietetic Association* 67: 17–21.

Saleh, S. A., T. A. El-Kemery, K. A. Farrag, M. R. Badawy, N. N. Sarkis, F. S. Soliman and

H. Mangoud. 2004. Ramadan fasting: relation to atherogenic risk among obese Muslims. *Journal of the Egyptian Public Health Association* 79: 461–83.

Sanchez, S., B. Sundermeier, K. Gray and R. Calin-Jagemanl. 2017. Direct replication of Gervais & Norenzayan (2012): no evidence that analytic thinking decreases religious belief. *Plos ONE* 12, no. 2: e0172636.

Sapp, S. 2010. Spiritual care of people with dementia and their carers. In *Supportive Care for the Person with Dementia*, eds. J. C. Hughes, M. Lloyd-Williams and G. A. Sachs, 199–206. Oxford: Oxford University Press.

Saroglou, V., O. Corneille and P. Cappellen. 2009. Speak, Lord, your servant is listening: religious priming activates submissive thoughts and behaviors. *International Journal for the Psychology of Religion* 19: 143–54.

Sarraf-Zadegan, N., M. Atashi, G. A. Naderi, A. M. Baghai, S. Asgary, M. R. Fatehifar, H. Samarian and M. Zarei. 2000. The effect of fasting in Ramadan on the values and interrelations between biochemical, coagulation and hematological factors. *Annals of Saudi Medicine* 20: 377–81.

Sartori, P. 2014. *The Wisdom of Near-Death Experiences*. London: Watkins.

Schaffer, O. 2013. *Crafting Fun User Experiences: A Method to Facilitate Flow*. Fairfield, IA: Human Factors International.

Schjødt, U., H. Stødkilde-Jørgensen, A. W. Geertz and A. Roepstorff. 2008. Rewarding prayers. *Neuroscience Letters* 443: 165–8.

Schjoedt, U. 2009. The religious brain: a general introduction to the experimental neuroscience of religion. *Method and Theory in the Study of Religion* 21: 301–39.

Schjoedt, U., H. Stødkilde-Jørgensen, A. W. Geertz et al. 2009. Highly religious participants recruit areas of social cognition in personal prayer. *Social Cognitive and Affective Neuroscience* 4: 199–207.

Schliermacher, F. 1799/1976. *On Religion: Speeches to Its Cultured Despisers*. Trans. Richard Crouter. Cambridge: Cambridge University Press.

Schmidt, A. A., K. K. Miller, M. Van Puymbroeck and N. Schalk. 2016. Feasibility and results of a case study of yoga to improve physical functioning in people with chronic traumatic brain injury. *Disability and Rehabilitation* 38: 914–20.

Schultz, W. 2002. Getting formal with dopamine and reward. *Neuron* 36: 241–63.

Schwanenflugel, P. J., K. K. Harnishfeger and R. W. Stowe. 1988. Context availability and lexical decisions for abstract and concrete words. *Journal of Memory and Language* 27: 499–520.

Sechehaye, M. 1970. *Autobiography of a Schizophrenic Girl*. New York: Signet.

Seiden, R. 1968. Where are they now? A follow-up study of suicide attempters from the Golden Gate Bridge. *Suicide and Life-Threatening Behavior* 8: 203–16.

Senders, A., D. Bourdette, D. Hanes, Y. Vijaysgree and L. Shinto. 2014. Perceived stress in multiple sclerosis: the potential role of mindfulness in health and well-being. *Journal of Evidence-Based Complementary and Alternative Medicine* 19: 104–11.

Shabtai, D. 2012. *Defining the Moment: Understanding Brain Death in Halakhah*. New York: Shoresh.

Shackman, A. J., T. V. Salomons, H. A. Slagter, A. S. Fox, J. J. Winter and R. J. Davidson. 2011. The integration of negative affect, pain and cogntive control in the cingulate cortex. *Nature Reviews Neuroscience* 12: 154–67.

Shanely, B. 2007. Beyond libertarianism and compatibilism: Thomas Aquinas on created freedom. In *Freedom and the Human Person*, ed. Richard Velkley, 70–89. Washington, DC: Catholic University of America Press.

Shanks, N. J., and D. Al-Kalai. 1984. Arabian medicine in the Middle Ages. *Journal of the Royal Society of Medicine* 77: 60–5.

Shapira, M. Y., M. Chelouche, R. Yanai, C. Kaner and A. Szold. 2001. Tai Chi Chuan practice as a tool for rehabilitation of severe head trauma: 3 case reports. *Archives of Physical Medicine and Rehabilitation* 82: 1283–5.

Shaw, A., S. Joseph and P. A. Linley. 2005. Religion, spirituality, and posttraumatic growth: a systematic review. *Mental Health, Religion, and Culture* 8: 1–11.

Sheehan, H. E., and S. J. Hussain. 2002. Unani Tibb: history, theory, and contemporary practice in South Asia. *Annals of the*

American Academy of Political and Social Science 583: 122–35.

Shehab, A., A. Abdulle, A. El Issa, J. Al Suwaidi and N. Nagelkerke. 2012. Favorable changes in lipid profile: the effects of fasting after Ramadan. *PLoS One* 7, no. 10: e47615.

Sheldin, M., D. Wallechininsky and S. Saunia. 1973. *Laughing Gas (Nitrous Oxide).* California: And/Or Press.

Shenhav, A., D. G. Rand and J. D. Greene. 2012. Divine intuition: cognitive style influences belief in god. *Journal of Experimental Psychology: General* 141: 423–8.

Shewmon, D. A. 1998. Chronic 'brain death': meta-analysis and conceptual consequences. *Neurology* 51: 1538–45.

Shisler-Marshall, R., J. Lores-Gore and K. Love. 2017. Brief mindfulness meditation group training in aphasia: exploring attention, language and psychophysiological outcomes. *International Journal of Language and Communication Disorders* 53: 40–54.

Shravat, A. 2014. The role of a Yoga group within a holistic rehabilitation setting for ABI using compassion focused therapy approach: a qualitative case illustration. *Neuro-disability and Psychotherapy* 2: 100–7.

Shreve-Neiger, A. K., and B. A. Edelstein. 2004. Religion and anxiety: a critical review of the literature. *Clinical Psychology Review* 24: 379–97.

Siddiqui, M. Z. 1928. *Firdausu'l Hikmat or Paradise of Wisdom of 'Ali b. Rabban-al-Tabari.* Berlin: Buch- u. Kunstdruckerei 'Sonne'.

Siegert, R., K. McPherson and W. Taylor. 2004. Toward a cognitive-affective model of goal setting in rehabilitation: is self-regulation theory a key step? *Disability and Rehabilitation* 26: 1175–83.

Silman, Y. D. 1999. *The Voice Heard at Sinai: Once or Ongoing?* Jerusalem: Magnes Press, Hebrew University.

Silverthorne, C., S. B. Khalsa, R. Gueth, N. DeAvilla and J. Pansini. 2012. Respiratory, physical, and psychological benefits of breath-focused yoga for adults with severe traumatic brain injury (TBI): a brief pilot study report. *International Journal of Yoga Therapy* 22: 47–51.

Simpson, R., J. Booth, M. Lawrence, S. Byrne, F. Mair and S. Mercer. 2014. Mindfulness based interventions in multiple sclerosis: a systematic review. *BMC Neurology* 14: 15.

Simpson, R., S. Byrne, K. Wood, F. S. Mair and S. W. Mercer. 2018. *Optimising Mindfulness-Based Stress Reduction for People with Multiple Sclerosis.* London: Sage.

Simpson, R., F. S. Mair and S. W. Mercer. 2017. Mindfulness-based stress reduction for people with multiple sclerosis – a feasibility randomised controlled trial. *BMC Neurology* 17: 141.

Smart, J. J. C. and J. J. Haldane. 2003. *Atheism and Theism.* 2nd edn. Hoboken, NJ: Blackwell.

Smith, A. 2009. Emotional empathy in autism spectrum conditions: Weak, intact, or heightened? *Journal of Autism and Developmental Disorders* 39: 1747–8.

Snowdon, D. A. 2003. Healthy aging and dementia: findings from the Nun Study. *Annals of Internal Medicine* 139: 450–4.

Snyder, R., and C. Snow. 1967. Fatal injuries resulting from extreme water impact. *Aerospace Medicine* 38: 779–83.

Soloveitchik, H. 2013. *Collected Essays.* Oxford: Littman Library of Jewish Civilization.

Spelke, E., A. Phillips and A. Woodward. 1995. Infants' knowledge of object motion and human action. In *Causal Cognition*, ed. D. Sperber, D. Premack and A. Premack, 44–78. Oxford: Clarendon Press.

Sperber, D. 1997. Intuitive and reflected beliefs. *Mind and Language* 12: 67–83.

Sperry, R. W. 1939. Action current study in movement coordination. *Journal of General Psychology* 20: 295–313.

Speth, J., C. Speth, M. Kaelen, A. M. Schloerscheidt, A. Feilding, D. J. Nutt and R. L. Carhart-Harris. 2016. Decreased mental time travel to the past correlates with default-mode network disintegration under lysergic acid diethylamide. *Journal of Psychopharmacology* 30: 344–53. doi:10.1177/0269881116628430.

Spetzler, R., M. Hadley, D. Rigamonti, P. Carter, P. Raudnes, S. Shedd et al. 1988. Aneurysms of the basilar artery treated with circulatory arrest, hypothermia, and barbiturate cerebral protection. *Journal of Neurosurgery* 68: 868–79.

Spillantini, M. G., M. L. Schmidt, V. M. Lee et al. 1997. Alpha-synuclein in Lewy bodies. *Nature* 388: 839–40.

Squire, L., B. Knowlton and G. Musen. 1993. The structure and organisation of memory. *Annual Review of Psychology* 44: 453–95.

Stadlan, N. 2010. Conceptual and logical problems arising from defining life by the presence or absence of circulation. *Meorot* 8: 1–11.

Stanley-Hermanns, M., and J. Engebretson. 2010. Sailing the stormy seas: the illness experience of persons with Parkinson's disease. *The Qualitative Report* 15: 340–69.

Stanovich, K. E., and R. F. West. 2003. Evolutionary versus instrumental goals: how evolutionary psychology misconceives human rationality. In *Evolution and the Psychology of Thinking: The Debate*, ed. D. E. Over, 1–53. New York: Psychological Press.

Starbuck, E. 1899. *The Psychology of Religion: An Empirical Study of the Growth of Religious Consciousness*. New York: Scribner.

Steinberg, A. 1998. Moment of death. In *Medicine and Jewish Law*, ed. Fred Rosen, 18–68. Lanham, MD: Jason Aronson.

Stender, J., O. Gosseries, M. A. Bruno, V. Charland-Verville, A. Vanhaudenhuyse, A. Demertzi et al. 2014. Diagnostic precision of PET imaging and functional MRI in disorders of consciousness: a clinical validation study. *Lancet* 384: 476–7.

Stern, M. B., A. Lang and W. Poewe. 2012. Toward a redefinition of Parkinson's disease. *Movement Disorders* 27: 54–60.

Sternberg, S. 1997. Review of 'Guide to Masechet Hullin and Masechet Bechorot' by I. M. Levinger. *Bekhol Derakhekha Daehu* 4: 81–102.

Stuckey, J. C., S. G. Post, S. Ollerton, S. J. Fallcreek and P. J. Whitehouse. 2002. Alzheimer's disease, religion, and the ethics of respect for spirituality: a community dialogue. *Alzheimer's Care Quarterly* 3: 199–207.

Sungkarat, S., S. Boripuntakul, N. Chattipakorn, K. Watcharasaksilp and S. R. Lord. 2017. Effects of tai chi on cognition and fall risk in older adults with mild cognitive impairment: a randomized controlled trial. *Journal of the American Geriatrics Society* 65: 721–7.

Surwillo, W. W., and D. P. Hobson. 1978. Brain electrical activity during prayer. *Psychological Reports* 43: 135–43.

Svedholm, A. M., and M. Lindeman. 2012. The separate roles of the reflective mind and involuntary inhibitory control in gatekeeping paranormal beliefs and the underlying intuitive confusions. *British Journal of Psychology* 104: 303–19.

Swanson, L. R. 2018. Unifying theories of psychedelic drug effects. *Frontiers in Pharmacology* 9: 172.

Swidler, L., and P. Mojzes. 2000. *The Study of Religion in an Age of Global Dialogue*. Philadelphia: Temple University Press.

Tabarī, Ai. S. R., A. N. Munzavī and M. I. Zākir. 2012. *Firdaws al-ḥikmah : Baḥr al-Manāfi' Va Shams al-Adāb*. 1391; repr., Tehran: Markaz-i Taḥqīqāt-i ⊠ibb-i Sunnatī va Mufradāt-i Pizishkī-i Dānishgāh-i 'Ulūm-i Pizishkī-i Shahīd Bihishtī.

Tagliazucchi, E., R. L. Carhart-Harris, R. Leech, D. Nutt and D. R. Chialvo. 2014. Enhanced repertoire of brain dynamical states during the psychedelic experience. *Human Brain Mapping* 35: 5442–56. doi:10.1002/hbm.22562.

Tagliazucchi, E., L. Roseman, M. Kaelen, C. Orban, S. Muthukumaraswamy and K. Murphy et al. 2016. Increased global functional connectivity correlates with LSD-induced ego dissolution. *Current Biology* 26: 1043–50. doi:10.1016/j.cub.2016.02.010.

Tallis, R. 2003. *The Hand: A Philosophical Inquiry into Human Being*. Edinburgh: Edinburgh University Press.

Tallis, R. 2004. *The Knowing Animal: A Philosophical Inquiry into Knowledge and Truth*. Edinburgh: Edinburgh University Press.

Tallis, R. 2005. *I Am: A Philosophical Inquiry into First-Person Being*. Edinburgh: Edinburgh University Press.

Tallis, R. 2011. *Aping Mankind: Neuromania, Darwinitis and the Misrepresentation of Humanity*. Durham, UK: Acumen.

Tang, V., W. S. Poon and P. Kwan. 2015. Mindfulness-based therapy for drug-resistant epilepsy: an assessor-blinded randomized trial. *Neurology* 85: 1100–7.

Tavee, J., M. Rensel, S. M. Planchon, R. S. Butler and L. Stone. 2011. Effects of meditation on pain and quality of life in multiple sclerosis and peripheral neuropathy. *International Journal of MS Care* 13: 163–8.

Taylor, C. 1989. *Sources of the Self*. Cambridge, MA: Harvard University Press.

Taylor, C. 2003. *Varieties of Religion Today: William James Revisited*. Cambridge, MA: Harvard University Press.

Taylor, E. and R. E. Taylor-Piliae. 2017. The effects of Tai Chi on physical and psychosocial function among persons with multiple sclerosis: a systematic review. *Complementary Therapies in Medicine* 31: 100–8.

Taylor, J. 2015. What did Jesus really look like? *Ancient Near East Today* 6: 1–16.

Taylor-Piliae, R. E., T. M. Hoke, J. T. Hepworth, L. D. Latt, B. Najafi et al. 2014. Effect of Tai Chi on physical function, fall rates and quality of life among older stroke survivors. *Archives of Physical Medicine and Rehabilitation* 95: 816–24.

Teasdale, J., and P. Barnard. 1993. *Affect, Cognition and Change*. Hillsdale, NJ: Erlbaum.

Tedeschi, R., and L. Calhoun. 1995. *Trauma and Transformation: Growing in the Aftermath of Suffering*. Thousand Oaks, CA: Sage.

Tedrus, G. M., L. C. Fonseca and G. C. Hoehr. 2014. Spirituality aspects in patients with epilepsy. *Seizure* 23: 25–8.

Teicher, M., and J. Samson. 2013. Childhood maltreatment and psychology: a case for ecophenotypic variants as clinically and neurobiologically distinct subtypes. *American Journal of Psychiatry* 170: 1124–33.

Tenke, C. E., J. Kayser, C. Svob, L. Miller, J. E. Alvarenga, K. Abraham, V. Warner, P. Wickramaratne, M. M. Weissman, and G. E. Bruder. 2017. Association of posterior EEG alpha with prioritization of religion or spirituality: A replication and extension at 20-year follow-up. *Biological Psychology* 124: 79–86.

Thompson, N. J., A. H. Patel, L. M. Selwa, S. C. Stoll, C. E. Begley, E. K. Johnson et al. 2015. Expanding the efficacy of Project UPLIFT: distance delivery of mindfulness-based depression prevention to people with epilepsy. *Journal of Consulting and Clinical Psychology* 83: 304–13.

Thonnard, M., V. Charland-Verville, S. Bredart et al. 2013. Characteristics of near-death experience memories as compared to real and imagined events memories. *PLOS One* 8: e57620.

Thornton, A. 2016. Varieties of animalism. *Philosophy Compass* 11: 515–26.

Tillich, P. 1967. *Systematic Theology*. Chicago: University of Chicago Press.

Todd, D., and M. Smith. Forthcoming. Acceptance and commitment therapy. In *Psychological Therapies in Neuropsychological Rehabilitation*, ed. G. N. Yeates and F. Ashworth. Hove, UK: Psychology Press.

Todman, D. 2008. Epilepsy in the Graeco-Roman world: Hippocratic medicine and Asklepian temple medicine compared. *Journal of the History of the Neurosciences* 17: 435–41.

Toh, S. F. M. 2013. A systematic review on the effectiveness of Tai Chi exercise in individuals with Parkinson's disease from 2003 to 2013. *Hong Kong Journal of Occupational Therapy* 23: 69–81.

Tomasino, B., D. Marin, M. Maieron, T. Ius, R. Budai, F. Fabbro and M. Skrap. 2013. Foreign accent syndrome: a multimodal mapping study. *Cortex* 49, no. 1: 18–39.

Tong, F. 2003. Out-of-body experiences: from Penfield to present. *Trends in Cognitive Sciences* 7: 104–6.

Trelles, J., and D. Lagache. 1932. Intoxication barbiturique recidivante s'accompagnant d'hallucinose pedoculaire. *Annales Médico-Psychologiques* 16: 565–72.

Tremlin, T. 2005. Divergent religion: a dual-process model of religious thought, behavior, and morphology. In *Mind and Religion: Psychological and Cognitive Foundations of Religiosity*, ed. H. Whitehouse and R. N. McCauley, 69–84. Walnut Creek, CA: AltaMira Press.

Tremlin, T. 2006. *Minds and Gods: The Cognitive Foundations of Religion*. New York: Oxford University Press.

Tremont, G., M. M. Smith, L. Bauer, M. L. Alosco, J. D. Davis, A. S. Blum, and W. C. LaFrance Jr. 2012. Comparison of personality characteristics on the bear-fedio inventory between patients with epilepsy and those with non-epileptic seizures. *Journal of Neuropsychiatry and Clinical Neuroscience* 24: 47–52.

Trimble, M., and A. Freeman. 2006. An investigation of religiosity and the Gastaut–Geschwind syndrome in patients with temporal lobe epilepsy. *Epilepsy and Behavior* 9: 407–14.

Trinh, J., and M. Farrer. 2013. Advances in the genetics of Parkinson disease. *Nature Reviews Neurology* 9: 445–54.

Tucker, D. M., R. A. Novelly and P. J. Walker. 1987. Hyperreligiosity in temporal lobe epilepsy: redefining the relationship. *Journal of Nervous and Mental Disorders* 175: 181–4.

Tyerman, A. and M. Humphrey. 1984. Changes in self concept following severe head injury. *International Journal of Rehabilitation Research* 7: 11–23.

Ullmann, M. 1978. *Islamic Medicine*. Edinburgh: Edinburgh University Press.

Unterrainer, H.-F., A. Lewis, J. Collicutt and A. Fink. 2013. Religious/spiritual well-being, coping styles, and personality dimensions in people with substance use disorders. *International Journal for the Psychology of Religion* 23: 204–13.

Urgesi, C., S. M. Aglioti, M. Skrap and F. Fabbro. 2010. The spiritual brain: selective cortical lesions modulate human self-transcendence. *Neuron* 65: 309–19. doi:10.1016/j.neuron.2010.01.026.

Vagg, D., R. Bandler and K. Keay. 2008. Hypovolemic shock: critical involvement of a projection from the ventro-lateral periaqueductal grey to the caudal midline. *Neuroscience* 152: 1099–109.

Valeo, T. 2012. Not just tremor: recognizing depression and other non-motor symptoms of Parkinson's disease. *Neurology Now Magazine* 8: 22–7.

Van Leeuwen, N. 2014. Religious credence is not factual belief. *Cognition* 13: 698–715.

van Lommel, P. 2010. *Consciousness beyond Life: The Science of the Near-Death Experience*. New York: Harper One.

van Lommel, P., R. van Wees, V. Meyers and I. Elfferich. 2001. Near-death experience in survivors of cardiac arrest: a prospective study in the Netherlands. *Lancet* 358: 2039–45.

van Veluw, S. J., and S. A. Chance. 2014. Differentiating between self and others: an ALE meta-analysis of fMRI studies of self-recognition and theory of mind. *Brain Imaging and Behavior* 8: 24–38. www.ncbi.nlm.nih.gov/pubmed/24535033.

Varela, F. J., E. Thompson and E. Kesch. 1993. *The Embodied Mind: Cognitive Science and Human Experience*. Cambridge, MA: MIT Press.

Visuri, I. 2012. Could everyone talk to God? A case study on Asperger's syndrome, religion and spirituality. *Journal of Religion, Health, and Disability* 16: 352–78.

Visuri, I. 2018. Rethinking autism, theism and atheism: bodiless agents and imaginary realities. *Archive for the Psychology of Religion* 1: 1–31.

Visuri, I. 2019. Sensory supernatural experiences in autism. *Religion, Brain, and Behavior*. Published online. doi:10.1080/2153599X.2018.1548374.

Visuri, I. Forthcoming. A room of one's own: autistic imagination as a stage for parasocial interaction and social learning. *Journal for the Cognitive Science of Religion*.

Von Steinbüchel, N., L. Wilson, H. Gibbons, G. Hawthorne, S. Höfer, S. Schmidt, J. Truelle et al. 2010. Quality of Life after Brain Injury (QOLIBRI): scale development and metric properties. *Journal of Neurotrauma* 27: 1167–85.

Wade, D. 1999. Goal planning in stroke rehabilitation: how? *Topics in Stroke Rehabilitation* 6: 16–36.

Wang, C., R. Bannuru, J. Ramel, B. Kupelnick, T. Scott and C. H. Schmid. 2010. Tai Chi on psychological well-being: systematic review and meta-analysis. *BMC Complementary Alternative Medicine* 10: 23.

Warrington, E. K., and T. Shallice. 1984. Category specific semantic impairments. *Brain* 107: 829–54.

Warrington, E., and L. Weskrantz. 1968. A study of learning and retention in amnesic patients. *Neuropsychologia* 6: 283–92.

Watt, W. M. 1953. His name is Ahmad. *The Muslim World* 43: 110–17.

Watts, F. 2002. *Theology and Psychology*. Aldershot, UK: Ashgate.

Waxman, S. G., and N. Geschwind. 1975. The interictal behavior syndrome of temporal lobe epilepsy. *Archives of General Psychiatry* 32: 1580–6.

Weaver, G. 2004. Embodied spirituality: experiences of identity and spiritual suffering among persons with Alzheimer's dementia. In *From Cells to Souls – and Beyond: Changing Portraits of Human Nature*, ed. M. A. Jeeves, 77–99. Grand Rapids, MI: Eerdmans.

Weintraub, D., and D. J. Burn. 2011. Parkinson's disease: the quintessential neuropsychiatric disorder. *Movement Disorders* 26: 1022–31.

Wexler, M., S. M. Kosslyn and A. Berthoz. 1998. Motor processes in mental rotation. *Cognition* 68: 77–94.

Whiting, D., G. Simpson, J. Ciarrochi and H. McLeod. 2012. Assessing the feasibility of acceptance and commitment therapy in promoting psychological adjustment after severe traumatic brain injury. *Brain Injury* 26: 588–9.

WHO. 2001. *International Classification of Functioning, Disability and Health*. Geneva: World Health Organization.

WHOQOL SRPB Group. 2006. A cross-cultural study of spirituality, religion, and personal beliefs as components of quality of life. *Social Science and Medicine* 62: 1486–97.

Whybrow, P. C. 1997. *A Mood Apart: Depression, Mania, and Other Afflictions of the Self*. New York: HarperCollins/Basic Books.

Widdershoven, G. A. M., and R. L. P. Berghmans. 2006. Meaning-making in dementia: a hermeneutic perspective. In *Dementia: Mind, Meaning, and the Person*, ed. J. C. Hughes, S. J. Louw and S. R. Sabat, 179–91. Oxford: Oxford University Press.

Wiech, K., M. Farias, G. Kahane et al. 2008. An fMRI study measuring analgesia enhanced by religion as a belief system. *Pain* 139: 467–76.

Wigger, J. B., K. Paxson and L. Ryan. 2013. What do invisible friends know? Imaginary companions, God, and theory of mind. *International Journal for the Psychology of Religion* 23: 2–14.

Wijdicks, E. F. M. 2001. The diagnosis of brain death. *New England Journal of Medicine* 344: 1215–21.

Wijdicks, E. F., P. N. Varelas, G. S. Gronseth and D. M. Greer. 2010. Evidence-based guideline update: determining brain death in adults: report of the Quality Standards Subcommittee of the American Academy of Neurology. *Neurology* 74: 1911–18.

Williams, D. 1956. The structure of emotions reflected in epileptic experiences. *Brain* 79: 29–67.

Williams, W. H. and J. J. Evans. 2003. Brain injury and emotion: an overview to a special issue on biopsychosocial approaches in neurorehabilitation. *Neuropsychological Rehabilitation* 13(1/12): 1–11.

Williams-Gray, C. H., J. R. Evans, A. Goris et al. 2009. The distinct cognitive syndromes of Parkinson's disease: 5 year follow-up of the CamPaIGN cohort. *Brain* 132: 2958–69.

Williams-Gray, C. H., S. L. Mason, J. R. Evans et al. 2013. The CamPaIGN study of Parkinson's disease: 10-year outlook in an incident population-based cohort. *Journal of Neurology, Neurosurgery, and Psychiatry* 84: 1258–64.

Wilson, B. 1987. *Rehabilitation of Memory*. New York: Guilford Press.

Wilson, I. 1997. *Life after Death*. London: Pan Books.

Winnicott, D. 1971. *Playing and Reality*. London: Tavistock.

Winser, S. J., P. Kannan, M. Pang, C. Smith and W. W. Tsang. 2018a. Potential benefits and safety of T'ai Chi for balance and functional independence in people with cerebellar ataxia. *Journal of Alternative and Complimentary Medicine* 24: 1221–3.

Winser, S. J., P. Kannan, M. Pang and W. W. Tsang. 2017. Tai Chi for improving balance in cerebellar ataxia: a feasibility. *Archives of Physical Medicine and Rehabilitation* 98, no. 10: e113–14.

Winser, S. J., W. W. Tsang, K. Krishnamurthy and P. Kannan. 2018b. Does Tai Chi improve balance and reduce falls incidence in neurological disorders? A systematic review and meta-analysis. *Clinical Rehabilitation* 32: 1157–68.

Wittgenstein, L. 1953. *Philosophical Investigations*. Trans. G. E. M. Anscombe. Oxford: Basil Blackwell.

Wood, P. 1980. *World Health Organization Classification of Impairments, Disabilities and Handicaps: A Manual of Classification Relating to the Consequences of Disease*. Geneva: World Health Organization.

Wu, S., J. Chen, S. Wang, M. Jiang, X. Wang and Y. Wen. 2018. Effect of Tai Chi exercise on balance function of stroke patients: a meta-analysis. *Medical Science Monitor Basic Research* 24: 210–15.

Wu, T. Q., Z. A. Miller, B. Adhimoolam, D. D. Zackey, B. K. Khan, R. Ketelle et al. 2013. Verbal creativity in semantic variant primary progressive aphasia. *Neurocase*, 12 December. www.ncbi.nlm.nih.gov/pubmed/24329034.

Wuerfel, J., E. S. Krishnamoorthy, R. J. Brown, L. Lemieux, M. Koepp, L. Tebartz van Elst and M. R. Trimble. 2004. Religiosity is associated with hippocampal but not amygdala volumes in patients with refractory epilepsy. *Journal of Neurology, Neurosurgery, and Psychiatry* 75: 640–2.

Wulff, D. 1996. *Psychology of Religion: Classic and Contemporary.* New York: John Wiley.

Wynn, M. 2005. *Emotional Experience and Religious Understanding: Integrating Perception, Conception and Feeling.* Cambridge: Cambridge University Press.

Wynn, M. 2013. *Renewing the Senses: A Study of the Philosophy and Theology of the Spiritual Life.* Oxford: Oxford University Press.

Xie, G. L., T. Rao, L. Lin, Z. Lin, T. Xiao, M. Yang, Y. Xu, J. Fan, S. Lin, J. Wu, X. Feng, L. Li, J. Tao and L. Chen. 2018. Effects of Tai Chi Yunshou exercise on community-based stroke patients: a cluster randomized controlled trial. *European Review of Aging and Physical Activity* 15: 17.

Yan Li, G., G. L. Liu and Y. Zhang. 2018. Effects of Tai Chi on balance and gait in stroke survivors: a systematic meta-analysis of randomized controlled trials. *Journal of Rehabilitation Medicine* 50: 582–8.

Yang, Y., X.-Y. Li, L. Gong, Y.-L. Zhu and Y.-L. Hao. 2014. Tai Chi for improvement of motor function, balance and gait in Parkinson's disease: a systematic review and meta-analysis. *PLoS ONE* 9(7): e102942.

Yeates, G. N. 2014. Using pagers and alerts as adjuncts to psychological therapies following acquired brain injury. In *Telerehabilitation and Adaptations: Assistive Technology for People with Neuropsychological Impairments*, ed. Anna Cantagallo. Milan: francoAngeli.

Yeates, G. N. 2015. Flow state experiences as a biopsychosocial guide for Tai Ji intervention and research in neuro-rehabilitation. *Neuro-disability and Psychotherapy* 3: 22–41.

Yeates, G. N. 2018. Flow state experiences as a biopsychosocial guide for Tai Ji intervention and research in neuro-rehabilitation. In *Neuro-disability and Psychotherapy, Specialist Topics: Vol. 1. Eastern Influences on Neuropsychotherapy: Accepting, Soothing and Stilling Cluttered and Critical Minds in Neurological Conditions*, ed. G. N. Yeates and G. Farrell, 210–19. Oxford: Routledge.

Yeates, G. N. Forthcoming. Mind–body interventions for neurological conditions. In *Psychological Therapies in Neuropsychological Rehabilitation*, ed. G. N. Yeates and F. Ashworth. Hove, UK: Psychology Press.

Yeates, G. N., and G. Farrell. 2014. Editorial for special issue: 'Accepting,soothing and stilling cluttered and critical minds in neurological conditions: The influence of Eastern practices'. *Neuro-disability and Psychotherapy* 2: 1–2.

Yeates, G. N., and G. Farrell. 2018. Editors' foreword. In *Neuro-disability and Psychotherapy, Specialist Topics: Vol. 1. Eastern Influences on Neuropsychotherapy: Accepting, Soothing and Stilling Cluttered and Critical Minds in Neurological Conditions*, ed. G. N. Yeates and G. Farrell, Oxford: Routledge.

Yeates, G. N., M. Hamill, L. Sutton, K. Psaila, S. Mohamed and J. O'Dell. 2008. Dysexecutive problems and interpersonal relating following frontal brain injury: reformulation in cognitive-analytic therapy. *Neuro-Psychoanalysis* 10: 43–58.

Yeates, G. N., M. Murphy, J. Baldwin, J. Wilkes and M. Mahadevan. 2015. A pilot evaluation of a yoga group for survivors of acquired brain injury in a community setting. *Clinical Psychology Forum* 267: 46–51.

Yeates, G. N., S. Nagrani, A. Smith, J. Dorney-Savage, J. Whitman and E. Khan. 2008. Diversity of needs Tai Chi (Taiji) group interventions following acquired brain injury: a mixed methods study. Unpublished manuscript.

Yeates, G. N., S. Nagrani, A. Smith, J. Dorney-Savage, J. Whitman and E. Khan. Forthcoming. Mind–body interventions following expressive aphasia and stroke a single case study. In *Neuro-disability and Psychotherapy, Specialist Topics: Vol. 2. Psychotherapy and Aphasia: Supporting Emotions and Relationships*, ed. G. N. Yeates & K. Meredith. Oxford: Routledge.

Yonker, J. E., L. R. O. Edman, J. Cresswell and J. L. Barrett. 2016. Primed analytic thought and religiosity: the importance of individual characteristics. *Psychology of Religion and Spirituality* 8: 298–308.

Zabeen, B., S. Tayyeb, B. Benarjee, A. Baki, J. Nahar, F. Mohsin, N. Nahar and K. Azad. 2014. Fasting during Ramadan in adolescents with diabetes. *Indian Journal of Endocrinology and Metabolism* 18: 44–7.

Zahavi, D. 2014. *Self and Other.* Oxford: Oxford University Press.

Zeeneldin, A. A., A. A. Gaber and F. M. Taha. 2012. Does fasting during Ramadan trigger non-adherence to oral hormonal therapy in breast cancer patients? *Journal of the Egyptian National Cancer Institute* 24: 133–7.

Zhang, L., C. Layne, T. Lowder and J. Liu. 2011. A review focused on the psychological effectiveness of Tai Chi on different populations. *Evidence-Based Complementary and Alternative Medicine*. Published online. doi:10.1155/2012/678107.

Zheng, G., W. Zhou, R. Xia, J. Tao and L. Chen. 2016. Aerobic exercises for cognition rehabilitation following stroke: a systematic review. *Journal of Stroke and Cerebrovascular Disease* 25: 2780–9.

Zhou, J., T. Yin, Q. Gao and X. C. Yang. 2015. A meta-analysis on the efficacy of Tai Chi in patients with Parkinson's disease between 2008 and 2014. *Evidence Based Complementary and Alternative Medicine* 2015: 593263.

Zigmond, A. S. and R. P. Snaith. 1983. The Hospital Anxiety and Depression Scale. *Acta Psychiatrica Scandinavica* 67: 361–70.

Zinnbauer, B. J., K. I. Pargament, B. Cole, R. S. Rye, E. M. Butter, T. G. Belavich, K. M. Hipp, A. B. Scott and J. L. Kadar. 1997. Religion and spirituality: unfuzzying the fuzzy. *Journal for the Scientific Study of Religion* 36: 549–56.

Zou, L., C. Wang, X. Chen and H. Wang. 2018a. Baduanjin exercise for stroke rehabilitation: a systematic review with meta-analysis of randomized controlled trials. *International Journal of Environmental Research and Public Health* 15: 600.

Zou, L., A. Yeung, N. Zeng, C. Wang, L. Sun, G. Thomas and H. Wang. 2018b. Effects of mind–body exercises for mood and functional capabilities in post-stroke patients: an analytical review of randomized controlled trials. *International Journal of Environmental Research and Public Health*, 15: 721.

Zuckerman, P. 2007. Atheism: contemporary numbers and patterns. In *The Cambridge Companion to Atheism*, ed. M. Martin, 47–65. New York: Cambridge University Press.

Index

Neurology and Religion

Edited by
Alasdair Coles
Department of Clinical Neuroscience, University of Cambridge
Joanna Collicutt
University of Oxford

CAMBRIDGE
UNIVERSITY PRESS

CAMBRIDGE
UNIVERSITY PRESS

University Printing House, Cambridge CB2 8BS, United Kingdom

One Liberty Plaza, 20th Floor, New York, NY 10006, USA

477 Williamstown Road, Port Melbourne, VIC 3207, Australia

314–321, 3rd Floor, Plot 3, Splendor Forum, Jasola District Centre, New Delhi – 110025, India

79 Anson Road, #06–04/06, Singapore 079906

Cambridge University Press is part of the University of Cambridge.

It furthers the University's mission by disseminating knowledge in the pursuit of education, learning, and research at the highest international levels of excellence.

www.cambridge.org
Information on this title: www.cambridge.org/9781107082601
DOI: 10.1017/9781316014165

© Cambridge University Press 2020

This publication is in copyright. Subject to statutory exception and to the provisions of relevant collective licensing agreements, no reproduction of any part may take place without the written permission of Cambridge University Press.

First published 2020

A catalogue record for this publication is available from the British Library.

Library of Congress Cataloging-in-Publication Data
Names: Coles, Alasdair, editor. | McGrath, Joanna Collicutt, editor.
Title: Neurology and Religion / edited by Alasdair Coles, Joanna Collicutt.
Description: Cambridge, United Kingdom ; New York, NY : University Printing House, [2019]
Identifiers: LCCN 2019021292 | ISBN 9781107082601 (hardback) | ISBN 9781107442962 (paperback)
Subjects: MESH: Neurology | Religion | Nervous System Diseases | Religion and Science
Classification: LCC RC346 | NLM WL 21 | DDC 616.8–dc23
LC record available at https://lccn.loc.gov/2019021292

ISBN 978-1-107-08260-1 Hardback

Cambridge University Press has no responsibility for the persistence or accuracy of URLs for external or third-party internet websites referred to in this publication and does not guarantee that any content on such websites is, or will remain, accurate or appropriate.

Every effort has been made in preparing this book to provide accurate and up-to-date information which is in accord with accepted standards and practice at the time of publication. Although case histories are drawn from actual cases, every effort has been made to disguise the identities of the individuals involved. Nevertheless, the authors, editors and publishers can make no warranties that the information contained herein is totally free from error, not least because clinical standards are constantly changing through research and regulation. The authors, editors and publishers therefore disclaim all liability for direct or consequential damages resulting from the use of material contained in this book. Readers are strongly advised to pay careful attention to information provided by the manufacturer of any drugs or equipment that they plan to use.

For EU product safety concerns, contact us at Calle de José Abascal, 56–1°, 28003 Madrid, Spain or eugpsr@cambridge.org.

www.ingramcontent.com/pod-product-compliance
Lightning Source LLC
LaVergne TN
LVHW011914200926
848484LV00002B/622
9781107082601